江苏省高等学校重点教材　编号 2014-2-031

EXPERIMENT FOR PHARMACOLOGY OF TRADITIONAL CHINESE MEDICINE

中药药理学实验

双语教材

主　编　马世平

副主编　刘　康　黄　芳

编　者　（以姓氏笔画为序）

马世平　马占强　刘　康

陈刚领　吴斐华　黄　芳

傅　强　谢　媛　魏志凤

主　审　刘保林

东南大学出版社
SOUTHEAST UNIVERSITY PRESS
·南京·

图书在版编目(CIP)数据

中药药理学实验/马世平主编. —南京:东南大学出版社, 2015.10(2022.12重印)

双语教材

ISBN 978-7-5641-5970-2

Ⅰ. ①中… Ⅱ. ①马… Ⅲ. ①中药学-药理学-双语教学-医学院校-教材 Ⅳ. ①R285

中国版本图书馆CIP数据核字(2015)第189384号

中药药理学实验双语教材

出版发行	东南大学出版社
出 版 人	江建中
责任编辑	褚　蔚(电话:025-83790586)
社　　址	南京市四牌楼2号
邮　　编	210096
经　　销	全国各地新华书店
印　　刷	江苏凤凰数码印务有限公司
开　　本	787 mm×1092 mm　1/16
印　　张	19.25
字　　数	433千字
书　　号	ISBN 978-7-5641-5970-2
版　　次	2015年10月第1版
印　　次	2022年12月第2次印刷
定　　价	49.00元

(本社图书若有印装质量问题,请直接与营销部联系,电话:025-83791830)

前　言
PREFACE

中药药理学实验是中药药理学课程的重要内容。近年来，中医药受到全世界关注，中药药理学发展迅速。为适应学科发展和教学需要，我们总结了多年本科生和研究生的教学经验，并借鉴相关实验书籍和文献，以中英文对照的方式，编写了这本《中药药理学实验双语教材》。

教材分两部分：第一部分介绍中药药理实验的基础理论和基本技能，帮助学生掌握和了解中药药理实验的基本要求和方法；第二部分是各类中药的主要实验项目，帮助学生掌握中药药理实验的具体操作技术。书后附录有常用生理溶液的成分和配制、常用实验动物的最大给药剂量等。

教材编写突出中医药传统特色，以传授中药药理学常用的经典实验方法为主，同时结合学科发展，精选了部分新的实验内容，体现出一定的创新性和时代气息。这既有利于培养学生的基本知识和基本技能，加深其对基本理论的理解，又有利于培养学生的创新能力，提高其专业素养，使之更好地适应中医药学走向世界的新形势。

本教材为江苏省高等学校重点教材，得到中国药科大学重点教材基金的资助。

本教材主要面向医药院校中药学、药学及其相关学科专业本科生及研究生，对从事中医药研究的科研人员也有一定的参考价值。

采用中英文双语编写中药药理学实验教材尚属首次，加上编者水平所限，不妥之处在所难免，恳请读者批评指正。

编者

2015 年 10 月

目 录
CATALOGUE

第一章　常用实验动物的选择、捉持和给药方法

实验动物的选择：小鼠是药理实验最常用的一种实验动物，常用于药物的筛选，LD_{50}、ED_{50} 的测定，中枢神经系统药实验，抗炎免疫药实验，避孕药、抗肿瘤药以及抗衰老药实验等。大鼠的用途与小鼠相似，常用作抗关节炎药物实验、血压测定、利胆药实验、子宫药实验和长期毒性实验等。豚鼠对组胺很敏感，研究平喘药和抗组胺药时常选用。家兔常用作观察药物对呼吸、心脏、血管、肠肌运动的影响，或用作解热药实验及热源检查。雌兔常用作避孕药研究及观察药物对子宫的影响。狗常用于慢性实验，如高血压实验、胃瘘、肠瘘，用于观察药物对冠脉血流的影响、利尿药实验以及长期毒性实验等。

Chapter 1　How to choice, catch, hold and administrate the experimental animals

The choice of experimental animals in pharmacology studies: mice are the most commonly used experimental animals for the screening of drug activity, as well as the determination of LD_{50} and ED_{50}. Mice are also widely used for the observation of the regulation of central nervous system, immunological system and inflammatory response and the evaluation of contraceptive agents, antineoplastic agents and anti-aging agents, and so on. The use of rats is similar to mice. Rats are usually used in antiarthritic experiments, determination of blood pressure, experiments of choleretic drugs, experiments of drugs' effect on metra, and long-term toxicity tests, and so on. Guinea pigs are sensitive to histamine, and are commonly used in studies of antasthmatic drugs and antihistamine drugs. Rabbits are usually used in studies of drugs' effects on respiration, heart, blood vessel, and enterokinesia. And rabbits are often used in antipyretic studies and determination of pyrogen. Female rabbits are usually used in studies of contraceptive agents and observation of drugs' effect on metra. Dogs are usually used in chronic experiments, for example: treatment test of hypertension, gastric fistula, and intestinal fistula, studies of the effects of drugs on coronary artery blood flow, experiments of emictory, and long-term toxicity tests, and so on.

实验一　小鼠的捉持和给药方法

【目的】学习并掌握正确的小鼠的捉持方法。学习并熟练掌握小鼠的不同给药方法。

【原理】用正确的方法捉持和给药可以防止动物过度挣扎或受损伤，并可避免人被咬伤，减少动物所受到的伤害，从而保证实验顺利进行。

【器材】小鼠笼；天平；1 mL 注射器；小鼠灌胃针；注射针头；小鼠尾静脉注射用固定箱。

【试剂】生理盐水。

【动物】小鼠，18~22 g。

【方法】

1. 捉持方法

（1）双手捉持法：右手拇指和食指提起小鼠尾巴，将小鼠放置于鼠笼盖或粗糙面上，向后轻拉小鼠尾巴，使小鼠身体伸展。当小鼠向前挣扎爬行时，迅速用左手的拇指、食指和中指捏住小鼠头颈部的皮肤，将小鼠身体紧贴左手大鱼际，无名指、小指按住小鼠尾巴根部，使头部朝上，颈部拉直但不宜过紧，以免动物窒息。

（2）单手捉持法：将小鼠置于鼠笼盖或粗糙面上，先用左手食指和拇指抓住小鼠尾巴，后用手掌及小指和无名指夹住其尾巴根部，向后轻拉，再以拇指及食指捏住其头颈部皮肤。

2. 给药方法

（1）灌胃：左手持鼠，使头颈部充分伸直，头部朝上。右手拿起装有灌胃针头的注射器，将针头自口角插入口腔，再从舌背面沿上颚进入食道。如插入正确，灌胃针头容易进入，如遇阻力，可能插入气管，则应退出再插。有落空感即可注射，灌胃液最多不超过 1.0 mL。

（2）皮下注射：通常选用颈背部皮肤。左手拇指及食指将皮肤提起，使注射针头与皮肤成一定角度刺入。把针头轻轻向左右摆动，容易摆动则表明已刺入皮下，然后轻轻抽吸，如无回流物，即缓慢注射药物。注射完药物之后，旋转出针，以免药液漏出。

（3）肌肉注射：左手拇指和食指抓住小鼠头部皮肤，小指、无名指和手掌夹住鼠尾及一侧后肢，将针头（选用 4 号或 5 号针头）刺入后肢外侧部肌肉。如两人合作，一人左手抓住小鼠头部皮肤，右手拉住鼠尾，另一人持注射器。注射量每腿不宜超过 0.2 mL。

（4）腹腔注射：左手持小鼠，方法同灌胃，小鼠头部朝下，右手持带有 5 号或 6 号针头的注射器，以 10° 角从下腹部腹中线稍向左或右的位置刺入皮下，继续进针 3~5 mm，再以 45° 角刺入腹腔，针尖有刺空感时表明已进入腹腔，回抽无液体即可缓缓注入药液。为避免刺破内脏，可将动物头部放低，尾部提高，使脏器移向横隔处。

（5）尾静脉注射：小鼠尾部有四根血管十分明显：背腹各一根动脉，两侧各有一根静脉，两侧尾静脉比较容易固定。将小鼠置于特制的铁皮固定器内，露出尾巴，用45~50 ℃温水浸泡半分钟或涂擦75%乙醇，使血管扩张，表皮角质软化。然后将尾部向左或向右转90°，将一侧尾静脉朝上，以左手食指和中指捏住鼠尾上下，使静脉充盈，用无名指从下面托起尾巴，以拇指和小指夹住尾巴末梢，右手持注射器，使针头与静脉平行进针，刺入后先缓注少量药液，如无阻力，表明针头已进入静脉，可继续注入。注射完毕后把尾巴向注射侧弯曲以止血。静脉注射尽量从近尾端静脉开始，这样可以重复注射数次，以便失败后可在第一次穿刺点的上方重新进行。

Experiment 1 How to catch, hold and administrate mice

【Purpose】To learn how to catch, hold and administrate mice.

【Principles】The right methods of catching, holding and administrating the experimental animals can prevent the over struggle of animals, and avoid the animals being harmed and operators being bitten by animals, so the experiment can be proceeded smoothly.

【Equipments】Mouse cage, balance, syringe, needle, and box for fixing mouse.

【Reagents】Saline.

【Animals】Mice, weighing 18~22 g.

【Methods】

1. Catch and hold

(1) Two hands catch and hold: The tail of the mouse is caught with right hand. The mouse is put on a rough object and is slightly pulled backward. And then, the two ears and head skin of the mouse are pinched with the thumb, the forefinger and the middle finger of the left hand. The dorsal and the tail skin of the mouse are clamped with the ring finger, the little finger and the center of the palm. The head of the mouse is kept forward and the neck is kept straight but not made the skin of the neck too tight avoiding asphyxiation.

(2) One hand catch and hold: The tail of the mouse is caught with the forefinger and the thumb of the palm. Then the tail of the mouse is clamped with the palm, the little finger and the ring finger. Two ears and the back skin of the mouse are caught with the thumb and the forefinger. The advantage of the former method is easily learnt, and that of the latter method is convenient for fast catching and administrating.

2. Methods of administration

(1) Intragastric administration: The mouse is held in the left hand with its head forward and neck fully straight, and the syringe with a needle for intragastric administration is held in the right hand. Then, the needle is inserted into the mouth and sent to the portio pharyngis along the upper palate. And then the needle is inserted into the gullet following swallowing act. Whether the needle enters smoothly indicates the correct route or incorrect one through which the needle may enter the air tube. The administrative volume is not more than 1.0 mL.

(2) Subcutaneous injection: The mouse is held with the left hand. The dorsal skin of the mouse is pinched up, and the syringe with a needle of 5# or 6# is taken in the right hand. The needle is inserted into the dorsal skin and the parenteral solution is injected. The syringe is rotated to prevent any leakage of the drug solution and then the needle is pulled out. Another

way can be adopted through two persons' cooperation. The head skin of the mouse is held by one person and the tail is pulled with the right hand. The dorsal skin is pinched up by the other person with left hand and the needle is inserted under the skin with the right hand.

(3) Intramuscular injection: The head skin is held with the thumb and the forefinger of the left hand. The tail and the hindlimb of one side are clamped with the little finger, the ring finger and the palm. And then the needle of 4# or 5# is inserted into the lateral muscle of the hindlimb with the right hand. If two persons cooperate, the head skin is held with the left hand by one person and the tail is pulled with the right hand. The needle is inserted into the lateral muscle of the back leg with the right hand by the other person. The administrative volume is not more than 0.2 mL.

(4) Intraperitoneal injection: The mouse is held in the left hand (the method is similar to intragastric administration) with its abdomen upward and head down. The syringe with a needle of 5# or 6# is taken in the right hand. The needle is inserted into the left or right inferior belly skin at an angle of 10 degree towards the head in order to avoid bladder. And then the needle is inserted into abdomen at an angle of 45 degree and the physic liquor is injected. The advantage of this method is that it can prevent the drug leaking outside. The angle of syringe needle is adjusted twice to avoid injecting the drug subcutaneously. Avoid inserting the needle from the middle belly in case the bladder is pierced. Avoid inserting the needle too deep or too close to the upper abdomen in case the internal organs are damaged. The usual administrative volume is 0.5 mL and not more than 1.0 mL.

(5) Intravenous injection from the caudal vein: The mouse is fixed into a special box with its tail outside and the tail is wiped with 75% alcohol solution to dilate the vein. An obviously dilated vein is selected and the tail tip is held with the thumb and the middle finger. And then the tail pressed with the forefinger to keep the vein dilated all the time. A needle of 4# is inserted into the vein at an angle of 3 to 5 degree, almost paralleling to tail, and the physic liquor is injected. That resisting force occurs and the tail becomes white locally when injecting the drug indicates that the needle is inserted subcutaneously instead of intravenously. The needle is inserted from the far end of the tail to ensure that the vein can be injected repeatedly for several times if the failure occurs.

实验二　大鼠的捉持和给药方法

【目的】学习大鼠的捉持和各种给药方法。

【原理】用正确的方法捉持和给药可以防止动物过度挣扎或受损伤，并可避免人被咬伤，从而保证实验顺利进行。

【器材】鼠笼；天平；注射器；注射针头；灌胃针头；大鼠尾静脉注射用固定箱；手套一副。

【试剂】生理盐水。

【动物】大鼠，体重 180~250 g。

【方法】

1. 捉持法　大鼠容易激怒咬人，一般左手戴防护手套，按照与捉持小鼠相同的方式捉持，对于较大的动物可用左手的拇指和中指分别放在大鼠的左右腋下，食指放于颈部，使大鼠伸开前肢，握住大鼠。

2. 灌胃法　与小鼠相似。一次给药量不超过 2 mL。

3. 腹腔注射法　同小鼠。

4. 静脉注射法　麻醉后大鼠可以从舌下静脉或尾静脉注射给药。要充分加温或用二甲苯涂擦使其尾静脉扩张，尾静脉注射才易成功。

Experiment 2　How to catch, hold and administrate rats

【Purpose】To learn how to catch, hold and administrate rats.

【Principles】The right methods of catching, holding and administrating the experimental animals can prevent the over struggle of animals, and avoid the animals being harmed and operators being bitten by animals, so the experiment can be proceeded smoothly.

【Experiments】Rat cage, balance, syringe, needle, needle for oral administration, box for fixing rat, a pair of operation glove.

【Reagents】Saline.

【Animals】Rats, weighing 180~250 g.

【Method】

1. Catch and hold　The rats have acute teeth and stronger than mice. A glove should be weared on the left hand. Other details can be referred to related contents in Experiment 1. As for bigger rats, the left hand is used to hold the rats by putting the thumb and the middle finger under the front oxters and the forefinger on the neck to make rats stretch their forelimbs.

2. Intragastric administration　Similar to the method used in mice. The administrative volume is not more than 2.0 mL.

3. Intraperitoneal injection　Similar to the method used in mice.

4. Intravenous injection　The anesthetized rat can be administrated from either the sublingual vein or the caudal vein. Intravenous administration from the caudal vein can be conducted successfully only when the caudal vein is dilated by sufficiently heating or wiping it with dimethylbenzene.

实验三　家兔的捉持和给药方法

【目的】学习家兔的捉持和各种给药方法。

【原理】用正确的方法捉持和给药可以防止动物过度挣扎或受损伤，并可避免人被咬伤，从而保证实验顺利进行。

【器材】兔固定箱；兔开口器；磅秤；导尿管；注射器。

【试剂】生理盐水。

【动物】家兔，2~3 kg，雌雄不限。

【方法】

1. 捉持法　一手抓住家兔颈背部皮肤，将兔轻轻提起，另一手托住其臀部，使兔呈坐位姿势。不要抓两耳，以防兔挣扎。

2. 固定　将兔仰卧，一手抓住其颈部皮肤，另一手顺其腹部摸至膝关节。另一人用绳带捆绑兔的四肢，将家兔腹部向上固定在兔手术台上。头部则用兔头固定夹固定。

3. 灌胃　将兔固定于兔箱内，用木制开口器由齿列间横插入口内，并向内上方转动直至兔舌被掩压出为止，然后将导尿管从开口器中的小孔插入，沿上腭后壁轻轻地送入食道，约 15~20 cm 左右，送达胃部。注意不能插入气管，可将导尿管的外端浸入水内，观察有无气泡放出。无气泡方能注入药液，药液推完后再注入 4~5 mL 水或少许空气，以便将导尿管中的药液全部推至胃中。而后紧捏导尿管迅速拔出，否则水可由导尿管中滴至气管内。

4. 静脉注射　将兔固定于兔箱内，先拔去耳背面外侧静脉处毛以便于辨认静脉，然后用左手拇指和中指捏住耳尖部，食指垫在兔耳注射处的下面。右手持安装有 6 号针头的注射器，先从耳尖端开始注射，约以 5° 角刺入，刺入后用左手拇指、食指及中指捏住针头接头处及兔耳加以固定，以防突然挣扎时针尖脱出血管。注射时，注意不能有气泡注入，否则兔会立即死亡。常用注射量为 10 mL 以下，应缓缓注射药液。如插入血管，药液推进容易，如插在血管外，则有丘状隆起，应拔出针头，在近心端重新注射。针头拔出时须用棉球压住注射部位以防出血。

5. 皮下、肌肉、腹腔注射　方法与小鼠同。惟针头选用粗的，给药量增加（皮下：2 mL；肌肉：2 mL；腹腔：5 mL）。

Experiment 3　How to catch, hold and administrate rabbits

【Purpose】To learn how to catch, hold and administrate rabbits.

【Principles】The right methods of catching, holding and administrating the experimental animals can prevent the over struggle of animals, and avoid the animals being harmed and operators being bitten by animals, so the experiment can be proceeded smoothly.

【Experiments】Box for fixing rabbit, mouth gag for rabbit, platform balance, bladder catheter, syringe.

【Reagents】Saline.

【Animals】Rabbits (male or female), 2~3 kg.

【Methods】

1. Catch and hold　The rabbit is raised slightly by holding the nuchal skin with one hand, and its buttock is supported with the other hand. you should not lift the rabbits by the ears because it cannot bear its own wight,causing struggle.

2. Fixation　The rabbit is laid on its back by holding the jugular skin with one hand and the knee joint with the other hand. Then the rabbit is fixed on the operation platform by binding the extremities with ropes by another person. The head of the rabbit is fixed with a special device for fixing the head of the rabbit.

3. Intragastric administration　The rabbit is fixed into the special box. The wood-made mouth gag is horizontally inserted into the mouth of the rabbit. The wood-made mouth gag is rolled upwardly until the tone of the rabbit is stretched out. The bladder catheter is slightly inserted into the stomach instead of air tube as long as 15~20 cm following the routine of small hole in the device, back upper palate, and gullet. The way to check whether or not the bladder catheter goes into the air track is to observe whether or not the air bubble goes out if put the other end of the bladder catheter into the water. Thirdly, injecting of drug or saline is followed by injecting 4~5 mL of water or air in order to push all of them inside into the stomach. Lastly, the bladder catheter is pulled fast out by holding tightly the end of the bladder catheter in case the water inside drops into the air tube.

4. Intravenous injection　The rabbit is fixed into a special box. The vein in the back and external ear is made be clearly seen by cutting the fur. The tip of the era is held with the thumb and the middle finger, and the vein is supported with the forefinger of the left hand. The syringe with a needle of 6# is taken in right hand. The needle is inserted into the vein from the tip at an angle of 5°. The needle is fixed inside by pressing it outside with thumb,

the forefinger, and the middle finger of the left hand in case the needle goes out of the vein when the rabbit moves its head. Pay attention to not injecting air bubble in to the vein, or the animal will die at once. The normal volume of injection is about 10 mL. The injection should be operated slowly. If the needle is inserted into the vein, it is smoothly to inject. If the needle is not in the vein, there will be a swelling, and you should pull out the needle and reinject at proximal part. Pull out the needle followed by pressing the vein with cotton to prevent bleeding.

5. Subcutaneous injection, intramuscular injection and intraperitoneal injection Similar to administration of mice in Experiment 1 except that a bigger needle is needed and more volume is available (2 mL for subcutaneous injection, 2 mL for intramuscular injection and 5 mL for intraperitoneal injection).

实验四 豚鼠的捉持和给药方法

【目的】学习豚鼠的捉持和各种给药方法。

【原理】用正确的方法捉持和给药可以防止动物过度挣扎或受损伤,并可避免人被咬伤,从而保证实验顺利进行。

【器材】鼠笼;天平;注射器;针头。

【试剂】生理盐水。

【动物】豚鼠。

【方法】

1. 捉持法 豚鼠胆小易惊,性情温和,抓取时,以右手抓住豚鼠,将前肢夹在右手拇指和食指之间,抓住整个颈胸部(不要抓得太紧以免窒息),左手抓住两后肢,使腹部向上进行操作。

2. 灌胃法、腹腔注射法、皮下和肌肉注射 方法基本上同小鼠,给药量需稍多。

3. 静脉注射 可选用后脚掌外侧的静脉或外颈静脉进行注射。做后脚掌外侧静脉注射时,由一人捉豚鼠并固定一条后腿,另一人剪去注射部位的毛,用酒精棉球涂擦后脚掌外侧,使皮肤血管显露,将连在注射器上的小儿头皮静脉输液针头刺入血管。外颈静脉注射时需先剪去一点皮肤,使血管暴露,然后将连在注射器上的头皮静脉输液注射针头刺入。豚鼠的静脉血管壁比较脆弱,操作时需特别小心。

Experiment 4 How to catch, hold and administrate guinea pigs

【Purpose】To learn how to catch, hold and administrate guinea pigs.

【Principles】The right methods of catching, holding and administrating the experimental animals can prevent the over struggle of animals, and avoid the animals being harmed and operators being bitten by animals, so the experiment can be proceeded smoothly.

【Experiments】Cage, balance, syringe, needle.

【Reagents】Saline.

【Animals】Guinea pigs.

【Methods】

1. Method of catching and holding Guinea pig is a sort of coward animal, mild and never attack people.The abdomen of the guinea pig is caught upward by holding the forelimbs, the neck and the chest with the right hand. The hindlimbs are catched with the left hand. Do not catch too tightly or the guinea pig will be asphyxia.

2. Intragastric administration, subcutaneous injection, intramuscular injection and intraperitoneal injection Similar to the administration of mice in experiment 1 except that more volume of the drug is available.

3. Intravenous injection Either the vein in lateral of the sole of the foot or the external jugular vein can be selected. The former method is as follows. One hind leg of the guinea pig is held by one person. The fur of the leg is cut and the vein is made be clearly seen by wiping it with alcohol cotton by another person. Then the small needle for children head injection is inserted into the vein. The latter method is adopted such as the following. Make the external jugular vein exposed by cutting a little skin and insert the small needle into it. Be careful when inserting the needle into the vulnerable vein for the vein of guinea pigs is fragile.

实验五　狗的捉持和给药方法

【目的】学习狗的捉持和各种给药方法。

【原理】用正确的方法捉持和给药可以防止动物过度挣扎或受损伤，并可避免人被咬伤，从而保证实验顺利进行。

【器材】特制铁钳夹；狗开口器；磅秤；导尿管；注射器；针头；绳索。

【试剂】生理盐水。

【动物】狗，5~10 kg。

【方法】

1. 捉持法　对于未经驯服的狗，需先以特制铁钳夹住头颈，将其按倒，以绳索捆扎狗嘴。用粗绳带从下颌绕到上颌打一结，最后将绳带索引到头后，在颈顶上打第三结，在这一结上再打一活结。捆绑过程中要求动作轻巧迅速。捆绑狗嘴的目的只是避免其咬人。对于已驯服（一般经一周左右训练）的狗，不必施以暴力，只需将狗嘴绑好，即可进行给药，不宜用铁钳夹头，否则狗的性情将由此变坏而不听指挥。

2. 灌胃、皮下、肌肉和腹腔注射　方法基本上同家兔。用具和给药量相应增大。

3. 静脉注射　常用的注射部位是后肢小隐静脉，该血管由外踝前侧走向外上侧。也可选用前肢的皮下头静脉，该血管在脚爪上方背侧的正前位。注射时先局部剪毛，以酒精涂擦皮肤，一人捏紧注射肢体的上端，阻断血液回流，使静脉充盈，以便看清走向，另一人持注射器进行静脉穿刺，将药液注入。

Experiment 5 How to catch, hold and administrate dogs

【Purpose】To learn how to catch, hold and administrate dogs.

【Principles】The right methods of catching, holding and administrating the experimental animals can prevent the over struggle of animals, and avoid the animals being harmed and operators being bitten by animals, so the experiment can be proceeded smoothly.

【Experiments】Special iron tongs, mouth gag for dog, platform balance, bladder catheter, syringe, needle, rope.

【Reagents】Saline.

【Animals】Dogs, 5~10 kg.

【Methods】

1. Method of catching and holding In order to prevent being bitten, the tameless dog is pushed down by holding the head and neck with special iron tongs and its mouth is tied quickly and delicately with rope as following routes: first node from lower jaw to upper jaws; second node from upper jaw to lower jaw and third node added another slipknot from lower jaw to neck. When the tame dog which was trained for about 1 week is administrated, only need to tie up its mouth with rope, and not need to treat it with violence. Do not clamp its head with special iron tongs, or the dog will be too irascible to do the experiment.

2. Intragastric administration, subcutaneous injection, intramuscular injection and intraperitoneal injection Similar to administration of rabbit in experiment 3 except that bigger equipment and more volume of the drug is available.

3. Intravenous administration Either the small saphenous vein of the hindlimb, which goes from the anterior of the lateral malleolus to the external upper side, or the subcutaneous cephalic vein of the forelimb, which is at the right anteposition of the upper of the claw at the back side, can be selected. The fur extremity of the leg for injection is cut by one person. And the small needle is inserted into the vein and the drug solution is injected by another person.

第二章　动物剂量换算的计算方法

1. 体形系数（K）的确定　动物的体表面积可根据体重和体型系数近似计算。

$$A=K \cdot W^{2/3}$$ ［A 为表面积（m^2），K 为体形系数，W 为体重（kg）］

表 2–1　不同动物的体形系数（**K**）

动物	小鼠	仓鼠	大鼠	豚鼠	兔	猫	狗	猴	成人
体形系数（新法）	0.089 9	0.086 2	0.086	0.092	0.101 4	0.108 6	0.107 7	0.118	0.105 7
体形系数（原法）	0.06	—	0.09	0.099	0.093	0.082	0.104	0.111	0.1~0.11

计算可知，20 g 小鼠表面积为 0.006 6 m^2，经实际测量小鼠表面积为 0.006 4~0.006 9 m^2。

2. 动物剂量换算的经典公式　由于动物剂量大致与体表面积成正比，而体表面积可用 $A=K \cdot W^{2/3}$ 估算。即：

$$D(a):D(b) \approx A_a:A_b \approx K_a \cdot W_a^{2/3}:K_b \cdot W_b^{2/3} \quad (1)$$

故动物剂量换算方式可表达如下：

每只动物剂量：$D(b)=D(a) \cdot (K_b/K_a) \cdot (W_b/W_a)^{2/3}$　（2）

千克体重计量：$D_b=D_a \cdot (K_b/K_a) \cdot (W_b/W_a)^{1/3}$　（3）

$D(a)$：已知 a 种动物的剂量（mg/ 只）；$D(b)$：欲求 b 种动物的剂量（mg/ 只）；D_a、D_b：千克体重剂量（mg/kg）；A_a、A_b：体表面积（m^2）；K_a、K_b：体形系数；W_a、W_b：体重（kg）（下标 a、b 分别表示已知动物和欲求动物，下同）。

3. 动物剂量换算表及例算　根据 $R_{ab}=(K_a/K_b) \cdot (W_b/W_a)^{1/3}$，$S=(W_{标准}/W_a)^{1/3}$ 计算换算系数（R_{ab}）及校正系数（S_a, S_b），设计成如下由动物 a 到动物 b 的剂量（mg/kg）换算表。

由标准体重到标准体重 $D_b=D_a \cdot R_{ab}$　（4）

由标准体重到非标准体重 $D_b'=D_a \cdot R_{ab} \cdot S_b$　（5）

由非标准体重到非标准体重 $D_b'=D_a' \cdot S_a \cdot R_{ab} \cdot S_b$　（6）

注：D_a 和 D_b 是标准体重剂量（mg/kg）；D_a' 和 D_b' 是非标准体重剂量。

表 2-2　标准体重动物由动物 a 到动物 b 的 mg/kg 剂量折算表（表中数值为换算系数 R_{ab}）

动物品种	小鼠 b	仓鼠 b	大鼠 b	豚鼠 b	家兔 b	家猫 b	猕猴 b	比格犬 b	狒狒 b	微型猪 b	成人 b
标准体重 W(kg)	0.02	0.08	0.15	0.4	1.8	2.5	3.0	10.0	12.0	20.0	60.0
表面积（m^2）	0.006 6	0.016	0.025	0.05	0.15	0.2	0.25	0.5	0.6	0.74	1.62
体重系数 K	0.089 8	0.086 2	0.088 6	0.092 1	0.101 4	0.108 6	0.120 2	0.107 7	0.114 5	0.100 4	0.105 7
系数 S	3	5	6	8	12	12.5	12	20	20	27	37
小鼠 a	1.00	0.600	0.500	0.375	0.250	0.240	0.250	0.150	0.150	0.111	0.081
仓鼠 a	1.67	1.00	0.833	0.625	0.417	0.400	0.417	0.250	0.250	0.185	0.135
大鼠 a	2.00	1.20	1.00	0.750	0.500	0.480	0.500	0.300	0.300	0.222	0.162
豚鼠 a	2.67	1.60	1.33	1.00	0.667	0.640	0.667	0.400	0.400	0.296	0.216
家兔 a	4.00	2.40	2.00	1.50	1.00	0.960	1.00	0.600	0.600	0.444	0.324
家猫 a	4.17	2.50	2.08	1.56	1.04	1.00	1.04	0.625	0.625	0.463	0.338
猕猴 a	4.00	2.40	2.00	1.50	1.00	0.960	1.00	0.600	0.600	0.444	0.324
比格犬 a	6.67	4.00	3.33	2.50	1.67	1.60	1.67	1.00	1.00	0.741	0.541
狒狒 a	6.67	4.00	3.33	2.50	1.67	1.60	1.67	1.00	1.00	0.741	0.541
微型猪 a	9.00	5.40	4.50	3.38	2.25	2.16	2.25	1.35	1.35	1.00	0.730
成人 a	12.33	7.40	6.17	4.63	3.08	2.96	3.08	1.85	1.85	1.37	1.00

表 2-3　非标准体重动物的校正系数（S_a、S_b）

$B=W/W_{标}$	0.3	0.4	0.5	0.6	0.7	0.8	0.9	1.0	1.1	1.2	1.3	1.4
$S_a=B^{1/3}$	0.669	0.737	0.794	0.843	0.888	0.928	0.965	1.0	1.032	1.063	1.091	1.119
$S_b=1/B^{1/3}$	1.494	1.357	1.26	1.186	1.126	1.077	1.036	1.0	0.969	0.941	0.916	0.894
$B=W/W_{标}$	1.5	1.6	1.7	1.8	1.9	2.0	2.2	2.4	2.6	2.8	3.0	3.2
$S_a=B^{1/3}$	1.145	1.17	1.193	1.216	1.239	1.26	1.301	1.339	1.375	1.409	1.442	1.474
$S_b=1/B^{1/3}$	0.874	0.855	0.838	0.822	0.807	0.794	0.769	0.747	0.727	0.709	0.693	0.679

例 1：已知 150 g（标准体重）大鼠用 5 mg/kg，求成人（标准体重）的用药剂量：查表 2-2，大鼠 a 行，成人 b 列的 R_{ab}=0.162，故成人的剂量为 $D_b \cdot R_{ab}=5 \times 0.162=0.81$ mg/kg。

例 2：已知 20 g（标准体重）小鼠用 4 mg/kg，求 8 kg（标准体重）犬的用药剂量：查表 2-2，小鼠 a 行，犬 b 列的 R_{ab}=0.150，故犬的剂量 = $D_b \cdot R_{ab}=4 \times 0.150=0.600$ mg/kg。

例 3：已知 8 kg（标准体重）比格犬用 0.68 mg/kg，求 22 g 小鼠、38 g 老龄鼠的用药剂量：

①查表 2-2，犬 a 行，小鼠 b 列的 R_{ab}=6.67，故 20 g 小鼠的剂量 = $D_b \cdot R_{ab}= 0.68 \times 6.67=4.536$ mg/kg。

② 38 g 老龄鼠：根据 B=38/20=1.9，查表 2-3，S_b=0.807，故剂量 = $D_b' \cdot R_{ab} \cdot S_b= 0.68 \times 6.67 \times 0.807=3.660$ mg/kg。

Chapter 2 The calculation method of animal dose conversion

1. The determination of shape coefficient (*K*) The animal's body surface area is difficult to measure directly, it can be approximately calculated according to the weight and animal shape coefficient. Shape coefficient $K=A/W^{2/3}$ (*A* is surface area value, m^2, *W* is weight value, kg, some literature use cm^2 with area, then *K* should multiplied by 100). The *K* value of sphere was 0.04 836, size is more approximate to a sphere, the smaller the *K* value. Have *K* then can use $A=K{\bullet}W^{2/3}$ to estimate the surface area.

Table 2-1 Shape coefficient (*K*) of different animals

Animal	Mouse	Hamster	Rat	guinea pig	Rabbit	Cat	Dog	Monkey	Adult
Shape coefficient (new method)	0.089 9	0.086 2	0.086	0.092	0.101 4	0.108 6	0.107 7	0.118	0.105 7
Shape coefficient (old method)	0.06	—	0.09	0.099	0.093	0.082	0.104	0.111	0.1~0.11

It can be seen by the table that in the new method, mouse and rat have same the shape coefficient , guinea pig's shape is close to a ball, the *K* value slightly smaller. In the old method , the *K* value of rat is big the *K* value of guinea pig is bigger than the *K* value of mouse. The surface area of 20 g mouse is 0.006 6 m^2 calculated by new method , by old method is 0.004 4 m^2, the actual measuring of 20 g mouse's surface area is 0.006 4 ~ 0.006 9 m^2.

2. Classic formula of animal dose conversion Animal dose is roughly proportional to surface area, the surface area can be estimated by $A=K{\bullet}W^{2/3}$. That is ,

$$D(a):D(b)\approx A_a:A_b\approx K_a{\bullet}W_a^{2/3}:K_b{\bullet}W_b^{2/3} \quad (1)$$

So the animal dose conversion formula can be expressed as follow:

The dose of each animal: $D(b)=D(a)\cdot(K_b/K_a)\cdot(W_b/W_a)^{2/3}$ (2)

kg dose: $D_b=D_a\cdot(K_b/K_a)\cdot(W_b/W_a)^{1/3}$ (3)

The above formula is a general formula, suitable for any animal, any weight. $D(a)$ is the dose of the known animal a (mg/each), $D(b)$ is the dose of the animal b you want to know (mg/each), D_a, D_b is the kg dose mg/Kg. A_a, A_b is surface area (m^2), K_a, K_b is shape coefficient, W_a, W_b is weight (kg) (subscript a represent the known animal, subscript b represent the animal want to know, same in the following).

When conversion in a same species, their shape coefficient ($K_b/K_a = 1$) is same, the formula can be simplified as the $D(b) = D(a)\cdot(W_b/W_a)^{2/3}$ and $D_b = D_a\cdot(W_b/W_a)^{1/3}$.

In pharmacological experiments, drug always be distributed into a certain concentration of solution, then in accordance with the number of milliliters per kilogram (or per 10 g) of solution administered. As long as the difference between animal body weight and standard weight was less than ± 20%,you can use the dose of medication of the same kilogram of body weight . Thus, formula kg dose (3) is more commonly used in dose conversion.

3. Animal dose conversion tables and calculate example It's more trouble that calculate according to formula (3) in every experiment. Now introduce animal shape coefficient and its standard weight into formula, calculate conversion coefficient (R_{ab}) and correction coefficient (S_a,S_b) (can be looked up in the table) in advance, $R_{ab}=(K_a/K_b)\cdot(W_b/W_a)^{1/3}$, $S=(W_{standard}/W_a)^{1/3}$, thus designed into dose (mg/kg) conversion table from animal a to animal b, D_a and D_b is standard weight dose mg/kg, D_a' and D_b' is non-standard weight dose. R_{ab}, S_a, S_b can be looked up in the table.

From standard weight to standard weight $D_b=D_a\cdot R_{ab}$ (4)

From standard weight to non-standard weight $D_b'=D_a\cdot R_{ab}\cdot S_b$ (5)

From non-standard weight to non-standard weight $D_b'=D_a'\cdot S_a\cdot R_{ab}\cdot S_b$ (6)

When animal is standard weight, S_a,S_b=1, then formula (6) changed into formula (4)、(5), use formula (3) for directly calculating. In designed pharmacological experiments mainly use standard weight, it is approximately applicable within ± 20%, so formula (4) is most common.

Dose (mg/kg) multiplied by the weight can calculate the dose of each animal.

Table 2–2 standard weight animal's dose (mg/kg) Conversion table—from animal a to animal b (the data in table is conversion coefficient R_{ab})

Animal spices	Mouse b	Hamster b	Rat b	guinea pig b	Rabbit b	Cat b	Macaqueb	Beagle b	Baboon b	miniature pig b	Adult b
Standard weight W (kg)	0.02	0.08	0.15	0.4	1.8	2.5	3.0	10.0	12.0	20.0	60.0
Surface area (m^2)	0.006 6	0.016	0.025	0.05	0.15	0.2	0.25	0.5	0.6	0.74	1.62
Weight Coefficient K	0.089 8	0.086 2	0.088 6	0.092 1	0.101 4	0.108 6	0.120 2	0.107 7	0.114 5	0.100 4	0.105 7
Coefficient S	3	5	6	8	12	12.5	12	20	20	27	37
Mouse a	1.00	0.600	0.500	0.375	0.250	0.240	0.250	0.150	0.150	0.111	0.081
Hamster a	1.67	1.00	0.833	0.625	0.417	0.400	0.417	0.250	0.250	0.185	0.135
Rat a	2.00	1.20	1.00	0.750	0.500	0.480	0.500	0.300	0.300	0.222	0.162
Guinea pig a	2.67	1.60	1.33	1.00	0.667	0.640	0.667	0.400	0.400	0.296	0.216
Rabbit a	4.00	2.40	2.00	1.50	1.00	0.960	1.00	0.600	0.600	0.444	0.324
Cat a	4.17	2.50	2.08	1.56	1.04	1.00	1.04	0.625	0.625	0.463	0.338
Macaque a	4.00	2.40	2.00	1.50	1.00	0.960	1.00	0.600	0.600	0.444	0.324
Beagle a	6.67	4.00	3.33	2.50	1.67	1.60	1.67	1.00	1.00	0.741	0.541
Baboon a	6.67	4.00	3.33	2.50	1.67	1.60	1.67	1.00	1.00	0.741	0.541
Miniature pig a	9.00	5.40	4.50	3.38	2.25	2.16	2.25	1.35	1.35	1.00	0.730
Adult a	12.33	7.40	6.17	4.63	3.08	2.96	3.08	1.85	1.85	1.37	1.00

Table 2–3 non-standard animal weight correction coefficient

$B=W/W_{standard}$	0.3	0.4	0.5	0.6	0.7	0.8	0.9	1.0	1.1	1.2	1.3	1.4
$S_a=B^{1/3}$	0.669	0.737	0.794	0.843	0.888	0.928	0.965	1.0	1.032	1.063	1.091	1.119
$S_b=1/B^{1/3}$	1.494	1.357	1.26	1.186	1.126	1.077	1.036	1.0	0.969	0.941	0.916	0.894
$B=W/W_{standard}$	1.5	1.6	1.7	1.8	1.9	2.0	2.2	2.4	2.6	2.8	3.0	3.2
$S_a=B^{1/3}$	1.145	1.17	1.193	1.216	1.239	1.26	1.301	1.339	1.375	1.409	1.442	1.474
$S_b=1/B^{1/3}$	0.874	0.855	0.838	0.822	0.807	0.794	0.769	0.747	0.727	0.709	0.693	0.679

Eg1. Known 150 g (standard weight) rats use 5 mg/kg, calculate the dose of adult (standard weight): look up at attached table 2-2, the cross of rat a and adult b is R_{ab}=0.162, so adult's dose=D_b•R_{ab}=5 × 0.162=0.81 mg/kg.

Eg2. Known 20 g (standard weight) mice use 4 mg/kg, calculate the dose of 8 kg dog (standard weight) :look up at attached table 2-2,the cross of mouse a and dog b is R_{ab}=0.150, so dog's dose=D_b•R_{ab}=4 × 0.150=0.600 mg/kg.

Eg3. Known 8 kg (standard weight) beagles use 0.68 mg/kg, calculate the dose of 22 g mouse and 38 g old mouse: ① look up at attached table 2-2, the cross of dog a and mouse b is R_{ab}=6.67, so 20 g mouse's dose=D_b•R_{ab}=0.68 × 6.67=4.536 mg/kg. ② the difference between 22 g mouse and standard weight mouse is less than 20%, so according to the weight, 4.536 mg/kg is basically feasible. According to the standard weight $W_{standard}$=20 g, actual weight W_b=22 g, B=22/20=1.1, look up at attached table 2-3, S_b=0.969, so the dose=D_b'•R_{ab}•S_b=0.68 × 6.67 × 0.969=4.395 mg/kg, the difference between two dose is less than 3%. ③ 38 g old mouse: according to B=38/20=1.9, look up at attached table 2-3, S_b=0.807, so the dose=D_b'•R_{ab}•S_b=0.68 × 6.67 × 0.807=3.660 mg/kg, this dose also can be used in 31~46 g old mice.

It's not strange that the smaller animal weight is, the bigger kg doses is.The kg dose of kid is bigger than adults' clinically.

The conversion dose is the starting dose values for reference only, and should be explored in the pre-trial. For the conversion dose should not be overly pursue their precision.

第三章　中药的毒性和制剂安全限度实验

开发中药新品种在临床试用前都必须进行安全性评价或危险性评价，还要尽可能地找出这些不良反应与剂量、疗程之间的关系以及毒性作用是否可逆和如何预防。新药安全性评价的内容包括急性毒性、亚慢性毒性和慢性毒性试验，也包括特殊毒性试验，如致畸、致癌试验、免疫毒性、遗传毒性及神经毒性试验。作用于中枢神经系统的新药应进行药物依赖性试验，通过皮肤给药的药物还需进行皮肤刺激性试验和皮肤过敏性试验。

Chapter 3　The experiments of toxicity of Chinese materia medica and the safety limit of preparation

Before a new kind of Chinese material medical is used in clinic, a serial study of toxicity must be done carefully and seriously. We must fully evaluate the safety of the new medicine and find the target organ and tissue for its adverse effect. It is necessary to find the relation between the adverse effect and the dose or the course of treatment, and to determine if the toxicity of the drug is reversible or not and how to preclude. The safety evaluation of new drugs includes acute toxicity test, long-term toxicity test and special toxicity test. The special toxicity test includes mutagenic test, reproductive toxicity test, and carcinogenesis test. The drug dependence should be examined in the new medicine which affects central nervous system. And the skin stimulus test and the skin hypersensitivity test are required for new medicine which is administrated per cutem.

实验一 急性毒性试验(半数致死量测定)

【目的】了解急性毒性试验的含义,掌握药物半数致死量(LD_{50})的计算方法。

【原理】急性毒性试验是指一次或在24小时内多次给予受试药物后,动物在短期内出现的毒性反应,包括致死和非致死的指标参数。衡量一个药物的急性毒性大小,一般是以该药物使动物致死的剂量(lethal dose)为指标。通常用LD_{50}来表示,因为LD_{50}是剂量反应曲线上最敏感的一点。

【器材】注射针头;一次性注射器。

【试剂】厚朴注射液。

【动物】小鼠。

【方法】小鼠雌雄分笼,称重,体重相近的小鼠放入一个笼内。然后将雌雄小鼠分别按体重大小,按照下列方式分层随机分为5个组,使不同性别和体重的小鼠能均匀分配于各组,每组均为10只。

组别	1#	2#	3#	4#	5#
每轮分配顺序	1	2	3	4	5
	5	1	2	3	4
	4	5	1	2	3
	3	4	5	1	2
	2	3	4	5	1

小鼠腹腔注射剂间比为1∶0.8的厚朴注射液,五组剂量分别为3.40 g/kg、4.25 g/kg、5.31 g/kg、6.64 g/kg、8.30g/kg。观察3天内各组小鼠死亡率。

【结果】实验报告应包括:药物的批号、规格、生产厂家、理化性状、溶液的浓度、实验室温度。实验动物和种系、性别、体重范围、分组情况、给药途径、剂量、给药时间、给药后见到的中毒症状、死亡时间和死亡率。LD_{50}的计算过程和结果(包括LD_{50}值的95%可信限范围)。

【注意事项】应挑选体重相近的健康小鼠[(20±2)g]。通常在正式试验前,先要摸索出合适剂量范围,即测定出能使小鼠出现接近0%和100%死亡的剂量。在预试验所获得的0%和100%死亡的剂量范围内,按等剂间比[一般取(1∶0.8)~(1∶0.7)]设4~5个剂量,尽可能使半数组的死亡率在50%以下,另半数组的死亡率在50%以上。小鼠分组时应先将不同性别分开,在将不同体重分开,然后随机分配,此法称为分层随机分组法。小鼠称重及给药剂量力求准确。动物的饥饱,实验室温度、实验时间等均会影响实验结果,应尽量保持一致。

计算方法:孙氏改进寇氏法。

（1）基本要求：数据符合或接近对数正态分析；相邻两剂量的比值应相等；各组动物数相等或相近，一般为 10 只；不要求死亡率必须包括 0% 和 100%，但最大剂量组的死亡率和最小剂量组的死亡率之和最好在 80%~120% 范围内。

（2）计算公式：当最小剂量组的死亡率为 0%，最大剂量组的死亡率为 100% 时，按下列公式计算：

$$LD_{50}=\lg^{-1}[X_m-i(\sum p-0.5)]$$

式中

X_m——最大剂量的对数；

p——每组动物的死亡率（以小数表示）；

$\sum p$——每组动物死亡率的总和（$p_1+p_2+p_3\cdots\cdots$）；

i——相邻两组对数剂量的差值。

当最小剂量组的死亡率大于 0% 而又小于 30%，或最大剂量组的死亡率小于 100% 而又大于 70% 时，可按下列校正公式计算：

$$LD_{50}=\lg^{-1}\left[X_m-i(\sum p-\frac{3-P_m-P_n}{4})\right]$$

式中

P_m——最大剂量组的死亡率；

P_n——最小剂量组的死亡率。

LD_{50} 的标准误按下式计算：

$$S_{\lg LD_{50}}=i\cdot\sqrt{\frac{\sum p-\sum p^2}{n-1}}$$

式中

n——每组的动物数。

LD_{50} 的 95% 可信区间按下式计算：

$$\lg^{-1}(\lg LD_{50}\pm 1.96S_{\lg LD_{50}})$$

表 3–1　小鼠腹腔注射厚朴注射液实验结果

组别	小鼠（只）	剂量（g/kg）	对数剂量	死亡动物（只）	死亡率（p）	p^2
1	10	3.40				
2	10	4.25				
3	10	5.31				
4	10	6.64				
5	10	8.30				
					$\sum p$:	$\sum p^2$:

【思考题】急性毒性试验的含义？如何计算 LD_{50}？

Experiment 1 Acute toxicity test (LD_{50} determination)

【Purpose】Study the method, procedure and calculation of LD_{50} determination.

【Principles】Acute toxicity test is the test of the rapid and severe toxic reaction in animals in a short term when animals are administrated with large dose once or several times within 24 h. The lethal dose is usually used to measure the acute toxicity of a drug. Because the 50% lethal dose (LD_{50}) is the most sensitive point in dose response curve, it is often used to express the acute toxicity of the drug.

【Experiments】Syringe and needle.

【Reagents】Magnoliae cortex injection.

【Animals】Mice.

【Methods】The male mice and the female mice are separated and weighed respectively. The mice of the same weight class are put into the same mouse cage. The mice are randomly divided into 5 groups with 10 mice in each group of same sex according to the weight class (from big to small or from small to big).

Number of group	1#	2#	3#	4#	5#
Number of mice	1	2	3	4	5
	5	1	2	3	4
	4	5	1	2	3
	3	4	5	1	2
	2	3	4	5	1

The mice are intraperitoneally injected with magnoliae cortex injection with a ratio of 1 : 0.8 between the adjacent doses. The doses of five groups are 3.40 g/kg, 4.25 g/kg, 5.31 g/kg, 6.64 g/kg and 8.30 g/kg, respectively. Then observe the death rate of each group within 3 days.

【Results】Experiment report should include the lot number of the drug, specification, manufacturer, physical and chemical properties, concentrations of the drug and the temperature in the laboratory. And the report should record the species, sex, weight range, groups, route of administration, dose, time of administration, toxic symptom, death time and death rate of the animals. The calculating process and the result of LD_{50} should be described in the report, and the result should include the value of LD_{50} and 95% confidence limit of LD_{50}.

【Notes】The mice selected should be healthy and in same weight (20 ± 2g).

The proper dose range of the certain drug should be tested before determining its LD_{50} accurately and several proper doses are chosen in the range of doses causing 0% and 100% mice dead in the preliminary test. Four to five doses with ratio of 1 : 0.8 to 1 : 0.7 between adjacent doses are usually used for mice. It is better to make over 50% death rate in half of the groups and below 50% death rate in another half of groups. When dividing the mice into groups, set apart the different sexes and then the different weights before grouping the mice at random. This is called stratified randomization. Try to weigh and administrate the mouse as accurate as possible. Try to maintain the fasting time, room temperature and experimental time as same as possible, because they can influence the results of the experiment.

Calculating method: Improved Kurber method by Sun.

(1) Basic requirements: Data should be consistent with or near logarithm normal distribution. The ratio of the adjacent doses should be equal. The number of animals in each group should be same or similar. 10 animals in one group are usually used. Death rate of 0% and 100% are not necessary, but the sum of the maximal death rate and the minimal death rate are preferably in the range of 80% to 120%.

(2) Calculating formula: The following formula can be used to calculate LD_{50} when the death rate of the minimal dose group is 0% and the death rate of the maximal dose group is 100%.

$$LD_{50}=\lg^{-1}[X_m-i(\sum p-0.5)]$$

X_m——the logarithm of highest dose;

p——death rate in each group (expressed with decimal);

$\sum p$——the sum of death rate of all groups ($p_1+p_2+p_3+\cdots\cdots$);

i——the difference between two logarithm doses in adjacent groups.

The following correcting formula can be used to calculate LD_{50} when the death rate of the minimal dose group is over 0% and below 30%, or when the death rate of the maximal dose group is below 100% and over 70%.

$$LD_{50}=\lg^{-1}\left[X_m-i(\sum p-\frac{3-P_m-P_n}{4})\right]$$

P_m——the death rate of the maximal dose group;

P_n——the death rate of the minimal dose group.

The standard error of LD_{50} can be calculated by following formula.

$$S_{\lg LD_{50}}=i\cdot\sqrt{\frac{\sum p-\sum p^2}{n-1}}$$

n——the number of animals in each group.

95% confidence interval of LD_{50} can be calculated by the following formula.

$$\lg^{-1}(\lg LD_{50} \pm 1.96S_{\lg LD_{50}})$$

Table 3–1　Effect of magnoliae cortex injection intraperitoneally injected on mice.

group	Mice number	Dose(g/kg)	Logarithm dose	Number of the dead	Death rate (p)	p^2
1	10	3.40				
2	10	4.25				
3	10	5.31				
4	10	6.64				
5	10	8.30				
					$\sum p$:	$\sum p^2$:

【Questions】What is acute toxicity test? And how to calculate LD_{50}?

实验二　升麻葛根颗粒小鼠灌胃给药最大给药量的测定

【目的】学习中药药物安全性评价方法；学习最大给药量的计算方法。

【原理】最大给药量测定是指在最大浓度，最大容积，单次或 24 小时内多次（2~3 次）给药的最大给药剂量。中药研究中往往存在受试物的毒性较低，或者因剂型关系，药物浓度或体积受到限制，选择最大给药量作为临床推荐方法，对药物安全性进行评估。升麻葛根颗粒因预实验灌胃未见动物死亡，从而选为受试物。

【器材】电子天平（*d*=0.01）；电子天平（*d*=1 mg）；小鼠灌胃针头；手术器械。

【试剂】升麻葛根颗粒提取物；蒸馏水。

【动物】小鼠 20 只，雌雄各半，体重 18~22 g。

【方法】

1. 分组　取健康小鼠 20 只，雌雄各半，体重 18~22 g，试验前小鼠禁食不禁水 16 小时，根据体重和性别随机分为对照组和给药组，每组 10 只。

2. 升麻葛根汤的制备　升麻葛根汤颗粒，加适量蒸馏水研磨均匀，配置成刚好能通过 12 号灌胃针的混悬液最大浓度。

3. 给药　对照组给蒸馏水。给药组给升麻葛根汤。一日之内灌胃给药两次，灌胃容积为 0.4 mL/10 g 动物体重（小鼠灌胃最大容积），间隔时间为 6 小时。给药后即刻开始观察药物的毒性反应情况，连续观察 14 天，计算最大给药量，并推算该剂量相当于临床每日推荐用药量的倍数。

【结果】

表 3-2　受试物性质

品　名	
批号	
规格	
生产厂家	
理化性质	
溶液浓度	
实验室温度	

表 3–3　实验记录表

分组		性别	体重（g）	平均体重（g）	剂量（mL）	给药时间	给药后现象	死亡时间	死亡率
对照组	1								
	2								
	3								
	4								
	5								
	6								
	7								
	8								
	9								
	10								
给药组	1								
	2								
	3								
	4								
	5								
	6								
	7								
	8								
	9								
	10								

$$\text{小鼠的最大给药量倍数} = \frac{\text{每只小鼠最大给药量（g）} \times \text{成人平均体重（60 000 g）}}{\text{小鼠平均体重（g）} \times \text{成人每日用量（生药 g）}}\text{（倍）}$$

【注意事项】

1. 实验动物应挑选体重相近（20 ± 2 g 为宜）的健康小鼠，最好雌雄各半或者同一性别，应剔除怀孕的雌鼠。

2. 实验动物应使用尽量少的动物数原则。最大给药量实验动物数一般每组使用 10~20 只动物。最大给药量实验动物数根据中药及复方中药的毒性资料情况，无明显毒性中药每组可用 10 只动物，而有可能出现毒性反应者，每组可 15~20 只。

3. 对照组给什么是根据试验药用什么溶解或助溶剂而定。

4. 最大给药量实验应根据急性毒性实验的一般观察结果与可能涉及的组织、器官、系统观察进行具体观察和描述。

5. 小鼠称重及给药剂量力求准确。药液的 pH 及渗透压在生理范围内。动物的饥饱,实验室温度,实验时间等均会影响实验结果,应尽量保持一致。

6. 应尽可能保持实验条件的一致性,如:禁食时间、室温等,因为这些因素均能影响实验结果。

【思考题】

1. 分析动物死亡的可能机制。

2. 如何改进实验方法?

Experiment 2　The Maximum Dose Determination of Cohosh Puerarin Particles

【**Purpose**】To learn the method of evaluation of TCM safety and how to calculate the maximum dose determination.

【**Principles**】For the low toxicity or the limitation of concentration or volume, in the research of novel drug of TCM, the maximum dose is usually used to evaluate the degree of acute toxicity of the drug rather than LD_{50}. The determination of the maximum dose refers to the largest drug dose by single or multiple administration at the maximum concentration and the maxium volume in 24 hours. As no animal death was observed in preliminary experiment, cohosh puerarin particles is chosen as the test drug in this experiment to determine the maximum dose.

【**Equipments**】Mouse cages, balance, and syringe.

【**Reagents**】Cohosh puerarin particles, distilled water.

【**Animals**】Mice (male or female) weighing 18~22 g.

【**Methods**】

1. Grouping　Take 20 healthy mice, half male and half female, and weigh them respectively. Divide the 20 mice into control group and drug group randomly according to weigh and sex, 10 in each group. All mice are fasted 16 hours with free access to water before the experiment.

2. Preparation of the Cohosh Puerarin suspension at maximum concentration　To prepare the suspension at the maximum concentration which is able to transmit through $12^{\#}$ needle tubing, grill cohosh puerarin particle uniformly and mix it with moderate distilled water.

3. Administration　Administrate the mice in the control group with distilled water and the drug group with the suspension twice a day with the interval time of 6 hours, at the volume of 0.4 mL/10 g (body weight). Immediately start to observe the toxicity response after administration and the observation is lasted for 14 days. Calculate the maximum dose and the equivalent of clinical recommended daily dose.

【Results】

Table 3–2 Properties of Cohosh Puerarin Particles.

Trade Name
Batch Number
Specification
Manufacture
Physical and Chemical Properties
Concentration
Temperature

Table 3–3 Experimental record sheet

Groups		Sex	Weight (g)	Average Weight(g)	Dose (mL)	Time of Administration	Toxic Symptom	Death Time	Death Rate
Control Group	1								
	2								
	3								
	4								
	5								
	6								
	7								
	8								
	9								
	10								
Drug Group	1								
	2								
	3								
	4								
	5								
	6								
	7								
	8								
	9								
	10								

Times of dose equivalent of clinical recommended daily dose =[every mouse maximum dose (g) × adult average weight (60 000 g)] ÷ [average of mice weight (g) × adult daily dose of crude drug (g)]

【 Notes 】

1. The mice selected should be healthy, in the similar weight (18~22 g), no pregnancy, and the sex should be half male and half female or of the same sex.

2. The number of experimental animals should be as few as possible. In maximum dose experiment, commonly use 10~20 animals in each group according to the background information on the toxicity of traditional Chinese medicine and Chinese medicine compound.

3. What fed in the control group depends on solvent and co-solvent which is used in drug group.

4. The maximum dose experiment should based on general observations of acute toxicity test which may involve observations and descriptions on tissues, organs, and system levels.

5. Try to weigh and administer the mouse as accurate as possible. The pH and osmotic pressure of the drug should be within in physiological range.

6. Try to maintain the experimental conditions, such as fasting times, room temperature etc. as same as possible, for these changes can influence the results of the experiment.

【 Questions 】

1. Analyze the possible causes for animal deaths.

2. How will you improve the experimental design?

实验三　苍耳子水煎剂的肝毒性实验

【目的】本实验通过对小鼠进行苍耳子水提物灌胃，观察小鼠给药后的症状及小鼠各脏器的变化，从而进行苍耳子对小鼠肝脏毒性的研究。

【原理】通过苍耳子的急性毒性实验来研究苍耳子对小鼠肝脏的毒害情况，即：研究动物 24 h 内一次或多次给予受试物后，一定时间内动物产生的毒性反应及其严重程度。

【器材】电子天平；剪刀；镊子；棉球；烧杯；小鼠笼；灌胃针头等。

【试剂】蒸馏水；苦味酸；70% 乙醇溶液；苍耳子水煎剂。

【动物】SPF 级小鼠，昆明种，20 只，雌雄各半，体重 18~22 g。

【方法】

1. 实验前动物在实验环境中适应性喂养 2 天，按体重及性别随机分成 4 组，分别为高、中、低、对照组，每组 5 只并编号。

2. 将苍耳子水煎剂干粉配成四种浓度，分别相当于生药量 210 g/kg，161 g/kg，112 g/kg 。

3. 采用等容灌胃给药，给药体积为 0.1 mL/10g。高、中、低剂量组分别灌胃给予生药量 210 g/kg，161 g/kg，112 g/kg 的苍耳子水提物混悬液，对照组给予相同体积的 0.9% 的氯化钠溶液，每次灌胃之前禁食 14~16 h，不禁水，给药后常规饲养。

4. 灌胃给药后各组小鼠自由摄取鼠料，自由饮水。密切观察小鼠的行为活动、精神状态、毛色光泽、摄食饮水，大小便情况，并如实记载。

5. 死亡动物即刻尸检，肉眼观察其主要脏器（心、肝、脾、肺、肾）的变化，发现肉眼可见的病变器官则进行组织病理学检查。

【结果】

1. 将各组小鼠的行为活动记录于表 3-4。

表 3-4　苍耳子水煎剂对小鼠行为活动的影响

组别	精神状态	毛色光泽	饮水摄食情况	大小便情况
高剂量组				
中剂量组				
低剂量组				
对照组				

2. 统计各组小鼠的死亡个数及死亡率，并记录于表 3-5。

表 3-5　苍耳子水煎剂对小鼠死亡个数及死亡率的影响

组别	动物死亡时间			
	0~30 min	30 min~1 h	1~2 h	2~4 h
高剂量组				
中剂量组				
低剂量组				
对照组				

3. 将死亡后小鼠的脏器变化记录于表 3-6。

表 3-6　苍耳子水煎剂对小鼠脏器变化的影响

组别	心	肝	脾	肺	肾
高剂量组					
中剂量组					
低剂量组					
对照组					

【注意事项】

1. 在对小鼠进行分组时，请注意要按照随机分组法进行分组。

2. 在设计给药量时要参照该药的 LD_{50}（死亡率 50%）、D_n（死亡率 0%）、D_m（死亡率 100%）数值，此给药量应处于 D_n 与 D_m 范围之内。

3. 在对小鼠灌胃给药时，应采取等容给药法。组别不同，给药浓度不同。

【思考题】

1. 在设计动物给药量时应注意哪些事项？

2. 根据死亡后解剖小鼠的脏器变化，分析苍耳子水煎剂对小鼠肝脏毒损伤程度及小鼠死亡原因？

Experiment 3 The hepatotoxicity of Fructus Xanthii's water decoction in mice

[Purpose]

In this study, mice were gavaged with aqueous extract of Fructus Xanthii's, then symptoms after the administration and the changes of various organs of mice were observed in order to find h the livertoxicity of Fructus Xanthii.

[Principles]

The research of mice liver poisoning of Fructus xanthii can be examined through acute toxicity experiment. This means that animals will be given the subject content at given concentration for once or several times within 24 h, and then toxic effects and the degree of severity after a certain time will be observed.

[Equipments] Electronic balance, scissors, tweezers, cotton balls, beaker, mouse cages, lavage needles.

[Reagents] Distilled water, picric acid, 70% ethanol solution, the water decoction of fructus xanthii.

[Animals] 20 SPF mice, kunming species, half male and half female, weighing 18~22 g

[Methods]

1. Before the experiment, animals are kept adaptively under the lab environment for two days, divide these mice into four groups randomly according to the weight and sex (high dose group, middle dose group, low dose group and the control group, 5 mice in a group).

2. Prepare the decoction powder of fructus xanthii into four concentrations equivalent to the amount of crude drug 210 g/kg, 161 g/kg, 112 g/kg.

3. According to the isometric gavage method (0.1 mL/kg), aqueous-extract suspension of fructus xanthii was given by gavage at doses of 210 g/kg, 161 g/kg, 112 g/kg respectively. The control group is given an equalan equal volume of 0.9% sodium chloride solution. Food, but not water, was deprived for 14~16 h before the gavage.

4. After treatment, mice were kept in the cage with free access to chow and water. The Observe behavior of the mice activities, mental state, color luster, food and water intake, stool and urineand make a descriptive record.

5. Dissect the dead animals immediately, and observe the changes of major organs (heart, liver, spleen, lung, kidney) by visual. Histopathological examination should be done after finding the macroscopic lesions tissues.

【Results】

1. Record mice's activities of each group in the table 3-4.

Table 3–4　The effects of Fructus Xanthii's water decoction on mice's activity

group	Mental state	Shiny coat	Water feeding conditions	Toilet case
High dose group				
Medium dose group				
Low dose group				
control				

2. Calculate the statistics of deaths and mortality for each group of mice, and record in the table 3-5.

Table 3–5　The effects of mice's mortality and death rate from Fructus Xanthii's water decoction

group	Animal dead time			
	0~30 min	30 min~1 h	1~2 h	2~4 h
High dose group				
Medium dose group				
Low dose group				
control				

3. Record organ changes of dead mice in the table 3-6.

Table 3–6　The effects of Fructus Xanthii's water decoction on changes inorgans

group	Heart	Liver	Spleen	Lung	Kidney
High dose group					
Medium dose group					
Low dose group					
control					

【Notes】

1. Please refer to the random grouping method in the grouping of mice.

2. Refer to the LD_{50} (mortality rate 50%), D_n (mortality rate 0%) and D_m (mortality rate 100%) of this drug when designing the dosage. Besides, the dosage should be in the range of D_n and D_m.

3. Constant volume dosing method should be used when the drug is given by gavage to the animals, different groups with different concentrations.

【Questions】

1. What tissues should be paid attention to when designing animal dosage?

2. According to the changes in the organsafter death, analysis the liver-toxic severity caused by water decoction of fructus xanthii and the reasons for damage.

实验四 关木通的急性肾毒性实验

【目的】

1. 学习掌握急性肾毒性实验的操作。

2. 了解不同剂量关木通水煎液对肾脏的急性毒性。

3. 了解急性肾毒性的一般检测指标。

【原理】

关木通中主要成分有马兜铃酸类成分,其具有较强的肾毒性作用。其对肾脏的毒性作用与剂量有一定的关系,通过对一些肾脏指标的测定与观察,与对照组比较可知其对肾脏的毒性作用的大小。

【器材】鼠笼;天平;电子秤;注射器。

【试剂】关木通水煎剂(3 g 生药 /mL);生理盐水。

【动物】SD 大鼠,体重 220 ± 10 g,雌雄各半。

【方法】

1. 将实验动物在实验前给予禁食 12 h,不禁水处理。

2. 将 SD 大鼠雌、雄分开,分别称重、标记。

3. 将 40 只 SD 大鼠随机分成 4 组,每组 10 只。

4. 按照如下情况给药:①低剂量组[15 g/(kg•d)];②中剂量组[30 g/(kg•d)];③高剂量组[60 g/(kg•d)];④正常对照组。前三组将关木通水煎液配成相应浓度给大鼠灌胃,每次 2.5 mL,每日两次,正常对照组,给予同体积生理盐水,连续灌胃 3 天。给药期间大鼠自由饮食、饮水。

5. 实验从首次给药后开始,分别于第 4 天、第 9 天、第 14 天从大鼠眶后静脉丛取血 1.5 mL,并用代谢笼留取大鼠 24 h 尿液。实验第 14 天各组分别处死大鼠,取肾脏组织,10% 中性福尔马林固定待进行病理学观察。

6. 实验期间,每日观察大鼠活动状况、饮食、饮水、毛色、粪便等一般情况变化,并作记录,在实验前、实验第 4 天、第 9 天、第 14 天时称取大鼠体重。

7. 观察检测 血液标本通过离心后,取血清以全自动生化分析仪检测尿素氮、肌酐含量。20 mL 量杯计 24 h 尿液总量、冰点渗量计测尿渗透压、比色法进行尿 NAG 酶的测定。

8. 将低、中、高剂量组与正常对照组进行比较,得出结论。

【结果】

将结果填入表 3-7 中。

表 3–7　关木通的急性肾毒性实验

分组	剂量[g/(kg·d)]	尿素氮(mmol/L)	肌酐(g)	尿液总量(mL)	尿渗透压(Osm/L)	尿 NAG 酶(U/mol)
正常组						
低剂量组						
中剂量组						
高剂量组						

【注意事项】

1. 实验动物应挑选体重相近的健康大鼠，最好雌雄各半或者同一性别，怀孕的雌鼠应剔除不用。

2. 大鼠分组时应先将不同性别分开，再将不同体重分开，然后随机分配。

3. 大鼠的称重及给药剂量力求准确。

4. 动物的饥饱、实验室温度、实验时间等均会影响实验结果，应尽量保持一致。

【思考题】

1. 什么叫急性毒性实验？急性毒性是如何分级的？

2. 马兜铃酸属于哪一类化合物？在体内的毒性机制是什么？

Experiment 4　Acute renal toxicity test of Caulis Aristolochiae Manshuriensis

【Purpose】

1. Learn the operation of acute renal toxicity experiment

2. Understand acute renal toxicity of Caulis Aristolochiae Manshuriensis in different water decoction dosages

3. Understand the general detection indexes of acute renal toxicity

【Principles】

The main component of Caulis Aristolochiae Manshuriensis is aristolochic acid, which has severe renal toxicity. Some renal parameters will be used to evaluate the dosagedependent toxicity, compared with the control.

【Equipments】Mouse cages, balance, electronic scale and syringe.

【Reagents】Water decoction (3 g powder/mL), normal saline (NS).

【Animals】SD rats, 220 ± 10 g, half male and half female.

【Methods】

1. The experimental animals were deprived of food with free access to water for 12 hour before the experiment.

2. Separate the male rats from the female, weight and mark them respectively.

3. Divide the rats into 4 groups randomly with 10 rats in each group.

4. Water decoction of Caulis Aristolochiae Manshuriensis is prepared in corresponding concentrations. Intragastric administrate corresponding water decoction to rats with the dose of 15 g/(kg•d), 30 g/(kg•d), 60 g/(kg•d) respectively in low group, middle group and high group. Treat the normal group with corresponding volume of normal saline in same way. Administrate the drug twice a day for three consecutive days. Rats have free access to water and food during the administration.

5. After 4 days, 9 days, 14 days of administration, collect 1.5 mL blood from the venous plexus of fundus of rats eye. 24 hours after administration, collect the urine from metabolic cages. On the fourteen day the rats are killed, and kidney tissues are fixed in 10% neutral formalin for pathological observation.

6. Record the general conditions (daily activities, food and , drinking intake, hair color, excrement, etc.) during the experiment and the body weights of the rats on day 0,day 4, day 9, day 14 during after administration.

7. Examinations Centrifuge blood samples and extract the serum. Detect blood urea nitrogen and creatinine by automatic biochemical analyzer. Measure 24 h urine volume with 20 mL cup. Measure urine osmotic pressure with freezing point osmometer, and detect urine NAG enzyme by colorimetric method.

8. Compare each group with normal group respectively, and then draw a conclusion.

【Results】

Write down your data in the table 3-7.

Table 3–7 Acute renal toxicity test of Caulis Aristolochiae Manshuriensis

分组	Dose [g/(kg · d)]	Blood urea nitrogen (mmol/L)	Creatinine (g)	24 h urine volume (mL)	Urine osmotic pressure (Osm/L)	Urine NAG enzyme (U/mol)
Normal						
Low dose						
Middle dose						
High dose						

【Notes】

1. The rats selected should be healthy, in similar weight, no pregnancy, and the sex should be half male and half female or of the same sex.

2. When dividing the rats, set apart the different sexes and then the different weights before dividing the rats at random.

3. Try to weigh and administer the rat as accurate as possible.

4. Try to maintain the hungry state of animals, temperature in the lab, experimental time as constant as possible, for they may influence the results of the experiment.

【Questions】

1. What is acute toxicity? How to classify the degree of acute toxicity?

2. What class of compounds does aristolochic acid belong to? What's the mechanism?

第四章　影响中药药理作用因素的实验

影响中药作用的因素概括起来有三方面，即药物、机体和环境因素。就药物因素而言，品种、产地、采收季节、采集部位、剂量、剂型、炮制、煎煮方法、煎煮火候和配伍等因素均影响药物作用。本章主要涉及炮制及配伍影响药效的实验。

Chapter 4　Experiments relevant to some factors influencing the pharmacological actions of TCM

In general, three factors affecting the pharmacological actions of TCM (traditional Chinese medicine) are drug itself, organism and environments. Concerning to the factor of drug itself, many aspects such as species, place of production, the season of collection, parts of plants or animals, doses, form of medication, processing method, decoction methods, timing in decoction to a proper degree and compatibility, affect the drug actions. In this chapter, the factors of processing method and compatibility are concerned.

实验一　附子炮制前后致小白鼠中毒死亡情况的比较

【目的】观察附子炮制前后毒性的不同。

【原理】附子有毒成分主要是乌头碱。它的性质不稳定，经长时间浸泡和加热煮制，都可使乌头碱水解成毒性较小的苯甲酰乌头胺和乌头胺。生附子中乌头碱含量高，经炮制后乌头碱含量减少，毒性也降低，引起动物中毒死亡的剂量较生附子大。

【动物】小白鼠。

【药品和试剂】生附子和熟附子水煎液各 1 g/mL；苦味酸。

【器材】小鼠笼；药物天平；注射器（1 mL）；小鼠灌胃针头。

【方法】小白鼠称重后用苦味酸标记后随机分为两组，分别用 20 g/kg 的生附子和炮制后的附子水煎液灌胃。30 min 后观察两组小鼠中毒症状和死亡数有无不同。

【结果】生附子灌服后约 20 min 动物出现腹部收缩，身体摇摆，步态不稳和不安静等现象；30 min 左右可能死亡。而炮制附子水煎液灌服后则无此中毒现象。结果记入表 4-1 内。

表 4–1　生附子和炮制附子毒性比较

分组	中毒动物数 / 动物数	死亡动物数 / 动物数
生附子		
制附子		

【注意事项】若用 30 mg/mL 的生川乌和制川乌的水煎液按 0.2 mL/10 g 给小鼠作腹腔注射，可见生川乌组小鼠迅速中毒而死亡，证明两者毒性有明显差异。

【思考题】

1. 中药经炮制后对临床用药有何意义？
2. 为预防附子中毒，应如何降低其毒性？

Experiment 1 Comparison of the changes of lethal toxicity in Aconite Root before and after preparation

【**Purpose**】To observe the difference of lethal toxicity between pre-preparing and post-preparing aconite root.

【**Principles**】Aconitine, the main toxic components of Aconite Root, can be hydrolyzed into less poisonous benzoyl aconine and aconine after long-time immersion in water or heat decoction because of its instable chemical property. After preparation, toxicity of Aconite Root decreases with a decrease in the content of aconitine, leading to an increased in its lethal dose.

【**Animals**】Mice.

【**Drugs and reagents**】Decoction of crude Aconite Root (1 g/mL), decoction of processed Acotine Root (1 g/mL), 2,4,6-trinitrophenol.

【**Equipments**】Mouse cages, balance for weighing medicine, syringes (1 mL), pinhead of intragastric administration for mouse.

【**methods**】Mice are weighed, marked with picric acid, divided into two groups at random, and orally administered with 20 g/kg of crude or processed Aconite Root decoction. The toxic symptoms and death number are compared between these two groups of mice after 30 minutes.

【**Results**】30 minutes after administration of crude Aconite Root, the symptoms of abdomen contraction, body rocking, instability of gait, and tension are observed in mice, while there are no abnormalities showed in mice treated with processed Aconite Root. Results are filled in the table 4-1.

Table 4–1 Toxicity comparison between crude and processed Aconite Root in mice.

Group	Animal number of being poisoned/ total animal number	Death animal number/total animal number
Crude Aconite Root		
Processed Aconite Root		

【**Notes**】If mice were intraperitoneally injected with 0.2 mL/10 g of crude or processed Common Monkshood Mother Root (30 mg/mL), the mice treated with the crude one would die quickly for the strong toxicity, which demonstrates the toxicity difference between these two preparation of the same drug.

【**Questions**】

1. What is the significance of the preparation of TCM to clinical medication?

2. How can we decrease the toxicity of Aconite Root in order to prevent body from being poisoned?

实验二　麻黄、麻黄配伍桂枝对大白鼠腋窝汗腺分泌的影响（组织形态观察法）

【目的】应用汗腺上皮组织形态法观察配伍用药对药效的影响。

【原理】利用光学显微镜观察汗腺活动。当汗腺兴奋、汗液分泌增加时，汗腺上皮细胞内空泡数目也相应增多并扩大。

【动物】雄性大白鼠。

【药品】1.6 g/mL 麻黄水煎液（麻黄 16 g，煎后浓缩成 10 mL）；10.7 g/mL 桂枝水煎液（桂枝 10.7 g，浓缩成 10 mL）；2.7 g/mL 麻黄加桂枝水煎液（麻黄 16 g、桂枝 10.7 g，共煎后浓缩成 10 mL）；10 mg/mL 毛果芸香碱溶液。

【器材】定时钟；手术剪；带塞玻璃瓶；棉手套；注射器（1 mL）；大鼠灌胃针头。

【方法】大白鼠 40 只，禁食 8 h，称重标记，随机分成 5 组。前 4 组分别灌服麻黄水煎液、桂枝水煎液、麻黄桂枝水煎液各 1 mL/100 g 体重和等容量生理盐水；第 5 组皮下注射毛果芸香碱溶液（3.5 g/kg）。给药后 1 h 处死大鼠，切取腋窝皮肤，甲醛固定，乙醇脱水，二甲苯透明，石蜡包埋，切片，HE 染色。用光学显微镜观察各组大鼠汗腺上皮细胞变化，记录汗腺总数和空泡汗腺数，并计算空泡发生率。

【结果】与空白对照组比较，阳性药组汗腺空泡发生率明显提高。受试药组大鼠汗腺空泡发生率均有不同程度提高，其中麻黄加桂枝组发汗作用最强。数据记录于表 4-2 内。

表 4–2　辛温解表药对大鼠腋窝汗腺上皮细胞形态学的影响

组别	动物数	剂量（g/kg）	观察汗腺数（个）	空泡汗腺数（个）	空泡发生率（%）
空白对照					
麻黄					
桂枝					
麻黄加桂枝					
毛果芸香碱					

【注意事项】取皮肤组织时动作应轻快。

【思考题】麻黄、桂枝和麻黄加桂枝水煎液对汗腺组织形态学的影响说明了什么？

Experiment 2　The effect of Ephedra Herb or Ephedra Herb compatible with Ramulus Cinnamomi on the secretion of armpit sweat glands in rats

【Purpose】 To observe the effect of drug compatibility on pharmacological action by the method of microscopic tissue morphology for the detection of sweat gland secretion.

【Principles】 The state of sweat glands is observed under the light microscope. When sweat gland is activated and the secretion increases, the vacuoles in epithelial cells of sweat gland become more and bigger.

【Animals】 Male rats.

【Drugs】 1.6 g/mL of Ephedra Herb decoction (16 g of Ephedra Herb, decocted with water and condesed to 10 mL), 10.7 g/mL of Ramulus Cinnamomi decoction (10.7 g of Ramulus Cinnamomi, decocted and condensed to 10 mL), 2.7 g/mL of Ephedra Herb compatible with Ramulus Cinnamomi (16 g of Ephedra Herb and 10.7 g of Ramulus Cinnamomi are decocted, condensed to 10 mL) and 10 mg/mL of pilocarpine solution.

【Equipments】 Timing clock, surgical scissors, glass bottles with stopper, cotton gloves, syringes and pinhead of intragastric administration for rats.

【Methods】 Rats are fasted for 8 h, weight, marked, and divided into 5 groups at random. The first 4 groups of rats are orally administered with 1 mL/100 g of Ephedra Herb decoction, Ramulus Cinnamomi decoction, Ephedra Herb compatible with Ramulus Cinnamomi and normal saline respectively, the 5th group of animals are subcontaneously injected with 3.5 g/kg of pilocarpine solution. After 1 h, rats are sacrificed, the skin of axillary fossa is obtained followed by formalin fixation, ethyl alcohol dehydration, dimethyl benzene clearing, slice and HE staining. Changes in epithelial cells of sweat gland are detected under light microscope. The number of sweat glands and the population of sweat glands containing vacuolated cells are recorded to calculate the percentage of vacuolated sweat glands.

【Results】 Compared with blank control, percentage of vacuolated cells of rats in positive drug group increases obviously. The tested drugs also show various degrees of perspiration effect, among which the action of Ephedra Herb compatible with Ramulus Cinnamomi is strongest. Data are filled in table 4-2.

Table 4-2 Effects of acrid-warm herbs relieving superficies on the morphology of epithelial cells of axillary fossa sweat gland in rats.

Group	Animal number	Dose (g/kg)	Number of observed Sweat glands	Number of sweat glands containing vacuolated cells	Rate of sweat glands containing vacuolated cells (%)
Blank control					
Ephedra Herb					
Ramulus Cinnamomi					
Ephedra Herb plus Ramulus Cinnamomi					
pilocarpine					

【**Notes**】The operation should be quick when the skin tissue is cut down.

【**Question**】What could be demonstrated from the effects of Ephedra Herb decoction, Ramulus Cinnamomi decoction, Ephedra Herb compatible with Ramulus Cinnamomi on the histomorphology of sweat glands?

第五章　中药药代动力学

实验一　液质联用法检测不同剂量丹酚酸 A 的狗的药代动力学及其生物利用度

【目的】研究服用不同剂量丹酚酸 A 的狗的药代动力学及在口服后，丹酚酸 A 的生物利用度。

【原理】丹参是多方面疗效的中药重要之一，根据植物化学研究报道，丹参的化学成分可分为两大类，亲脂性和亲水性，丹酚酸 A 是丹参中主要的有效丹参水溶性酚酸。本实验采用 LC-MS 法测定犬血浆中丹酚酸 A 的浓度，具有较高的灵敏度和分辨率。

【器材】安捷伦 1200 液相 -6110 质谱仪；G1379B 真空除气器；G1311A 季梯度泵；G1329A 自动进样器；G1316A 柱加热炉和电喷雾接口，用于 LC-MS 分析。数据采集与处理是采用 LC / MSD 化学工作站软件 versionB.04.02 来完成。

【试剂】丹参；以丹参的干燥根为原料，经过粉碎，溶剂萃取，大孔吸附树脂柱分离，浓缩，干燥，用 HPLC 分析纯度达 98% 以上。尼泊金丁酯；乙腈和甲醇（色谱纯）；甲酸（色谱纯）；其他试剂均为分析纯；盐酸和乙酸乙酯；坏血酸（维生素 C，VC）；肝素抗凝管；蒸馏水。

【动物】六只健康比格犬［雌雄各半，（7.5 ± 1.5）kg］。

【色谱条件】液相色谱分离，在 30 ℃柱温的 3.5 μM Agilent ZORBAX SB-C18 柱执行（100 mm × 2.1 mm，内径），分析柱前用 Agilent ZORBAX SB-C18 作保护柱。色谱条件为：两种溶剂进行梯度洗脱：溶剂 A，0.05% 甲酸水溶液和溶剂 B，0.05% 甲酸的乙腈溶液。从 15%~75% 的 B 进行梯度洗脱 5 min，然后在 5.01 min 返回到初始状态，总运行时间为 10 min，流速 0.3 mL/min。注射量为 20 μL。

ESI 是用氮气雾化进行协助；负离子模式下的 SIM。典型参数：喷雾室参数，包括毛细管电压，雾化压力，干燥气体流速和干燥气体温度分别为 −3 000 V，35 Psig，10 L/min，350 ℃；复合参数，包括碰撞诱导解离，增益和停留时间丹酚酸 A 和 IS 的分别都是 −75 V，1.5 和 144 ms。对 M / z 在 493 的丹酚酸 A 及 193 的 IS 目标离子监测。

【方法】

1. 原液和标准溶液的准备　丹酚酸 A 储备液用甲醇 - 水（50:50，V/V，含 VC100 μg/mL）制备为 100 μg/mL 浓度，用相同的溶剂稀释得到标准工作溶液。丹酚酸 A 母液在 −80 ℃存储。

内标尼泊金丁酯储备液（1 mg/mL）用甲醇为溶剂制备。内标母液（1 μg/mL）是用甲醇稀释储备液而得。在不使用时内标储备液在 −20 ℃储存。工作液浓度在 2.5~500 mg/L 范围内，取 20 μL 丹酚酸 A 工作溶液加到 180 μL 空白血浆中来制备。丹酚酸 A 的质量控制（QC）血浆样品按 5，50 和 250 mg/L 制备。

2. 血浆样品的准备　Beagle 犬禁食过夜（约 12 h），在整个实验期间自由饮水。丹酚酸 A 溶于生理盐水。给六只犬灌胃丹酚酸 A 5，10 和 20 mg/kg，或静脉注射丹酚酸 A 50 μg/kg。所有动物通过口服和静脉给药途径接受单剂量的丹酚酸 A，在经过一周消除干净。从前肢静脉取血液样本（500 μL）到肝素管，取样时间点为给药前以及口服给药后 0.083，0.167，0.25，0.333，0.5，0.75，1，2，4，8，12 和 24 h 或注射给药后 0.033，0.083，0.167，0.25，0.333，0.5，0.75，1，1.5，2，4，8，12 和 24 h。血液样本在 4 ℃，4 500 rpm 离心 15 min，用于 200 μL 的血浆样品。这些样品储存在 −80 ℃用于分析。

处理前血浆样品在室温下解冻。在 200 μL 的部分血浆样品中，加入维生素 C 10 μL（10 mg/mL）和 10 μL 的内标溶液（尼泊金丁酯，1 μg/mL）。然后，混合物用 100 μL 的 1 M HCl 酸化并用 800 μL 乙酸乙酯涡流混合为 3 min。在 13 400 rpm 离心 10 min 后，上层的有机层被转移到一个干净的离心管。在下层水相用 800 μL 乙酸乙酯再次提取，提取过程重复。结合上面的两个有机层相，并在 30 ℃氮气下蒸干。将残渣溶于 100 μL 甲醇 - 水（50 : 50，V/V，含 VC 100 μg/mL）中。在 13 400 rpm 离心 5 min 后，取 20 μL 上清液进样，LC-MS 分析。

3. 药代动力学分析　采用 DAS 药代动力学软件数据分析系统 3 版从血浆浓度 - 时间数据由非房室模型计算药代动力学参数：C_{max}、相应的时间（T_{max}）及 AUC。

4. 统计分析　对总结丹酚酸 A 的药代动力学参数进行统计学分析（SPSS）。

【结果】

1. 记录所取血浆样品的 LC-MS 结果，记录峰面积、保留时间。对六个不同大小的犬的空白血浆及用 IS 和 SAA 加标后的血浆的结果进行比较，计算 SAA 在血浆样品中浓度，绘制血浆浓度 - 时间曲线。

2. 采用 DAS 药代动力学软件数据分析系统 3 版从血浆浓度 - 时间数据由非房室模型计算药代动力学参数：C_{max}、相应的时间（T_{max}）及 AUC，并将结果填于表 5-1。

3. 基于幂模型评估 SAA 的剂量比例，将结果填于表 5-2。

表 5-1　SAA 在猎犬体内的药动学参数（$n=6$）

参数	单位	口服（mg/kg）			静脉注射（μg/kg）
		5	10	20	50
AUC（0-t）	μg/（L·h）				
C_{max}	μg/L				
T_{max}	h				
$t_{1/2}$	h				
MRT0-t	h				
F	%				

表 5-2　基于幂模型评估 SAA 的剂量比例

参数	作用范围	SAA	
		β_1	90% 置信区间
C_{max}	μg/L		
AUC（0-t）	h		

【注意事项】

1. 实验用 Beagle 犬应是健康的，并且在开始之前和实验结束之后进行寄生虫检查。

2. 试验前和试验时，狗被保存在有空调，光 / 暗循环交替 12 h，在（22 ± 2）℃温度和相对湿度 50% ± 10% 的房间的动物区。

【思考题】根据是实验结果分析服用不同剂量 SAA 的狗的药代动力学并分析剂量比例。

Chapter 5 Pharmacokinetics of TCM

Experiment 1 Pharmacokinetic study of salvianolic acid A in beagle dog after oral administration by a liquid chromatography-mass spectrometry method: A study on bioavailability and dose proportionality

【**Purpose**】To study the pharmacokinetics of different doses of SAA in beagle dogs and figure out the absolute bioavailability and dose proportionality of SAA after oral administration.

【**Principles**】Salvia miltiorrhiza Bunge (Lamiaceae), also known as Danshen, is one of the most used traditional Chinese drugs with multyfunctions. According to phytochemical reports, chemical constituents of Danshen can be classified into two major categories: the lipophilic and the hydrophilic. Salvianolic acid A is the main effective, water-soluble polyphenolic acid of Danshen, which was found to have various curative activities after intravenous injection.

For quite a long time, the administration route of SAA was limited to intravenous injection. However, compared with the pharmaco-logical research, reports regarding the pharmacokinetic study of SAA were scarce.Preclinical pharmacokinetic study of innovative drugs should be tested in two or more animal species (one being a rodent and another being a non-rodent) and the bioavailability means a lot to the clinical research and development of an oral drug. Assessment of dose proportionality can help predict patient's response to changes in dose.

Single quadrupole mass spectrometry (LC-MS) has a high sensitivity, a good resolution and a moderate price, which is undoubtedly more suitable for the application of our research and becomes an alternative to LC/MS/MS.

【**Equipments**】An Agilent 1,200 liquid chromatography-6110 mass spectrometer (SantaClara,CA,USA) equipped with a G1379B vacuum degasser,a G1311A quaternary gradient pump, a G1329A autosampler, a G1316A column oven and an ESI interface, was used for LC-MS analyses.The data acquisition and processing were accomplished using the LC/MSD Chemstation software, versionB.04.02.

【**Reagents**】Salvia miltiorrhiza Bunge, taking the dried roots of Salvia miltiorrhiza as raw material, after crushing, solvent extraction, macroporous resin column separation,concentration, and drying processes, SAA was isolated from the roots of Salvia miltiorrhiza by our laboratory, with a purity of over 94% by HPLC analysis. Butyl paraben; Acetonitrile (CH3CN, LC-MS-grade) and methanol (MeOH, LC-MS-grade); Formic acid (HCOOH,HPLC-grade); All the other reagents were of analytical grade. Hydrochloric acid (HCl) and ethylacetate (EtOAc); Ascorbic acid (VitaminC, VC);Anticoagulation tubes with heparin; Watsons distilled water was used through out the study.

【**Animals**】Six healthy ,intact beagle dogs [male and female, (7.5 ± 1.5) kg]

【**Chromatographic conditions**】LC separations were performed on a 3.5 μm Agilent Zorbax SB-C18 (1002.1mm2, i.d.) at 30 ℃ with an Agilent Zorbax SB-C18 guard column used before the analytical column.Chromatographic conditions were as follows: gradient elution was performed with two solvents:solvent A, 0.05% HCOOH in water and solvent B, 0.05% HCOOH in CH3CN. The program was initiated with a linear gradient from 15%~75% B for 5min,then returned to the initial state at 5.01 min.The total run time was 10 min with a constant flow rate of 0.3mL/min.The injection volume was 20 μL.

The ESI was performed using nitrogen to assist nebulization. SIM with negative ion mode was used.Typical parameters were used: the spray chamber parameters,including capillary voltage, nebulizer pressure,drying gas flow rate and drying gas temperature were −3 000 V, 35 psig, 10 L/min and 350 ℃ , respectively; the compound parameters, including fragmentor, gain and dwell time were −75 V, 1.5and144ms for both SAA and IS.Target ions were monitored at m/z493 for SAA and 193 for IS.

【**Methods**】

1. Preparation of stock solutions and standards The stock solution of SAA was prepared in MeOH–H_2O (50 : 50, V/V, containing VC 100 μg/mL) to be 100 μg/mL and diluted with the same diluent to obtain working standard solutions. Stock solution of SAA was stored at −80 ℃ . The IS stock solution was prepared using MeOH as the solvent at 1 mg/mL. The IS spiking solution (1 μg/mL) was prepared from the stock solution using MeOH for dilution.Stock solutions of IS was stored at −20 ℃ when not in use.Calibrators, ranging from 2.5~500 mg/L, were prepared by adding 20 μL SAA working solutions to180 μL blank plasma. Quality control (QC) samples of SAA in plasma were prepared at 5, 50 and 250 mg/L, respectively.

2. Preparation of plasma samples The dogs were fasted over night (12 h) and had free access to water throughout the experimental period. SAA was dissolved in normal saline. In order to avoid the influence of enzyme induction as a contributing factor with plasma drug levels at subsequent dosage, a Latin square design was used in the oral administration experiment. Six dogs were given an oral administration of SAA at 5, 10 and 20 mg/kg in random orde rusing the Latin square design and an intravenous dose of SAA at 50 μg/kg. All

animals received a single dose of SAA via both oral and i.v. routes, with a 1-week washout period between dosing. The blood samples (500 μL) were drawn from the fore vein into tubes with heparin before dosing and subsequently at 0.083, 0.167, 0.25, 0.333, 0.5, 0.75, 1,2, 4, 8, 12 and 24 h postdosing in the oral experimentor 0.033, 0.083, 0.167, 0.25, 0.333, 0.5, 0.75, 1, 1.5, 2, 4, 8, 12 and 24 h postdosing in the i.v. experiment.The blood samples were centrifuged at 4,500 rpm for 15 min at 4 1C to get 200 μL plasma samples. These samples were stored at −80 1C for analysis.

Plasma samples were thawed at room temperature before processing. To a 200 μL aliquot of plasma sample,10 μL of vitamin C (10 mg/mL) and 10 μL of the IS spiking solution (Butylparaben, 1 μg/mL) were added.Then, the mixture was acidified with 100 μL of 1M HCl and vortex-mixed with 800 μL EtOAc for 3 min. After centrifugation at 13,400 rpm for 10 min, the upper organic layer was transferred to a clean Eppendorf tube. To the lower aqueous phase 800 μL EtOAc was added again and the extraction process was repeated. The two upper organic layers were combined and evaporated to dryness under nitrogen at 30 ℃. The residue was reconstituted in 100 μL of MeOH–H_2O (50 : 50, V/V, containing VC 100 μg/mL). After centrifugation at 13,400 rpm for 5min, 20 μL of the supernatant was injected to the LC-MS system.

3. Pharmacokinetics analysis Pharmacokinetic parameters were calculated from plasma concentration-time data using the DAS pharmacokinetic software Data Analysis System Version3.0 by a non-compartmental model. C_{max}, the corresponding time (T_{max}) and AUC could all be obtained.

4. Statistical analyses Descriptive statistics were used to summarize the pharmacokinetic parameters for SAA. Dose proportionality for AUC (0-t) and C_{max} was assessed by linear regression of ln-transformed parameters on the natural ln- transformed dose [$\ln(PK)=\beta_0+\beta_1\ln(\text{dose})$]. Values of the proportionality constant, β_1, and its corresponding 90% confidence interval were estimated with the SPSS 13.0 software.The primary methodology used to assess dose proportionality from 5~20 mg/kg was a comparison of the 90% confidence interval (CI) of the slopes with the modified acceptance range [$1+(\ln(\theta L)/\ln(r)$, $1+\ln(\theta H)/\ln(r)$] based on a power model, where θL and θH are the lower and upper limits of the confidence interval and r is the maximal dose ratio for the study. Dose proportionality was concluded if the plot of pharmacokinetic parameter vs. dose indicated linearity (i.e.,slope=1) and the 90% CI for the slope fell within the modified acceptance range.

【Results】

1. Analyzing six different lots of beagle dog blank plasma and compared with those results obtained from spiking the blank plasma with SAA and IS, and calculate the concentrations of SAA in plasma samples to make up the plasma concentration-time curve.

2. Pharmacokinetic parameters were calculated from plasma concentration-time data using the DAS pharmacokinetic software Data Analysis System Version3.0 by a non-

compartmental model. C_{max}, the corresponding time (T_{max}) and AUC could all be obtained.Fill in the table 5-1.

3. Assess the dose proportionality of SAA based on power model, fill in the table 5-2.

Table 5-1　Pharmacokinetics parameters of SAA in beagle dogs (n=6).

parameters	Unit	Oral (mg/kg)			i.v. (mg/kg)
		5	10	20	50
AUC (0-t)	μg/ (L · h)				
C_{max}	μg/L				
T_{max}	h				
$t_{1/2}$	h				
MRT0-t	h				
F	%				

Table 5-2　Assessment of dose proportionality of SAA based on power model.

Parameters	Acceptance range	SAA	
		β_1	90% confidence interval
C_{max}	μg/L		
AUC (0-t)	h		

[Notes]

1. The dogs were considered to be healthy and free from disease and parasites based on physical examination before initiation and after completion of the study.

2.The dogs were maintained in air-conditioned animal quarters with alternating 12h light/dark cycles at a room temperature of (22 ± 2) ℃ and a relative humidity of 50% ± 10% before and during the trial.

[Questions] Analysis the Pharmacokinetic of SAA in beagle dog and study its dose proportionality based on the datas.

实验二　快速敏感的液相色谱－质谱法串联法测定大鼠血浆中的人参皂苷 Rb1，Rb2 和 Rb3 方法学建立及在药代动力学研究中的应用

【目的】掌握 LC-MS/MS 方法，比较三种人参皂苷药代动力学行为的相似性和差异。

【原理】人参皂苷已被视为三七药材的药理作用的主要活性成分。三七提取物中，人参皂苷 Rb1、Rb2 和 Rb3 是主要的皂苷成分。这三种人参皂苷均为 20（S）- 原人参二醇皂苷（PPD），并具有相同的糖基化位点（C-3 位点，C-20 位点）。区别仅在于连接到 C-20 位点的糖苷。皂苷 Rb1 连接有两个葡萄糖，RB2 连接有一个葡萄糖和一个 α-L-吡喃阿拉伯糖基，和 Rb3 连接有一个葡萄糖和一个 β-D- 木糖。由于紫外检测方法不适合于人参皂苷的测定，因此液相色谱－质谱（LC-MS）和液相色谱－串联质谱（LC-MS/MS）的方法被广泛用于分析人参皂苷。

【试剂】人参皂苷 Rb1，Rb2、Rb3 和 Rg2（内标）（99%）；甲酸铵；试剂为色谱纯。

【动物】SD 大鼠（200~220 g）。

【仪器和色谱条件】Agilent 1200 快速分离 HPLC 系统与配有电喷雾电离（ESI）的安捷伦 6 410 三重四极杆质谱仪串联色谱。Agilent ZORBAX SB-C 18 柱（50 mm × 4.6 mm，1.8 ≤ M）。流动相：甲醇和 1 mM 甲酸铵（74∶26，体积 / 体积，pH 值 6.0），流速为 0.4 mL/min。对 Rb1，Rb2，Rb3 和 IS 分别在 M / Z1107.7 → M / Z 178.9，M / Z1077.7 → M / Z 148.6，M / Z1077.7 → m/z783.4，和 m / z783.6 → M / Z475.1 的负多反应监测来进行定量。Rb1，Rb2，和 Rb3 的裂解 / 碰撞能量的值分别在 250 V/55 V，210 V/67 V，200 V/58 V。流速，9 L/min；雾化压力，40 磅；气体温度，350 ℃。

【方法】

1. 校准曲线和血浆样品的制备　标准曲线的制备用原液对空白大鼠血浆加标至浓度：Rb1 和 Rb2 为 20，50，100，500，1 000 ng/mL，Rb3 为 50，100，500，1 000 和 2 500 ng/mL。样品（100 μL）与 IS 溶液（1 μg/mL，10 μL）混合，用 900 μL 饱和的正丁醇萃取。以 13 000 × g 的离心 10 min 后，将上清液在氮气流中蒸发浓缩至干。将残余物溶解在 100 μL 流动相中，离心 10 min。取 20 μL 上清液进样分析。

2. 在大鼠体内的药代动力学研究　大鼠随机分为六组：三组分别经尾静脉静脉注射（10 mg/kg）Rb1，Rb2、Rb3，另外三组分别口服人参皂苷 Rb1，Rb2、Rb3（50 mg/kg）。血液样品在 0.083，0.25，0.5，1，2，4，6，8，12，24 和 36 h 收集（iv），和 0.25，0.5，0.75，1，1.5，2，3，4，6，8，10，12，24，和 36 h（po）。血液样品立即离心（4 000 rpm），取上清，置于 –20 ℃条件下存储。

【结果】

1. 根据所取血浆样品的 LC-MS/MS 测定结果计算血浆样品中皂苷浓度,采用 DAS2.0 软件的非房室模型计算药代动力学参数,并将结果填在表 5-3 中。

2. 绘制口服 10 mg/kg 和静注 50 mg/kg 剂量后(n = 6),Rb1、Rb2、Rb3 的血浆浓度–时间的曲线。

表 5-3　经静脉注射(10 mg/kg)和口服(50 mg/kg)的大鼠体内,人参皂苷 Rb1,Rb2、Rb3 的药代动力学参数(n = 6)

参数	Rb1		Rb2		Rb3	
	i.v.	p.o.	i.v.	p.o.	i.v.	p.o.
AUC0-t(mg · h / L)						
AUC0-∞(mg · h / L)						
$t_{1/2}$(h)						
MRT0-t(h)						
T_{max}(h)						
C_{max}(mg/L)						

【注意事项】大鼠分组按照随机分组原则进行。

【思考题】根据实验结果分析 Rb1,Rb2、Rb3 在大鼠的药代动力学的区别。

Experiment 2 Determination of ginsenosides Rb1, Rb2, and Rb3 in rat plasma by a rapid and sensitive liquid chromatography tandem mass spectrometry method: Application in a pharmacokinetic study

【Purpose】To study to use LC-MS/MS method to determine plasma concentrations of Rb1, Rb2, and Rb3 after oral and intravenous administration and to systematically compare their similarities and differences in pharmacokinetic behaviors.

【Principles】Ginsenosides have been regarded as the main active components responsible for the pharmacological activities of Panax herbs. Ginsenoside Rb1 is the main saponin,while Rb2 and Rb3 as the other minor chief constituents in Panax extract. The three ginsenosides all are 20(S)-protopanaxadiol saponins (PPD) and have the same glycosylation site (C-3 site, C-20 site). The difference only lies in glycoside connected to the C-20 site. Rb1 connects with two glucoses, Rb2 connects with one glucose and one α-L-arabinopyranosyl, and Rb3 connects with one glucose and one β-d-xylose.

Although the pharmacokinetic characteristic of Rb1 is known, the information of Rb2 and Rb3 are rare. Therefore, pharmacokinetic studies of Rb2 and Rb3 are necessary and could help clarify the relationship between pharmacokinetics and structural preference of ginsenosides. Since ginsenosides have poor UV radiation in maximum absorption of 203 nm. The liquid chromatography mass spectrometry (LC-MS) and liquid chromatography–tandem mass spectrometry (LC-MS/MS) method are widely used for analyzing ginsenosides.

【Reagents】Ginsenoside Rb1, Rb2, Rb3 and Rg2 (internal standard, IS) (99.0%); Ammonium formate; All other reagents were of HPLC grade.

【Animals】Sprague Dawley rats (200~220 g)。

【Equipments and analytical conditions】The Agilent 1,200 rapid resolution HPLC system was interfaced with an Agilent 6,410 triple quadrupole mass spectrometer equipped with an electrospray ionization (ESI). The column was an Agilent Zorbax SB-C18 column (50 mm × 4.6 mm, 1.8 vm).The mobile phase was methanol and 1 mM ammonium formate (74:26, V/V, pH 6.0), the flow rate was 0.4 mL/min. Quantitation was performed in negative multiple reaction monitoring of m/z 1107.7 → m/z 178.9, m/z 1077.7 → m/z 148.6, m/z 1077.7 → m/z 783.4, and m/z783.6 → m/z 475.1 for Rb1, Rb2, Rb3, and IS,respectively. The values of fragmentation/collision energy were at 250 V/55 V, 210 V/67 V, 200 V/58 V for Rb1, Rb2, and Rb3, respectively. Flow rate, 9 l/min; nebulizer pressure, 40 psi; gas temperature, 350 ℃.

【 **Methods** 】

1. Preparation of calibration curve and plasma samples　Calibration curve were prepared by spiking blank rat plasma with the stock solution to the concentrations: 20, 50, 100, 500, 1,000 ng/mL for Rb1 and Rb2; 50, 100, 500, 1,000, and 2,500 ng/mL for Rb3. The sample (100 μL) was mixed with the IS solution (1 μg/mL, 10 μL) and extracted with 900 μL saturated N-butanol. After centrifugation at 13,000 × g for 10 min, the supernatant was evaporated to dryness under a stream of nitrogen. The residue was dissolved in 100 μL mobile phase and centrifuged for 10 min. 20 μL of the supernatant was injected into the LC-MS/MS.

2. Pharmacokinetics study in rats　The rats were randomLy assigned into six groups: three groups were intravenous administered of Rb1, Rb2, and Rb3, respectively through tail vein (10 mg/kg), the three other groups were orally administered of Rb1, Rb2, and Rb3, respectively (50 mg/kg). Blood samples were collected at 0.083, 0.25, 0.5, 1, 2, 4, 6, 8, 12, 24, and 36 h (iv) and 0.25, 0.5, 0.75, 1, 1.5, 2, 3, 4, 6, 8, 10, 12, 24, and 36 h (p.o.). Blood samples were centrifuged immediately and stored at –20 ℃ until analysis.

【 **Results** 】

1. Record the LC-MS/MS results of the plasma samples obtained, calculate the plasma concentration, and calculate Pharmacokinetic parameters by the non-compartmental mode using DAS2.0 software.Fill in the table 5-3.

2. Make up plasma concentration–time curve of Rb1 (A), Rb2 (B) and Rb3 (C) after oral dose of 50 mg/kg and i.v. dose of 10 mg/kg ($n = 6$).

Table 5–3　Pharmacokinetic parameters of Rb1, Rb2, and Rb3 after i.v. (10 mg/kg) and oral (50 mg/kg) administration in rats (n =6)

parameters	Rb1		Rb2		Rb3	
	i.v.	p.o.	i.v.	p.o.	i.v.	p.o.
AUC0-t (mg · h / L)						
AUC0-∞ (mg · h / L)						
$t_{1/2}$ (h)						
MRT0-t (h)						
T_{max} (h)						
C_{max} (mg/L)						

【 **Notes** 】Make sure that the rats were randomly assigned into six groups.

【 **Questions** 】Analysis the pharmacokinetics of Rb1, Rb2, and Rb3 in rats and the pharmacokinetic preference behaviors of ginsenosides based on the datas.

实验三 人参皂苷 compound K 在 Caco-2 细胞的吸收机制

【目的】在 Caco-2 细胞上考察人参皂苷 compound K 的转运机制。

【原理】许多研究显示，大多数的人参皂甙由于其高极性在人体肠道的吸收较差。人参皂苷 compound K 是二醇型人参皂苷在人体肠道内的主要代谢产物和最终吸收形式。由于其表现了与人类小肠上皮细胞在形态和功能上的相似性，Caco-2 单层细胞已被公认为一个用于预测人类肠道的药物吸收和用于肠道药物转运的机制研究的体外模型。

【器材】Transwell 细胞培养室（孔径，0.4 μm；直径，24 mm）；ERS 伏欧表；酶标仪。

【试剂】Caco-2 细胞；DMEM；非必需氨基酸；青霉素 – 链霉素（10 000 IU /μL）；Hank's 平衡盐溶液（HBSS）；EDTA；磷酸盐缓冲盐水（PBS）溶液；胎牛血清（FBS）；甘露醇；维拉帕米和 MK-571。

【方法】

1. Caco-2 细胞培养　Caco-2 细胞在含胎牛血清（10%，V / V），NEAA（1%，V / V），青霉素（100 U /mL），链霉素（0.1 μg/mL），和谷氨酰胺（0.29 g/L）的 DMEM 培养基中培养，放置在含 5% 的 CO_2 的湿空气中 37 ℃培养。培养基每 2 天更换，细胞在约 90% 用胰蛋白酶 / EDTA 溶液（0.25% / 0.02%）以 1~4 的分流比汇合中传代。

2. Caco-2 单层的跨膜运输实验

（1）在运输实验中，Caco-2 细胞接种到涂有密度为 4×10^5 cells/cm^2 的 I 型胶原的 6- 孔的 Transwell 小室上以生成 Caco-2 单层细胞。每 2~3 天更换培养基，传代后 21~27 天进行实验。细胞层的完整性和紧密连接在每个实验前用 ERS 式设备测量细胞单层的电阻（TEER）来测定。TEER 值超过 300 Ω•cm^2 的适用于转运实验。

（2）在实验前单层用 HBSS（pH 值 7.4，37 ℃）轻轻漂洗两次。细胞单层细胞在 37 ℃转运缓冲液中孵育 30 min。测量 AP-BL 渗透性，取含 CK 的缓冲液 0.5 mL，添加到 AP 侧的 Transwell 小室，另 1.5 mL 的溶液添加到 BL 室。然后将该板置于 37 ℃环境中。在相应时间点从 BL 侧收集 0.4 mL 溶液，并用等体积的 HBSS 更换。BL-AP 方向的渗透性，取含 CK（50 μM）的缓冲液 1.5 mL，添加到 BL 侧，另 0.5 mL 的 HBSS 加到 AP 侧。所有的孵育重复 3 次。

3. CK 的细胞摄取　依照描述制备细胞单层。将 CK 溶液加在单层细胞的 AP 侧于 37 ℃孵箱放置 2 h。在各个时间点收集 AP 和 BL 侧的溶液，然后测定 CK 的含量。用冰 HBSS 将单分子膜洗五次，用含 1% Triton X-100 的甲醇室温提取 1 h。在 10 000 g 将细胞裂解液离心 5 min，用高效液相色谱分析上清液。采用 BCA 蛋白检测试剂盒以牛血清白蛋白为标准测定细胞裂解液中的蛋白质浓度。待测化合物的吸收表示为 nmol / mg protein。

4. 高效液相色谱分析

（1）高效液相色谱系统：高压液相色谱与二极管阵列检测器（DAD）。检测波长为203 nm。Hypersil ODS 柱（150 mm × 3.9 mm，水域，米尔福德，MA）进行样本分析。流动相为乙腈 / 水（85 : 15，V/V），流速为 1 mL/min。

（2）HPLC 测定 CK 的浓度（0.05~50 μM），测量峰面积以生成用于样本定量的校准曲线。

【结果】

1. 测量每个时间间隔的待测化合物的累计量并绘制成时间曲线。
2. 计算表观渗透系数（Papp，cm/s）。
3. 计算（B-A）和（A-B）的渗透系数比来测定流出率（Re）。
4. 用 SPSS 13 软件进行 *t* 检验。

【注意事项】注意细胞培养过程中的无菌操作。

【思考题】

1. 分析 CK 在 Caco-2 细胞模型的转运机制。
2. 如何改进 CK 在 Caco-2 细胞模型的跨膜吸收及转运？

Experiment 3 Absorption Mechanism of Ginsenoside Compound K and Its Butyl and Octyl Ester Prodrugs in Caco-2 Cells

【Purpose】To examine the transport mechanisms of CK, CK-B, and CK-O using human Caco-2 cells; To find the method to improve the transport of CK across Caco-2 cells.

【Principles】Panax ginseng C.A. Meyer, the active components of ginsenosides, is frequently utilized as a herbal drug in traditional oriental medicine. These ginsenosides, which belong to the class of triterpene saponins, have been reported to exhibit various biological and pharmacological activities such as antiaging, antiinflammation and antioxidation in central nerve system, cardiovascular system and immune system. Previous studies have shown that the pharmacological actions of ginsenosides was relative with t their metabolites through biotransformation by human intestinal bacteria. Compound K（CK）is one of the main pharmacologically active metabolites of protopanaxadiol ginsenosides（e.g., Rb1, Rb2 and Rc）. More studies revealed that most of the ginsenosides are poorly absorbed along the human intestinal tract due to a high polarity. The biological activities of drugs depend not only on their chemical structures, but also on their degree of lipophilic and membrane permeation, which could enhance their transport across the cell membrane or influence their interaction with proteins and enzymes.

Recently, considerable attention has been paid to the development of ester prodrugs, which is a widely used approach to improving overall lipophicity, membrane permeability and oral absorption of poorly absorbed drugs. Mannich bases and N-masked prodrugs of norfloxacin（NFX）have been reported to enhance its lipophilicity, bioavailability and in vivo activity. To increase the oral absorption of CK, esterification provides a route to obtain more lipophilic derivatives.

Caco-2 cell monolayers have been generally accepted as an in vitro model for prediction of drug absorption across human intestine and for mechanistic studies of intestinal drug transport since these cells show morphological and functional similarities to human small intestinal epithelial cells.

【Equipments】Transwell cell culture chambers（pore size, 0.4 μm; diameter, 24 mm）; Millicell-ERS voltohmmeter; Microplate reader.

【Reagents】The human colon adenocarcinoma cell line, Caco-2; Dulbecco's modified Eagle's medium（DMEM）; nonessential amino acids（NEAA）; penicillin-streptomycin

(10 000 IU/mL); Hank's balanced salt solution (HBSS); trysin and ethylenediaminetetraacetic acid (EDTA) (0.25%/0.02%) in Phosphate Buffer Saline (PBS); Fetal bovine serum (FBS); Mannitol;verapamil and MK-571; The CK and its ester derivatives CK-B and CK-O.

【Methods】

1. Caco-2 Cell Culture Caco-2 cells are cultured in DMEM containing FBS (10%, v/v), NEAA (1%, V/V), penicillin (100 U/mL), streptomycin (0.1 mg/mL), and glutamine (0.29 g/L) in a humidified atmosphere with 5% CO_2 at 37 ℃ . The medium is replaced every 2 days and the cells are passaged at approximately 90% confluence using a trypsin/EDTA solution (0.25%/0.02%) at a split ratio of 1~4.

2. Transepithelial Transport Experiments across Caco-2 Monolayer

(1) For transport experiments, Caco-2 cells are plated onto the 6-well transwell inserts coated with type-I collagen at a density of 4×10^5 cells/cm^2 to generate Caco-2 monolayers. Medium is changed every 2~3 days and the monolayers used for the experiments were left to differentiate for 21~27 days after postseeding. The integrity of the cell layer and the full development of the tight junctions are monitored before every experiment by measurement of transepithelial electrical resistance (TEER) of filter-grown cell monolayers with millicell-ERS equipment. Only a monolayer with a TEER value of more than 300 $\Omega \cdot cm^2$ is used for the transepithelial transport experimnets.

(2) The monolayers were gently rinsed twice with warm HBSS (pH 7.4, 37 ℃) prior to the experiments. Cell monolayers are then incubated for 30 min at 37 ℃ in the transport buffer. To measure the apical-to-basolated (AP-BL) permeability, 0.5 mL of mixture containing CK, CK-B or CK-O over 10~50 μM in transport buffer is added to the AP side of the transwell insert and 1.5 mL of HBSS is added to the BL chamber. The plates are then put in an incubator at 37 ℃ . At designated time intervals, 0.4 mL of aliquots of solution is collected from the BL side and then replaced with an equal volume of HBSS. In the direction of BL-AP, CK, CK-B or CK-O in 1.5 mL of transport buffer over 10~50 μM is added to the BL side, and 0.5 mL of the HBSS to AP side. All incubations were performed in triplicates.

3. Cellular Uptake of CK Cell monolayers are prepared as described for the transport studies. Test compound (CK) is loaded onto the AP side of the cell monolayer over 2 h at 37 ℃ . At the selected time point, the solutions in the AP and BL side are collected and the amounts of the test compounds are then measured. The monolayers are washed five times with icecold HBSS and extracted with methanol containing 1% Triton X-100 for 1 h at room temperature. Cell lysates are centrifuged at 10 000 g for 5 min and the supernatants are analyzed using HPLC. The protein concentration in cell lysates is determined using the BCA protein assay kit (Pierce, Rockford, IL) with bovine serum albumin as the standard. The uptake of the test compounds is expressed as nmoL/mg protein.

4. Analysis by HPLC

(1) The HPLC system: Agilent HPLC series 1100; Diode array detector (DAD);

Detection Wavelength: 203 nm; Hypersil ODS column (150 mm × 3.9 mm, Waters, Milford, MA); Mobile phase: acetonitrile/water (85 : 15, V/V); flow rate: 1.0 mL/min.

(2) The standard concentrations (0.05~50 μM) of CK and ester derivatives are analyzed by HPLC and peak area measurement is used to generate calibration curves for the quantification of samples. The corresponding standards of CK, CK-B and CK-O for identification and quantification are prepared in methanol solution.

【Results】

1. The cumulative quantity of test compound permeated at each time interval is measured and plotted against time.

2. Calculate the apparent permeability coefficients (Papp, cm/s).

3. Determine the efflux ratio (Re) by calculating the ratio of Papp (B-A) versus Papp (A-B).

4. Student's t test is conducted with a P-value of less than 0.05 as statistically significant. All statistical analyses are carried out using SPSS 13.0 software for Windows.

【Notes】Pay attention to the aseptic operation during the Cell culture process.

【Questions】

1. Analyze the absorption mechanism of Ginsenoside Compound K in Caco-2 Cells.

2. How to improve the transport of CK across Caco-2 cells?

第六章　解表药实验

凡能发散表邪，解除表证的药物称为解表药。表证是由六淫之邪或疫疠邪气从人体皮毛或口鼻侵入；病位在表，引起恶寒发热、头痛身疼、无汗或有汗、舌苔薄、脉浮等症状。以感受风邪为主，兼夹寒邪侵犯人体所致者，称为风寒表证；若兼夹热邪侵犯人体所致者，称风热表证。根据药物的性能特点和功效主治，解表药可分为发散风寒药和发散风热药两类。

发散风寒药，性味多为辛温，发汗作用较强。主要药物有：麻黄、桂枝、紫苏、荆芥、防风等。发散风热药，性味多为辛凉，发汗作用较为缓和，重在透表而导热外出。主要药物有：菊花、薄荷、柴胡、牛蒡子、葛根等。

现代药理研究表明，解表药具有发汗、解热、抗炎、抗病原微生物、抗过敏、免疫调节等作用，此外还有镇痛、镇静、止咳祛痰、利尿等作用。

在研究解表药的药理作用时，要结合表证的病因（外感六淫的性质）、主要症状（出汗、发热、头身疼痛、咳嗽等）、药物的性味与功效，设计研究指标与方法。现对目前常用的实验方法简介如下：

1. 发汗实验　有些解表药能使机体汗腺分泌活动增强，兴奋体温调节中枢，扩张周围血管，促进体表的血液循环，表现为汗液分泌增加。其作用机理可能是兴奋外周的 α 受体，抑制汗腺导管对 Na^+ 的重吸收，以及拟肾上腺素作用。常用的实验方法有：汗液着色法、汗液定量测定法、汗腺上皮组织形态观察法、皮肤电生理技术法和腋窝部皮肤汗腺导管内径测定法等。

2. 解热实验　发热是表证的常见症状，多数解表药具有散热功效，对异常升高的体温有明显降温作用。作用机理比较复杂，可能是抑制发热的多个环节，如降低机体的产热、抑制内生性致热源的生成等相关。常通过对正常动物（大鼠或家兔）皮下或静脉注射一定量的致热源（伤寒、副伤寒菌苗、内毒素、啤酒酵母液、细菌培养液、松节油、二硝基苯酚等），造成发热病理模型，在此模型上观察药物的解热作用。

3. 抗菌（抗病毒）实验　细菌及病毒作为六淫外邪之一，使机体产生表证，解表药对多种细菌及病毒有较强的体内外抑制作用。该实验方法常包括体外实验和体内实验（整体动物实验）两种。

（1）体外实验：测定药物的体外抗菌能力又有两大类方法：琼脂渗透法和试管稀释法。琼脂渗透法可将细菌混入琼脂培养基中，制成平板，或将细菌涂于琼脂平板的表面，再采用打洞法、滤纸片法、管碟法、挖沟法等不同的方法将药物置于琼脂平板中，置 37 ℃孵箱中培养 18~24 h，利用药物能渗透至琼脂培养基的性能，观察药物周围形成的抑菌圈，以测定药物的抗菌性能。试管稀释法是将药物提取液按倍比稀释法与肉汤培养基混匀成各种浓度，然后在各管中接种等量的细菌，培养 18~24 h，观察各管内细菌生长情况。

（2）体内实验（整体动物实验）：在体外实验中呈现抗菌作用的药物，还需利用整体动物实验做进一步的验证。对小鼠腹腔注射一定致病力的细菌进行感染，感染后给予药物治疗，观察实验小鼠的死亡率，评价药物的抗感染效果。

抗病毒实验常用体外实验有组织培养法，鸡胚培养法和整体动物实验法，观察药物对体内、外病毒感染的影响。

4. 镇咳、祛痰、平喘实验　咳、痰、喘是表证的常见症状，解表药大多具有镇咳、祛痰和扩张支气管作用。常见镇咳实验有氨水引咳法、SO_2 引咳法和电刺激法等；祛痰实验有气管酚红排泌法、气管纤毛运动法、毛细玻璃管法等；平喘实验有喷雾致喘法和肺溢流法等。通过上述实验可以观察药物的镇咳、祛痰和平喘作用。

5. 抗炎实验　呼吸道炎症是咳、痰、喘的根本原因，也是表证的临床表现，多数解表药能抑制炎症早期的白细胞游走、毛细血管通透性的升高和炎症后期肉芽组织的形成。具体实验方法参见祛风湿药。

有些解表药还具有镇痛、抗过敏、免疫调节等作用，其实验方法参见其他相关章节。总之，要了解一味药的药理作用及作用机理，应根据药物的特点、结合中医药理论对其所治疗病证的病因，发病机制的认识，合理设计实验内容，通过实验结果正确评价药物的主治功效及临床应用。

Chapter 6 Experiments on exterior-relieving herbs

Herbs that chiefly disperse the exterior evils and relieve exterior syndrome are called exterior-relieving herbs. The exterior syndromes, which display symptoms as chills and fever, headache and pain, no sweating or profuse sweating, thin tongue coating, floating pulse etc., are caused by the Six Exogenous Factors or infectious damp heat which invade the body from skin or mouth and nose. The exterior syndrome, caused mainly by wind pathogenic factor, if cold evil involved, is called wind-cold exterior syndrome; if heat evil involved, is called wind-heat exterior syndrome. According to their property, characteristics, functions and indications, exterior-relieving herbs can be classified as wind-cold-dispersing herbs and wind-heat-dispersing herbs.

Wind-cold-dispersing herbs are usually acrid in flavor and warm in nature. They promote sweating strongly. This family mainly includes Mahuang (Ephedra), Guizhi (Cinnamoni Twig), Zisu (Perillae), Jingjie (Hb Schizonepetae), Fangfeng (Hb Ledebourielliae). Wind-heat-dispersing herbs are usually acrid in flavor and cool in property. They promote sweating mildly and their therapy effects are principally due to the leading out of fever. Juhua (FI Chrysanthemi), Bohe (Hb Menthae), Chaihu (Rx Bupleuri), Niu Bangzi (Fr Arctii), Gegen (Rx Puerariae) are mainly included in this class.

Modern pharmacology researches indicate that these exterior-relieving herbs exhibit many activities, such as sweat-promoting, fever-relieving, anti-inflammation, anti-pathogenic microorgnism, anti-anaphylaxis, immunoregulation, analgesia, sedative, cough-stopping, phlegm-expelling, diuresis, etc..

The etiopathogenisis of exterior syndrome (nature of the Six Exogenous Evils), main symptoms (sweating, fever, headache, pain, coughing, etc.); the taste, property and functions of the herbs, all of which should be kept in mind when designing the experiment protocols and choosing index if one conducts studies focusing on pharmacology of exterior-relieving herbs. Here, we generally introduce some common experiments adopted at present.

1. The test of sweat-promoting Some exterior-relieving herbs can enhance the secretory activities of coil gland, stimulate the thermolytic center of the thermoregulation system of the body surface, resulting in increased sweat secretion. The mechanism of this phenomenon may be that these exterior-relieving herbs stimulate peripheral α-receptor, inhibit the re-absorption of Na^+ by ducts of coil gland and show adrenaline-like effects. The common experiments used include sweat-staining, sweat-quantitation, observation of epithelium tissure-morph, technology in the electronic physiology of skin, measurement of the inside diameter of coil gland duct in the skin of axillary fossa.

2. The test of fever-relieving Fever is a common symptom of exterior syndrome. Most of the exterior-relieving herbs have fever-dispersing activity, thus show obvious cooling effects for the abnormal fever. The mechanism is complicated; possibly by blocking the process of fever generation. For example, decrease the heat production of the body, or inhibit the formation of endogenous pyrogens. Commonly adopted experiments may as follows: to create a fever-model by subcutaneous or intravenous injecting a fixed amount of pyrogens (typhobacterin, paratyphoid vaccine, endotoxin, beer yeast liquid, bacteria-culture-medium, abies oil, dihitrophend) and evaluate the fever-relieving effects of herbs using this fever model.

3. Determination of anti-bacteria (anti-virus) activity Bacteria and virus are considered as one of the Six Exogenous Evils, and may cause exterior-syndrome. Exterior-relieving herbs show potent inhibitory effects on many kinds of bacteria and virus both in vivo and in vitro. Tests may be conducted in in vitro or in in vivo.

(1) In vitro experiments: There are two methods in vitro to determine the anti-bacteria activity of herbs: agar diffusion technique and tube dilution technique. Agar diffusion technique can be performed as follows: add bacteria into the agar medium and spread them out onto a plate or spread bacteria out on the surface of a plate coated with agar; then add tested herbs into the plate by any of the hole-digging method, filter-paper method, cylinder plate method and ditch-digging method; incubate the plate at 37 ℃ for 16~18 h and determine the anti-bacteria activity by measurement of the inhibition zone diameter. The test is based on the diffusion ability of herbs in the agar medium. Tube dilution technique may be performed as follows: dilute herb solution to different concentrations and mix them with broth culture medium; inoculate same amount of bacterium in each tube and incubate for 16-18 h; observe the growth of bacterium in all tubes.

(2) In vivo experiments: Functions of herbs that exhibited anti-bacteria effects in vitro should be further verifiated in in vivo. We may evaluate the anti-infection effects of herbs according to the mortality of mice which received herb therapy after i.p with some virulencous bacteria.Common protocols used in anti-virus experiments are tissure-culture, embryonated egg-culture and in vivo. All these protocols can be used to demonstrate the effects of herbs on virus-infection in vivo and in vitro.

4. Cough-stopping, phlegm-expelling, wheeze-stopping tests Cough, phlegm and wheeze are common symptoms of exterior syndrome. Most exterior-relieving herbs show ability of cough-stopping, phlegm-expelling and bronchi dilation. Ammonia water induced cough, SO_2-induced cough and electronic-stimulation are commonly used cough-stopping experiments. Trachea secretion of phenolsulfonphthalein, movement of trachea cilia, glass capillary techniques are included in phlegm-transformation experiments. Wheeze-stopping experiments include spray-induced cough and overflow of lung. We can evaluate the effects of herbs on cough-stopping, phlegm-expelling, wheeze-stopping by the experiments mentioned above.

5. Determination of anti-inflammation activity Respiratory inflammation is the main cause for cough, phlegm and wheeze, and it is also the clinical main festation of exterior syndrome. Most exterior-relieving herbs can inhibit the transmigration of leucocytes and the up-regulation of capillary vascular permeability at the early stage of inflammation. These herbs can also inhibit the formation of granulation tissure at the later stage of inflammation. Details are showed in the chapter of "rheumatism-driving herbs" .

Some exterior-relieving herbs have other activities, such as anti-anaphylaxis, immuno-regulation, and the experiments are seen in relative chapters. In a word, one should design experiments properly according to the characteristics of herbs, the etiological factors and the pathogenesis of syndromes these herbs treated. The functions, indications and clinical usage of herbs can only be evaluated by the results of related experiments. Remember that all the research should be conducted under the theory of traditional Chinese medicine.

实验一　麻黄配桂枝对大白鼠足跖汗液分泌的影响（着色法）

【目的】观察辛温解表药对汗液分泌的影响，掌握麻黄、麻黄配桂枝发汗作用的异同。

【原理】大鼠足跖部肉垫上有汗腺分布，可利用碘与淀粉遇汗液产生紫色反应的机理，观察和测定药物对大鼠汗液分泌的影响。

【器材】大鼠固定器；大鼠灌胃器；固定架；医用胶布；注射器（2.5 mL）；放大镜；秒表；棉签；针头等。

【试剂】麻黄水煎液（1 g/mL）；麻黄配桂枝水煎液（1 g/mL）；毛果芸香碱溶液（3.5 mg/mL）；苦味酸液；蒸馏水；无水乙醇；和田 - 高垣氏液等。

【动物】大鼠，体重 180~200 g。

【方法】

1. 药液的制备

麻黄桂枝水煎液：取麻黄 30 g、桂枝 20 g，共煎成 50 mL，即 1 g/mL 溶液。

麻黄水煎液：取麻黄 50 g，常规制备，浓缩成 1 g/mL 溶液。

和田 - 高垣氏液：

A 液：取碘 2 g 溶于 100 mL 无水乙醇，振荡混匀即可。

B 液：取可溶性淀粉 50 g，蓖麻油 100 mL，两者混匀即成。

2. 实验操作及观察　取健康大鼠 12 只，称重，用苦味酸液标记，随机分为 4 组，每组 3 只。

用棉签蘸无水乙醇擦干净大鼠足底部，甲组大鼠灌服蒸馏水（1 mL/100 g）、乙组大鼠腹腔注射毛果芸香碱溶液（3.5 mg/100 g）、丙组大鼠灌服麻黄水煎液（1 mL/100 g）、丁组大鼠灌服麻黄配桂枝水煎液（1 mL/100 g），给药后分别将大鼠固定于大鼠固定器中，暴露双下肢，并用医用胶布轻轻缚住，防止大鼠活动时下肢回缩到固定器中。

给药后 30 min 棉签拭干大鼠足跖部原有汗液，然后在大鼠足跖部皮肤涂上和田—高垣氏试剂 A 液，待干燥后，再薄薄涂上 B 液，然后用放大镜观察深紫色着色点（即汗点）出现时间、颜色和数量。待汗点出现后，连续观察 30 min，每 5 min 观察记录一次。

【结果】按表 6-1 记录。

表 6–1　麻黄、麻黄配桂枝水煎液对大鼠足跖部汗液分泌的影响

组别	剂量（g/kg）	给药途径	汗点出现时间（min）	给药后 1 h 汗点数
甲组				
乙组				
丙组				
丁组				

【注意事项】

1. 固定大鼠时操作应轻柔,尽量避免挣扎出汗而影响药效评价。

2. 为避免影响实验结果的准确性,观察大鼠足跖部汗点出现时间,在同一批实验中务必一致。

3. 实验室温度控制在(26 ± 1)℃左右,实验室相对湿度控制在 65% ± 5%。

【思考题】

1. 麻黄、麻黄配桂枝发汗作用有何特点?

2. 麻黄配桂枝为何有协同发汗的作用?

Experiment 1 The effects of Mahuang coupled with Guizhi on the sweat secretion at toes of rat (staining method)

【Purpose】To observe the effects of acrid-warm exterior-relieving herbs on sweat secretion; to know the commons and differences of the effects of Mahuang and Guizhi on sweat secretion.

【Principles】There are sweat glands at toes of rats, thus we may observe and determine the effects of herbs on sweat secretion by staining sweat with iodine and starch based on the colorable reaction among sweat, iodine and starch.

【Equipments】Rat fixing apparatus, needle for rat intragastric administration, fixing shelf, medicinal rubber cement, injector (2.5 mL), magnifier, second-counter, cotton bud, needle, etc..

【Reagents】Decoction of Mahuang (1 g/mL), decoction of Mahuang coupled with Guizhi (1 g/mL), solution of carpiline (3.5 g/mL), solution of trinitrophenal, distilled water, absolute alcohol, solution of Hetian-Gaoyuan-Shi, etc..

【Animals】Rat, weighing 180~200 g.

【Methods】

1. Preparation of reagents solution

Decoction of Mahuang coupled with Guizhi (1 g/mL): Mahuang 30 g and Guizhi 20 g together are decocted to 50 mL.

Decoction of Mahuang (1 g/mL): Mahuang 30 g prepared in routine way and is concentrated to 1 g/mL

Solution of Hetian-Gaoyuan-Shi:

Solution A: 2 g iodine dissolved in 100 mL absolute alcohol

Solution B: 50 g dissolvable starch and 100 mL castor oil are mixed together

2. The operation and observation of experiment 12 healthy rats, weighed, marked with trinitrophenal solution and randomly divided into four groups, three rats in each group

First, clean the paws of rats with cotton bud which had been dipped in absolute alcohol, then treat four groups with different reagents: Group A: intragastricly administrate distilled water (1 mL/100 g); Group B: intraperitonealy inject solution of carpiline (3.5 mg/100 g); Group C: intragastricly administrate decoction of Mahuang (1 mL/100 g); Group D: intragastricly administrate decoction of Mahuang coupled with Guizhi (1 mL/100 g). After the herb treatment, fix rats in rat fixing apparatus and let two legs outside, gentle tie the legs with medicinal rubber cement in case that the legs turn into the fixing apparatus.

30 min after the herbs treatment, wipe out the original sweat on the paws, smear solution A on the skin of rat toes, if dried, smear a thin layer of solution B, then observe the time point, color and amount of intense violet colored plaques by magnifier. Continuously observe for 30 min from the first plaque, and record each 5 min.

【Results】Results are recorded in the table 6-1.

Table 6–1　The effects of Mahuang coupled with Guizhi on the sweat secretion at the rat paws ($\bar{x} \pm SD$)

Group	Dose (g/kg)	Administration pathway	Turned-out time of sweat	Amount of sweat plaques 1 h after the herbs treatment
A				
B				
C				
D				

【Notes】

1. Be gentle when fixing the rats in case of sweat secretion because rats struggle would affect the results of experiment.

2. The time for observing the sweat plaques should be the same in one batch test in order to assure the accuracy of the results.

3. The environmental temperature should be kept (26 ± 1) ℃ , humidity 65% ± 5%.

【Questions】

1. What are the characteristics of the sweat-promoting activity of Mahuang and Guizhi?

2. Why do Mahuang and Guizhi show synergism sweat-promoting effects?

实验二　柴胡对发热家兔的解热作用

【目的】观察柴胡对家兔体温的影响；了解柴胡解热作用的特点。

【原理】本实验采用伤寒、副伤寒甲乙三联菌苗作为致热原，此三联菌苗注射家兔机体后很快诱生内生性致热源，内热源作为发热的信息分子，把信息传递到视前区丘脑下部的前部体温调节中枢，使机体体温调节中枢对体温的调节功能失常，产热大于散热，体温调定点上移，导致家兔体温升高，从而造成家兔发热模型。实验以正常兔作为对照，观察柴胡的解热作用及其解热特点。

【器材】数字显示测温计；磅秤；家兔固定架；注射器等。

【试剂】伤寒；副伤寒甲乙三联菌；柴胡注射液（2 g/mL, 10 mL/ 支）；氨基比林注射液（2 mL/ 支）；生理盐水；液体石蜡；苦味酸等。

【动物】家兔。

【方法】

1. 取健康家兔 4 只，称重后用苦味酸标记，随机分为 4 组，每组 1 只，兔架上固定。

2. 分别测肛温 2 次，以均值作为正常体温。

3. 甲、乙、丙 3 只家兔耳缘静脉注射伤寒、副伤寒甲乙三联菌（1 mL/kg），每隔 30 min 测体温一次。待体温升高超过 1 ℃后，分别按步骤 4 安排给药。

4. 甲组兔（发热兔）：耳缘静脉注射生理盐水 2 mL/kg；
乙组兔（发热兔）：耳缘静脉注射柴胡注射液 2 mL/kg；
丙组兔（发热兔）：耳缘静脉注射氨基比林注射液 60 mg/kg；
丁组兔（未发热兔）：耳缘静脉注射柴胡注射液 2 mL/kg。

【结果】给药后 30、60、90、120 min 分别测试肛温一次，结果记入表 6-2。

表 6-2　柴胡对家兔体温的影响（$\bar{x}\pm SD$）

组别	动物数	正常（℃）	致热后 1 h	给药后不同时间点家兔的体温（℃）			
				30	60	90	120
甲组							
乙组							
丙组							
丁组							

【注意事项】

1. 健康家兔，雌性未孕，体温正常（38.5~39.5 ℃）。

2. 每次测肛温前体温计前部涂少量液体石蜡，测温时操作尽量轻柔。

3. 体温计前部 3~3.5 cm 处用胶布固定若干圈，保证每次测肛温的位置尽可能恒定。

4. 使用体温计时先按下开关，插入肛门深处。当显示器上的“℃”标志停止闪烁时（1 min 左右）取出。记录体温后关闭开关。注意勿使任何液体接触显示器和开关等部位，以防损坏。实验结束后用中性洗涤剂浸过的抹布拭净感温探头。待温度计干燥后在放回盒内保存。

【思考题】

1. 根据实验验结果，试分析柴胡解热作用的特点及其解热作用的机理。

2. 解表药和清热药解热各有什么特点，为什么？

3. 柴胡与氨基比林解热有何异同？

Experiment 2 The fever-relieving effects of Chaihu on fever rabbit

【Purpose】To observe the effects of Chaihu on the body temperature of rabbit; to understand the characteristics of the fever-relieving activity of Chaihu.

【Principles】Typhoid vaccine and paratyphoid vaccine A B are used as pyrogen. Endopyrogens are soon induced after injecting the three combined vaccines to rabbit. The endopyrogen acts as signal molecule and transfers the signal to the front center of body temperature accommodation located at the thalamus of preoptic region, which makes the body temperature accommodation center works in an abnormal way. As heat produced is more than the heat lost, the set-point of body temperature accommodation center is up-regulated and leads to an increase of the rabbit body temperature. The rabbit with abnormal increased body temperature is used as a fever model whereas the rabbit with normal body temperature is chosen as the control to observe the effects and characteristics of the fever-relieving activity of Chaihu.

【Equipments】Digital display thermograrhy, platform scale, rabbit fixing shelf, injector, etc.

【Reagents】Typhoid vaccine and paratyphoid vaccine A B, parenteral solution of Chaihu（2 g/mL, 10 mL each bottle）, parenteral solution of aminophenazone（2 mL each bottle）, saline, liquid paraffin, solution of trinitrophenol, etc.

【Animals】Rabbit.

【Methods】

1. 4 healthy rabbits, weighed, marked with trinitrophenol solution and randomly divided into 4 groups, 1 rabbit in each group. Fix the rabbits on the shelf.

2. Determine rectal temperature twice and use the average of the two as the abnormal body temperature.

3. Inject typhoid vaccine and paratyphoid vaccine A B by vein in ear edge to rabbit A, B, C, the dose is 1 mg/kg. Determine rectal temperature each 30 min. When the increase in body temperature achieves to 1 ℃, the rabbit can be treated with herbs according to protocols in Step 4.

4. Rabbit A（fever rabbit）: inject saline by vein in ear edge（2 mL/kg）; Rabbit B（fever rabbit）: inject parenteral solution of Chaihu by vein in ear edge（2 mL/kg）; Rabbit C（fever rabbit）: inject parenteral solution of aminophenazone by vein in ear edge（60 mg/kg）;

Rabbit D (normal rabbit) : inject parenteral solution of Chaihu by vein in ear edge (2 mL/kg) .

【Results】 Determine rectal temperature 30, 60, 90, 120 min after the herb treatment and record the results in the table 6-2.

Table 6–2　Effects of Chaihu on the body temperature of rabbit ($\bar{x} \pm SD$)

Group	No. of mice	Normal (℃)	1 h after vaccine injection	The body temperature of rabbit at different time point after herb treatment			
				30	60	90	120
A							
B							
C							
D							

【Notes】

1. The rabbit should be health, no pregnancy in female, with normal body temperature (38.5~39 ℃)

2. Smear a little liquid paraffin on the front of thermograph each time before determining the ractal temperature and be gently as possible

3. Tie the front of thermograph (3~3.5 cm) with rubber cement to keep the site the same in each rectal temperature determination

4. Press the switch before using the thermograph and then insert the thermograph deeply to rectal, take it out when the sign of "℃" stops twinking. Shut the switch after recording the temperature. Take care that the display and switch of the thermograph do not touch any liquid as that will do damage to the thermograph. When the experiment is over, clean the temperature probe with neutral detergent and put it in box when it becomes dry.

【Questions】

1. Try to interpret the characteristic and mechanism of the fever-relieving effects of Chaihu.

2. What are the relative characteristics of the fever-reliving activity of exterior-relieving herbs and heat-clearing herbs? Why?

3. What is the common and difference between the fever-relieving effects of Chaihu and aminophenazone?

第七章　清热药实验

凡以清解里热为主要作用的药物称为清热药。根据药物功效和主治不同，清热药分为清热泻火、清热凉血、清热燥湿、清热解毒、清虚热药五类。临床常用的清热药有黄芩、黄连、黄柏、石膏、知母、玄参、丹皮、银花、连翘、板蓝根等。现代医学认为病人发热多因感染所致，中医的里热证主要是多种病原体感染所致的急性传染性、感染性疾病，急性感染性疾病是清热药的主要适应证，因此这类药物多具有抗病原微生物、抗毒素、解热、抗炎等作用，此外尚有免疫调节、保肝、抗肿瘤等作用。在研究清热药时，一般从抗病原微生物、解热、抗炎等方面设计实验指标，并结合药物的具体功效和临床应用选择其他项目和指标进行实验。常用的实验方法如下：

1. 抗病原微生物实验　病原微生物是临床感染性疾病的主要病因，常见病原微生物包括病毒、细菌、真菌、螺旋体或原虫等，研究清热药的抗病原微生物作用时，可根据研究目的及药物性质选择合适的病原微生物进行实验。可用体外实验观察药物的抗病原微生物的敏感谱，再用敏感微生物感染动物，观察药物的体内抗病原微生物的效果。

（1）抗菌实验：细菌感染是临床最常见的病原微生物感染，对清热药比较敏感的革兰氏阳性菌主要有金黄色葡萄球菌、肺炎球菌、化脓性链球菌、粪链球菌；革兰阴性菌有大肠杆菌、肺炎杆菌、绿脓杆菌、痢疾杆菌等。

①体外抗菌：体外试验方法简便，用药量少，实验条件可控，准确性高，实验周期短，实验结果具有参考价值。但中药的体外实验也具有一定的局限性，易受多种因素的影响，尤其是中草药中杂质较多，一些非抗菌性成分（如鞣质）可通过物理原因或非特异性抗菌原理抑制细菌生长，因此体外筛选阳性的药物必须通过体内实验验证后方可肯定。

②体内抗菌实验：主要是观察药物与宿主相互作用，不仅可以反应药物对细菌的固有直接作用，而且可以反应药物对机体反应性的影响，特别是非特异抗感染力的影响、药物到达感染部位的能力、机体对药物的灭活与代谢等。实验结果可以通过半数有效量、治疗指数等反映，是最重要的抗菌研究方法，是判定药物有无临床价值的抗菌作用的最主要指标。

（2）抗病毒实验：病毒因结构简单，不能单独进行物质代谢，必须在易感的活细胞中寄生繁殖，且只对一定的细胞有亲和力。由宿主细胞供给其合成的原料、能量与场所才能增殖。常用的病毒培养方法有动物接种、鸡胚培养及组织（细胞）培养三种。

动物接种是分离病毒较早应用的方法，常用的动物有小白鼠、大白鼠、豚鼠、家兔等。接种时要根据病毒对动物及组织细胞的亲嗜性而选择特定的部位，如鼻腔、皮内、皮下、腹腔、脑内、静脉等。实验动物在病毒学研究中的用途主要有：分离与鉴定病毒、制备疫苗及诊断抗原、制备免疫血清、研究病毒的致病性、免疫性、发病机理及有效药物疗法等。

鸡胚培养为常用的病毒培养法之一，它的主要优点是鸡胚来源充分，操作简便，管理容易，本身带病毒的情况少见，只要选择适当的接种部位，病毒很容易增殖，目前主要用于黏病毒、疱疹病毒的分离、鉴定、制备抗原和疫苗的生产等。

组织培养法是目前培养病毒应用最广的一种方法，其优点是一般没有隐性感染，没有免疫抵抗力，便于选择易感细胞，实验条件易于控制，成本便宜，经济适用。组织培养法多应用于病毒的分离、鉴定、病毒感染细胞的机制研究、生产疫苗和抗原等。组织培养法的组织来源多种多样，如各种动物组织、鸡胚组织、人胚羊膜组织或人胚组织等，主要根据细胞对病毒的敏感性选择适宜细胞株。人类病毒用人或猴的组织较敏感，因此研究人的病毒性疾病常用人胚肾、人胚肺或人羊膜细胞。

抗其他病原微生物如真菌、支原体、钩端螺旋体、阿米巴原虫等实验方法基本同抗菌和抗病毒实验。

2. 抗内毒素实验　对内毒素致病机理的研究表明，内毒素与单核细胞、巨噬细胞的表面受体结合，通过信号转导、基因激活、mRNA 转录，翻译成蛋白质，前体蛋白质成熟完成细胞因子的分泌。内毒素诱发的炎性细胞因子对组织细胞的损害远远超过内毒素本身对机体的直接影响，过量的细胞因子形成瀑布样连锁反应，引起脓毒血症、休克或死亡，其中以 TNF-α、IL-1 等最为严重。

抗内毒素作用研究常用的方法是体外鲎试验、半体内中和内毒素试验及动物保护试验相结合。体外鲎试验操作简单，可用定性或定量试剂进行，适用于大批样品初筛研究。半体内试验是将药物与内毒素体外孵育一段时间后再注射到小鼠、家兔或鸡胚以检测内毒素毒性的变化。上述两种试验都可以测定药物的最低抗度浓度，研究药物对内毒素的直接解毒效果。体内试验是观察药物对内毒素休克所致死亡的影响，是检测抗内毒素作用最终效果的可靠方法。

3. 解热实验　发热是各种刺激因子影响机体产生内热源所引起的中枢体温调定点上调所致，因此发热模型常采用致热源如：伤寒、副伤寒菌苗、细菌培养液，酵母液、松节油、二硝基苯酚等，皮下或静脉注射给予动物（常用家兔和大鼠），引起动物体温升高，然后给予药物，观察药物的退热作用。

4. 抗炎实验　清热药物主要对炎症的早、中期有较好的抑制作用，有些药物对免疫性炎症也有一定的治疗作用。因此通常选择毛细血管通透性测定，鼠耳肿胀法、大鼠足肿胀法，胸膜炎试验及大鼠气囊滑膜炎等炎症模型，考察清热药物的抗炎作用。免疫性炎症模型有小鼠迟发性超敏反应，小鼠接触性皮炎、大鼠佐剂性关节炎试验等。此外，还可根据药物的临床适应证选用其他炎症模型，如板蓝根常用于治疗呼吸道感染，研究其药理作用时可选择小鼠流感、副流感病毒性肺炎模型。

5. 免疫功能测定试验　免疫包括特异性免疫和非特异性免疫。

（1）非特异性免疫实验：常用的方法有免疫器官称重法和细胞吞噬功能测定法两种，前者是在给药一定时间后观察动物免疫器官（胸腺、甲状腺、脾脏等）重量的变化，后者主要观察给药后动物体内吞噬细胞吞噬异物的功能，以评价药物对非特异性免疫功能的影响。

（2）特异性免疫实验：常用的方法有玫瑰花环形成试验，淋巴细胞转化试验，皮肤迟发型过敏反应试验，溶血空斑测定、血清溶血素测定、血清凝集素测定等。

由于清热药临床上主要用于里热证的治疗，研究清热药的药理作用时，应根据传统中医药理论，结合现代医学对该病的病因、病机的认识，合理设计研究内容，还应根据清热药个体性味、功效、主治的不同，进行其他相关实验，如降压、保肝等。

Chapter 7　Experiments on heat-clearing drugs

Herbs which are chiefly able to clear interior heat are known as heat-clearing herbs. They can be divided into five classes depended on different efficacies and indications: heat-clearing and fire-clearing drugs, heat-clearing and blood-cooling drugs, heat-clearing and damp-drying drugs, heat-clearing and detoxicating drugs and deficient heat clearing drugs. Commonly used heat-clearing herbs in clinical include Huang Qin (Rx Scutellariae), Huang Lian (Rz Coptidis), Huang Bo (Cx Phellodendri), Shi Gao (Gypsum Fibrosum), Zhi Mu (Rz Anemarrhenae), Xuan Shen (Rx Scrophulariae), Dan Pi (Cortex Moutan), Yin Hua (Fl Lonicerae), Lian Qiao (Fr Forsythiae), Ban Lan Gen (Rx Isatidis) et al. Fever is considered to be mainly caused by infection in modern medicine science. The interior heat syndrome in traditional Chinese Medicine Science is mainly acute infectious diseases caused by many pathogens. The main indication of heat-clearing herbs is acute infectious diseases. Thus most of the herbs exhibit extensive activities as anti-pathogens, anti-toxin, fever-relieving, anti-inflammation, immuno-regulation, liver-protecting et al. Individuals who conduct studies on heat-clearing herbs may choose experimental index that is relative to the activities mentioned above as well as other index at the background of the specific efficacy and clinical applications. Commonly adopted experiments are as follows:

1. Determination of anti-pathogen activities　Pathogens, the main etiopathogenisis of infectious diseases commonly include virus, bacteria, fungus, helicoids and ectosarc et al. One may choose proper pathogen according to the purpose of the test and the herbal properties when conducting studies on the anti-pathogen activities of heat-clearing herbs. Protocols can be as follows: first, find out the sensitivity spectrum of herbs in vitro experiments; second, inject animals with the sensitive pathogens to infect them and then observe the anti-pathogen effects of herbs.

(1) Determination of anti-bacteria activity: Bacterial infection is the most common pathogen infection in clinical. The Gram-positive bacterium that are sensitive to heat-clearing herbs include Staphyloccus Aureus, Micrococcus Pneumoniae, Streptococcus Pyogenes, Streptococcus Faecium. The Gram-negative bacterium that are sensitive to heat-clearing herbs include E coli, Bacillus Pneumoniae, Bacillus Pyocyaneus, Bacillus Dysenteriae et al.

Ⅰ. Determination of anti-bacteria activity in vitro: In vitro tests have the advantages of easy performance, less cost of drugs, controlled experimental conditions, high accuracy, short experimental period and valuable results. However, in vitro tests of herbs have its limitations. The results are easy to be affected by many factors such as much foreign matter in traditional Chinese medicine which can inhibit the growth of bacterium through physical path or nonspecific anti-bacterium path (For example, tannin). So the herbs that show positive results in vitro anti-bacteria tests should be further certificated by in vivo tests.

Ⅱ. Determination of anti-bacteria activity in vivo: In vivo tests, we mainly focus on the interactions between herbs and the hosts. From the interactions, we may get information not only about the direct effect of herbs on bacterium but also the effect of herbs on the reactivity of the host, especially the effect of herbs on nonspecific anti-infection ability of the host, the ability of herbs arriving at the infection sites and the inactivation and metabolism fate of herbs in host et al. The results of the tests can be evaluated by the parameters as IC50, therapeutic index et al. The in vivo anti-bacteria test is the most important method in the determination of anti-bacteria ability and also the most important indicator to evaluate whether the herbs exhibit clinically valuable anti-bacteria activity.

(2) Determination of anti-virus activities: Virus can only survive and breed in susceptible live cells because their structures are too simple to accomplish substance metabolism alone. Viruses show affinity only to certain cells which can provide them with the raw materials, energy and place for multiplication. Commonly used virus culture methods include animal-inoculating, embryonated-egg culture and tissue (cell) culture.

Animal-inoculation is an early used method to isolate virus, and frequently used animals include mouse, rat, cavia cobaya, rabbit et al. According to the affinity that virus exhibits to the animals and the cells, one should choose specific site to perform the inoculation, for example, nasal cavity, intradermally, subcutaneously, abdominal cavity, brain, vein et al. The main usage of experimental animals in the research of virology are as follows: virus isolation and identification, vaccine preparation and antigen diagnosis, immune serum preparation, studies on pathogenicity, immunity, pathogenesis and effective drug therapy of virus.

Embryonated-egg culture is one of the commonly used virus-culture protocols which has the main advantages of easy availability, easy performance, less complicated management, rare carriage of virus, easy multiplication if the inoculation site is proper. Nowadays, this method is mainly used in the isolation, identification, antigen preparation and vaccine manufacturing of paramyxovirus and herper virus.

Tissue-culture is the most widely adopted method of virus-culture which has the advantages of no recessive infections, convenient sensitive cells selection, no immune-resistance, easily controlled experimental conditions and low cost. This method is used in the isolation, identification, the mechanisms involved in cell infection, preparation of vaccine and antigen of virus. The tissues used are from many resources, such as tissues of animals, embryonated-eggs, amnion or other tissues of human-embryo. One may choose proper cell lines according to the sensitivities of cells to virus. Human-embryoed lung cells or ammion cells are often employed in the study of human virus because of the more sensitivity of tissues from human beings or monkeys.

The determination of anti-fungus, anti-mycoplasma anti-leptospire, anti-amebic-protozoa activities are similar to the determination of anti-bacteria and anti-virus activity.

2. Determination of anti-endotoxin activity The researches aiming at the mechanisms of how endotoxin leads to diseases indicate that the precursor proteins which accomplish the cytokine secretion after maturation are translated through signal transduction, gene activation and mRNA transcription after the binding of endotoxin and the surface receptor of monocytes and macrophages. The damage cytokines induced by endotoxin do to the tissue cells are far more serious than the direct damage endotoxin itself does to the body. Waterfall-like chain reactions caused by excess amount of cytokines, especially TNF-α、IL-1, results in pyemia, shock or even death.

Tests usually used in the studies of anti-endotoxin are combinations of the limulus test in vitro, neutralization of endotoxin partly in vivo and the protection of animals. The limulus test in vitro is suitable for the prescreening of samples in great numbers due to its easy conduction and the usage of quantitative or qualitative reagents. Partly in vivo experiments are performed by injecting the endotoxin to mice, rabbits or embryonated-eggs after the incubation of herbs and endotoxin for a certain time in vitro and then observe the changes of toxicity of endotoxin. These two experiments both can determine the lowest anti-toxin concentration and demonstrate direct detoxication effects of herbs. In vivo experiments can be used to observe the effects of herbs on death caused by endotoxin-induced shock, thus it is a reliable method to determine the final detoxication effects of herbs.

3. Tests of fever-relieving The up-regulation of the central body temperature set-point caused by different cytokines-induced endogenous pyrogen leads to fever. Commonly used pyrogens in fever model include Typhoid Vaccine, Paratyphoid Vaccine, bacterium culture medium, yeast liquid, turpentine, dinitrophenol. First, prepare a fever model by subcutaneous or intravenous injection of the pyrogens to animals (usually rabbits and rats), then treat the animals with herbs to observe the fever-relieving effects of herbs.

4. Determination of anti-inflammation activity Heat-clearing herbs show good inhibitory effects in the early and middle stages of inflammation. Some herbs have therapeutic effects on immune-related inflammation. Determination of blood capillary permeability, swelling of ear or toes of rats, inflammation models as pleurisy and air sac synovitis of rats are usually employed methods to evaluate the anti-inflammation effects of heat-clearing herbs.

Inflammation models of studies focusing on immuno-related inflammation include tardive hypersensitivity reaction of mice, contact dermatitis of mice, adjuvant-induced arthritis of rats et al. In addition, one may choose other inflammation models according to the clinical indications of herbs. For example, flu of mice models and parainfluenze-virus-induced pneumonia inflammation models are employed when researching the pharmacology activities of radix as its main clinical indication is respiratory tract infection.

5. Determination of immune function Immunity includes specific immunity and nonspecific immunity.

(1) Nonspecific immunity tests: Methods often used include weighting the immuned organ and the determination of the phagocytosis function of cells. The index of the former method is the change of immune organ weight before and after the herb treatment. The latter pays close attention to the phagocytosis function of phagocytes after herb treatment. From these tests, we may evaluate the effects of herbs on nonspecific immune function.

(2) Specific immunity tests: Methods often used include formation of rose-like chaplet, transformation of lymphocytes, test of skin tardive hypersensitive reaction, determination of hemolysis lacunae, determination of serum hemolysin, determination of serum agglutinin.

Heat-clearing herbs are used to treat internal heat syndrome in clinical. One should design experiments properly according to the theory of traditional Chinese medicine as well as modern views on the etiological factor and pathogenesis of the diseases herbs treated. Other related experiments, for example, depressurization and liver-protection, should also be performed according to the nature and flavor, efficacy, indications of herbs.

一、抗感染实验

实验一 黄连解毒汤对金黄色葡萄球菌感染小鼠的影响

【目的】学习药物的体内抗菌实验方法，观察黄连解毒汤的抗感染效应。

【原理】给小鼠腹腔注射金黄色葡萄球菌培养液，造成动物感染，以感染动物的死亡率为指标，观察药物的抗感染作用。

【器材】灭菌试管；试管架；吸管；培养皿；注射器；灭菌牛肉膏汤。

【药品】黄连解毒汤水煎液（3 g/mL）；胃膜素悬液（5 g/mL）。

【动物】小鼠。

【方法】

1. 药液的制备　黄连解毒汤水煎液：取黄连 90 g，黄芩 60 g，黄柏 60 g，栀子 90 g，常规制备，浓缩成 100 mL，即 3 g/mL。5 g/mL 胃膜素悬液的配制：称取胃膜素 5 g，放于研钵中，加少量生理盐水研磨，随研随加水，最后定容至 100 mL，于 10 磅加压灭菌 10 min 即可。

2. 菌液的制备　将金黄色葡萄球菌接种于肉汤培养基中，37 ℃培养 16~18 h，用平皿表面计数法测定实验感染用的活菌数。将上述菌液用 5 g/mL 胃膜素悬液以 10 倍顺序稀释为 10^{-1}、10^{-2}、10^{-3}……不同浓度菌液备用。

3. 预试　将不同浓度的细菌混液分别腹腔注射于 5 只小鼠，每只 0.5 mL，观察小鼠的死亡情况。正式试验时选用能引起小鼠 80%~100% 死亡的菌液浓度进行。

4. 实验治疗　取同性别小鼠 20 只，按体重随机分为 2 组，每组 10 只，用预试中选定浓度的细菌悬液每鼠腹腔注射 0.5 mL 以感染各组小鼠，第 1 组于感染的同时及感染后每日 2 次灌胃给予黄连解毒汤 0.2 mL/10g 体重，第 2 组作空白对照组，灌胃给予等容量的生理盐水。

【结果】连续观察 2~3 天，记录各组小鼠死亡情况于表 7-1 内。

表 7-1　黄连解毒汤对金黄色葡萄球菌感染小鼠的影响

组别	动物数（只）	动物死亡数（只）
空白对照组		
黄连解毒汤组		

附: 活菌的测定方法

将培养基的菌悬液,依10倍顺序稀释其浓度为10^{-1}、10^{-2}、10^{-3}……(即以9 mL无菌生理盐水加1 mL菌悬液为10^{-1},依次类推)。选取适当浓度的菌悬液0.1 mL放在肉汤琼脂平板上,轻轻推开菌液,注意不要碰到平皿边缘,以免影响计数。共做3个平板,放入37 ℃培养18~20 h后计算菌落群数。挑选生长30~300个菌落的平板计数。一般取两个平板的平均数进行计算。根据细菌稀释浓度算出每毫升菌液的活菌数。

Test of ant-infection activity

Experiment 1　The effect of Huang-Lian-Jie-Du-Tang on mice infected by Staphylococcus aureus

【Purpose】To study the method of determination of anti-bacteria activity in vitro;to observe the anti-infection activity of Huang-Lian-Jie-Du-Tang.

【Principles】Inject Staphylococcus aureus to mice by intraperitoneal injection, then choose the death rate of infectious mice as the index to evaluate the anti-infection activity.

【Equipments】Sterilized tube, tube-carrier, pipette, Petri dish; injector, sterilized beef broth

【Reagents】Decoction of Huang-Lian-Jie-Du-Tang (3 g/mL); suspension of gastric mucin (5 g/mL)

【Animals】Mice.

【Methods】

1. Preparation of drugs solution　Decoction of Huang-Lian-Jie-Du-Tang: Huanglian 90 g, Huangqin 60 g, Huangbo 60 g, Zhizi 90 g, the preparation is as the routine method, then concentrate it to 100 mL, thus the concentration is 3 g/mL.

Suspension of gastric mucin: put the weighed 5 g gastric mucin in a mortar, add in saline when grinding to 100 mL and sterilize under ten pounds for 10 min.

2. Preparation of bacterium cultures　Inoculate the Staphylococcus aureus to broth culture, then incubate it at 37 ℃ for 16~18 hours and measure the number of viable organism by cultural plate counting method. Dilute the bacterium cultures with sterilized suspension of gastric mucin (5 g/mL) to concentrations of 10^{-1}, 10^{-2}, 10^{-3}……

3. Pretesting　Inject different concentrations of bacterium cultures to five mice intraperitoneally, 0.5 mL per mouse, and then observe the death rate of mice. Choose the concentrations that cause 80%~100% death when conducting the formal test.

4. Herb treatment　Twenty mice of same gender are randomly divided into two groups according to the weight. Inject 0.5 mL the bacterium cultures of the chosen concentration in pretest to every one of these twenty mice intraperitoneally. Administrate Huang-Lian-Jie-Du-Tang to mice twice a day in one group from the time of infection. The dosage of HLJDT is 0.2 mg/kg. Mice in the other group, which are administrated with an equal an equal volume of saline at the same time, is designed as the control group.

【**Results**】Observe 2~3 days and record the death rate of mice in the table 7-1.

Table 7–1 The effect of Huang-Lian-Jie-Du-Tang on mice infected by Staphylococcus aureus

Group	*n*(mice)	*n*(dead mice)
Control		
HLJDT-treated		

Appendix: Method of the determination of viable organism

Dilute the bacterium cultures to concentrations of 10^{-1}, 10^{-2}, 10^{-3}……(If add 9 mL sterilized saline to 1 mL bacterium cultures, the concentration is 10^{-1}, the rest may be deduced by analogy). Add 0.1 mL bacterium cultures of a proper concentration to a plate coated with broth agar, spread out the cultures lightly. Make sure that you don't touch the edge of the plate for which will affect the count. Prepare three plates and incubate the plates at 37 ℃ for 18~20 hours. After the incubation, count the number of colonies. Choose plates that have 30~300 colonies. Generally, the average of colonies of two plates are used to do the calculation. Calculate the concentration of viable organism in the original suspension according to diluted times.

二、对免疫功能影响实验

实验二 金银花对小鼠腹腔巨噬细胞吞噬鸡红细胞能力的影响

【目的】观察金银花对巨噬细胞吞噬功能的影响。

【原理】巨噬细胞吞噬能力是机体非特异性免疫机能的一项主要指标。药物如能提高吞噬细胞的吞噬能力表明药物能增强机体的防御能力。

【器材】显微镜；高压锅；离心机；孵箱；小鼠固定板；搪瓷盆；载玻片；注射器（2 mL，1 mL）；手术剪；镊子；纱布；棉花；擦镜纸。

【试剂】金银花水煎液（1 g/mL）；5% 鸡红细胞（CRBC）悬液；生理盐水；4% 姬姆萨 - 瑞特氏染色液；Alsever's 液；松柏油；2% 碘酊；75% 乙醇；苦味酸液。

【动物】小鼠；公鸡。

【方法】取小鼠 10 只，随机分成 2 组，即金银花水煎液组和空白对照组，分别每天灌胃给药 0.2 mL/10 g 体重，对照组为等容积生理盐水，共 4 天。停药后 2 h 每鼠腹腔注射 5% 鸡红细胞 0.4 mL，6~8 h 后动物脱颈椎处死，仰位固定于鼠板上。剪开腹部皮肤，经腹腔注射生理盐水 2 mL，转动固定板 1 min，然后抽出腹腔洗液 1 mL，滴涂于干净载玻片上，每片 0.2 mL，共 2 片，放在垫有湿纱布的搪瓷盒中，置于 37 ℃孵箱中温育 30 min 后取出玻片，用生理盐水漂洗，以除去未贴壁的细胞。晾干，以 1∶1 丙酮 - 甲醇液固定 5 min，再用 4% 姬姆萨 - 瑞特氏染色液染色 3 min 后用蒸馏水漂洗，晾干。在油镜下每片计数巨噬细胞 200 个，按下式计算其吞噬指数与吞噬百分率：

$$吞噬百分率=\frac{吞噬鸡红细胞的巨噬细胞数}{200个巨噬细胞}\times 100\%$$

$$吞噬指数=\frac{被吞噬的鸡红细胞总数}{200个巨噬细胞}$$

【结果】按上面公式计算，填于下表 7-2 中。

表 7-2 金银花对小白鼠腹腔巨噬细胞吞噬功能的影响（$\bar{x}\pm SD$）

组别	吞噬百分率	吞噬指数
金银花水提液		
生理盐水		

【思考题】试述中药清热解毒的意义是什么。

附：鸡红细胞悬液的制备

在无菌操作下，自鸡翼下静脉采血，置于三角烧瓶中，加入相当于血液量 5 倍的 Alsever's 溶液（枸橼酸钠 · $2H_2O$ 8.0 g，枸橼酸 0.5 g，无水葡萄糖 18.7 g，NaCl 4.2 g，蒸馏水加至 1 000 mL 后过滤，常规高压蒸气 20 min 灭菌，4 ℃冰箱保存）。摇匀，4 ℃贮存，可用 2~4 周。临用时用生理盐水洗涤 3 次，前两次用 1 500 rpm 分离红细胞，最后一次为 2 000 rpm 各 5 min，直至红细胞压积恒定。然后按此压积量，用生理盐水配成 2%~5%（V/V）浓度。

Effect of herbs on immune function

Experiment 2 The effect of Jin Yin Hua on the chicken red blood cell (CRBC) phagocytosis ability of macrophages

【Purpose】To observe the effect of Jin Yin Hua on the phagocytosis function of macrophages.

【Principles】The phagocytosis ability of macrophages is a major index of nonspecific immune function of the body. It may be concluded that the herbs can strengthen the body's immunity if it can enhance the phagocytosis function of the macrophages.

【Equipments】Microscope, autoclave sterilizer, centrifuge, incubator, mice fixing plate, enamel basin, slide, injector (1 mL, 2 mL), surgical scissors, nipper, bandage, cotton, lens wiping paper.

【Reagents】Decoction of Jin Yin Hua (1 g/mL), suspension of CRBC (5%), saline, JiMuSa-RuiTeShi staining (4%), Alsever's solution, pine and pitch oil, iodine tincture (2%), alcohol, trinitrophenol solution.

【Animals】Mice, cock.

【Methods】Ten mice are randomly divided into two groups as the decoction-treated group and control group. Mice in two groups are administrated with decoction and saline (0.2 mL/10 g) every day, respectively. The administration lasts for four days.

Mice are treated by intraperitoneal injection of I 0.4 mL of 5% CRBC 2 h after the administration of decoction and the mice are killed by cervical dislocation 6~8 h after the injection of CRBC.

Mice are fixed in supine position on the fixed plate and 2 mL of saline was injected intraperitoneally. Intraperitoneally inject 2 mL saline to the dead mouse which is fixed in supine position on the fixed plate. After opening the abdominal cavity, 1 mL of washing solution is collected and spreaded it on two clean slides after rotating the plate for one minute, each 0.2 mL. The two slides are put in the enamel basin with wet gauze at the bottom and incubated at 37 ℃ for thirty minutes. Wash the slides with saline to remove the cells that haven't adhered on the slides after the incubation and dry them in the open air. Fix the cells with acetone and methanol which is mixed by 1 : 1 for 5 min, and colour the cells with 4% JiMuSa-RuiTeShi solution for 3 minutes. Then wash the slides with distilled water and dry them in the open air.

Count each slide for 200 macrophages by immersion objective, calculate the index and rate of phagocytosis according to the following formula:

$$\text{The phagocytosis rate}=\frac{\text{the number of macrophages that phagocytosis CRBC}}{\text{200 macrophages}}\times 100\%$$

$$\text{The phagocytosis index}=\frac{\text{the number of CRBC that are phagocytosised}}{\text{200 macrophages}}$$

【Results】 Add your results to the table 7-2 as to the formulation.

Table 7–2 The effect of Jin Yin Hua on the phagocytosis function of macrophages ($\bar{x}\pm SD$)

group	The phagocytosis rate (%)	The phagocytosis index (%)
Jin Yin Hua-treated		
control		

【Question】 Try to describe the significance of the detoxication activity of heat-clearing herbs.

Appendix: Preparation of suspension of CRBC

Put the blood sample collected from the inferior vein in the cock wing under asepsis condition into a conical flask, add in five times of the volume of the blood of Alsever's solution (natrium citricum with two crystal water molecules 8.0 g, citric acid 0.5 g, anhydrous dextrose 18.7 g, NaCl 4.2 g, add 1,000 mL distilled water, then sterilize it for 20 min by routine high pressure vapor method after filtration. The solution is stored at 4 ℃ before use). Shake the mixture to be well–distributed, store at 4 ℃ . The solution should be used in 2~4 weeks. Before use, wash it with saline for three times, 15,000 rpm centrifuge for 5min to isolate red blood cells for the first two times, 20,000 rpm for 5 min the last time. The process can be terminates when the hematokrit remained constant. Then dilute the solution to the concentration of 2%~5% (V/V) with saline according to the constant hematokrit.

实验三　改良四妙散对急性胰岛素抵抗小鼠糖耐量的影响

【目的】学习炎症相关性急性胰岛素抵抗模型的制备方法；观察改良四妙散的降糖作用。

【原理】口服葡萄糖后血糖升高，致胰岛素分泌增加，后者作用于相应靶组织（肝、骨骼肌、脂肪等），促进血糖转运到靶器官储存、利用，从而降低血糖。炎症刺激可以降低机体对胰岛素的敏感性，导致靶器官转运、利用血糖能力降低，表现为血糖升高或/和恢复到正常血糖的时间延长。改良四妙散具有明显抗炎作用，能提高组织器官对胰岛素的敏感性。

【器材】6孔；96孔平底细胞培养板；移液器（1 mL, 200 μL）及相应吸头；常规手术器械；细胞培养箱；酶标仪。

【试剂】LPS；PBS；高糖DMEM；改良四妙散（黄连：黄柏：薏苡仁：苍术＝0.3：0.6：1：1）；二甲双胍片剂；葡萄糖测试盒（氧化酶法）。

【动物】雄性小鼠，体重22~24 g。

【方法】

1. 炎性巨噬细胞条件培养液的制备　取成年雄性小鼠（8~10周）数只，脱颈椎处死，全身浸泡于75%的乙醇中2 min，取出置于平皿中，腹腔注射5 mL PBS（磷酸盐缓冲液，pH 7.2），轻按摩腹部2 min，剪开腹部皮肤，在暴露出的腹肌上作一个小切口，用移液器吸头吸出腹腔液，内含腹腔巨噬细胞。将腹腔液于1 000 rpm离心5 min，收集细胞，接种于6孔（2×10^6孔）培养板中（一只小鼠腹腔细胞可接种1~2孔，以PBS培养），置细胞培养箱内培养2 h后，用PBS轻轻洗弃未贴壁细胞，已贴壁细胞绝大多数为巨噬细胞。更换培养液为无血清高糖DMEM，每孔2 mL，再加入LPS，使其终浓度为5 μg/mL。置于培养箱内培养24 h，收集并合并细胞培养液，3 000 rpm离心5 min，取上清，以0.22 μm孔径滤膜滤菌后，−70 ℃分装保存。此为巨噬细胞条件培养液。

2. 造模并观察药效　小鼠禁食12小时，随机分为5组，四妙散组灌胃给予改良四妙散5 g（生药量）/20 mL/ kg，阳性对照组灌胃二甲双胍200 mg/20 mL /kg，完全空白组、灌糖空白组及模型组给予等体积水。30 min后模型组、用药组及慢性药组小鼠腹腔注射稀释的巨噬细胞条件培养液（原上清：PBS =1：1，V/V）0.2 mL/只，其余小鼠腹腔注射等量生理盐水。30 min后，完全空白小鼠灌胃给予20 mL/ kg水，其余小鼠均灌胃葡萄糖4 g/20 mL/ kg，再经30 min，眼静脉丛取血于小离心管内，3 000 rpm离心10 min，取血清测定其中葡萄糖浓度（比色法，5 μL血清与200 μL试剂混匀，37 ℃保温10 min，酶标仪上测500 nm吸收度，再与标准比较，求出糖浓度）。

【结果】将结果填入表7-3中。

表 7–3　改良四妙散对巨噬细胞条件培养液刺激小鼠糖耐量的影响

分组	剂量（g/kg）	动物数	血糖浓度（mmol/L）
完全空白			
灌糖空白			
模型			
改良四妙散			
二甲双胍			

【注意事项】

1. 小鼠需禁食 12 h。
2. 取血点准确。
3. 取血时防溶血。

【思考题】

1. 分析造模原理及药物作用的可能机制。
2. 如何改进方法?

Experiment 3　The effect of modified Si-Miao-San on glucose tolerance in insulin resistant mice

【Purpose】To learn the method how to prepare insulin resistance in mice and observe the effects of modified Si-Miao-San on glucose tolerance.

【Principles】Blood glucose level increases after oral glucose load, leading to increased insulin secretion. Insulin then binds to the receptors in its target tissues such as liver, muscle and fat, promotes blood glucose transport and application, and then decreases the blood glucose. Inflammation impairs insulin sensitivity, leading to the decrease of insulin action, which is evidenced by delayed glucose disposal. Modified mSMS has significant anti-inflammatory activity, thereby can improve the sensitivity of target tissue to insulin under inflammatory conditions.【Equipments】6-, 96-well culture plates, transferpettors（10 μL-1,000 μL）, plastical tubes（1.5 mL, 5 mL）, water bath, syringes, surgical scissors, cell incubator, spectrophotometer.

【Reagents】Dulbecco's modified eagle's medium（DMEM, high glucose of 25 mmol/L）, lipopolysaccharide（LPS）, commercial glucose kit based on oxidase peroxidase（GOD-POD）method, modified SiMiaoSan（mSMS, coptis chinensis：cortex phellodendri：coicis semen：atractylodes rhizome = 0.3：0.6：1：1）, metformin.

【Animals】Mice（male or female）weighing 18~22 g.

【Methods】

1. Preparation of macrophages-derived conditioned medium　Mice are killed by cervical dislocation and 5 mL of PBS is injected intraperitoneally. After abdominal massage for 2 min, PBS containing peritoneal macrophages is collected, washed with PBS, then cultured in 6-well plates（2×10^6/well）for 2 h, after washed twice with PBS, adherent cells are cultured in serum-free DMEM, and stimulated by 5 μg/mL LPS for 24 h. Then, culture medium is centrifuged and the supernatant is collected as conditioned medium（CM）. TNF-α and IL-6 in CM were assayed using enzyme-linked immunosorbent assay（ELISA）kits（R&D, USA）, and the supernatant is filtered through a 0.22 μm filter and stored at −70 ℃.

2. Effect of mSMS on macrophage-CM induced oral glucose intolerance in mice　Mice are fasted for 12 h and treated by gavage with either vehicle, or mSMS（0.5, 1 and 5 g/kg）, dianoguanil（0.2 g/kg）or sodium salicylate（0.5 g/kg）. Thirty minutes after the treatment, the mice are intraperitoneally injected with 0.2 mL of diluted macrophage-CM（1：1, V/V）. Then, 30 min later, the animals are oral administered with glucose solution（4 g/kg）. Blood

is collected from orbital sinus at 0, 0.5, 1 and 2 h after oral glucose challenge. Levels of blood glucose are measured by using a commercial kit based on glucose oxidase peroxidase (GOD-POD) method.

【 Results 】Write down your data in the table 7-3.

Table 7–3 Effects of mSMS on CM–induced glucose intolerance in mice.

Group	dose (g/kg)	Animal number	Serum glucose (mmol/L)
Completely blank			
Blank-ig glucose			
model			
Modified Si-Miao-San			
metformin			

【 Notes 】

1. Mice should be fasted over-night.
2. The time points of blood collection should be exact.
3. Be careful when collect the blood to avoid haemolysis.

【 Questions 】

1. Analyze the mechanisms of the preparation of model and the effect of mSMS on glucose intolerance.
2. How will you improve the experimental design?

实验四 黄芩汤及黄芩苷急性给药对行为绝望模型小鼠的抗抑郁作用研究

【目的】学习小鼠行为绝望抑郁模型的造模方法；观察黄芩汤及黄芩苷的抗抑郁作用。

【原理】悬尾模型是固定动物的尾端，将其倒悬，让它们的活动受到限制，而产生类似行为绝望的不动性。强迫游泳中动物被迫在一个局限性的圆柱形容器内游泳而不能逃脱，开始时游泳运动剧烈试图逃脱，但无法逃脱，接着停止逃脱的企图，进入一种特征性的不动状态，这种不动状态反映了动物的一种绝望状态。绝大多数抗抑郁药可改善行为绝望模型中小鼠的不动时间，故行为绝望模型可作为抗抑郁药的筛选和评价。黄芩汤及黄芩苷可明显改善小鼠悬尾模型及游泳模型的不动时间，具有抗抑郁作用。

【器材】灌胃针；小鼠矿场行为测试仪；悬尾装置；小鼠强迫游泳测试仪；计时器。

【试剂】黄芩苷溶液；黄芩汤（黄芩：炙甘草：白芍：大枣 =3：2：2：16）；盐酸氟西汀；生理盐水。

【动物】雄性小鼠，体重 18~22 g。

【方法】

1. 分组与给药　将小鼠随机分为 4 组，每组 10 只，分别为对照组，阳性药组（盐酸氟西汀：20 mg/kg, ig.）、黄芩苷组（40 mg/kg, ig.）、黄芩汤组（15.2 g/kg, ig.）。各给药组按 0.2 mg/10 g 灌胃，阳性药组进行等容氟西汀灌胃，对照组给予生理盐水灌胃。灌胃每日一次，连续给药 7 天后进行检测。

2. 开野实验　末次给药 1 h 后进行实验。将小鼠置于开野测试仪中间，记录 6 min 内后 4 min 小鼠自发活动，在安静地环境下进行此项实验观察。观察指标：穿格（底部格子穿行数）得分和垂直活动（两前肢离地 1 cm 以上次数）得分。两次实验之间将开野测试仪彻底清理，以免影响下一只动物实验结果。每只动物测定一次。

3. 悬尾实验　末次给药 1 h 后进行实验。将小鼠倒置，距尾尖 1 cm 处用胶布粘贴于悬尾装置，头部距台面 15cm，每两只小鼠之间用挡板隔开动物视线，以免互相干扰，记录 6 min 内后 4 min 累计不动时间（小鼠在空中停止挣扎，或仅有细小的肢体运动）。

4. 强迫游泳　末次给药 1 h 后进行实验。将小鼠置于强迫游泳行为测试仪中，水深 10 cm，水温（25 ± 1）℃，每两只小鼠之间用挡板隔开动物视线，以免互相干扰，记录 6 min 内后 4 min 累计不动时间（小鼠停止挣扎，浮在水中保持不动，或仅做一些必要的轻微动作，保持头部浮在水面上）。

【结果】将结果填入表 7-4、表 7-5 及表 7-6 中。

表 7–4　黄芩汤及黄芩苷对小鼠自发活动的影响（$\bar{x}\pm SD$）

组别	剂量	动物数	穿格	站立
对照组	—			
氟西汀组	20 mg/kg			
黄芩苷组	40 mg/kg			
黄芩汤组	15.2 g/kg			

表 7–5　黄芩汤及黄芩苷对小鼠悬尾绝望模型的影响（$\bar{x}\pm SD$）

组别	剂量	动物数	不动时间（s）
对照组	—		
氟西汀组	20 mg/kg		
黄芩苷组	40 mg/kg		
黄芩汤组	15.2 g/kg		

表 7–6　黄芩汤及黄芩苷对小鼠强迫游泳绝望模型的影响（$\bar{x}\pm SD$）

组别	剂量	动物数	不动时间（s）
对照组	—		
氟西汀组	20 mg/kg		
黄芩苷组	40 mg/kg		
黄芩汤组	15.2 g/kg		

【注意事项】

1. 实验时应保持安静，以免对实验产生干扰。
2. 强迫游泳保持水温 25 ℃左右。

【思考题】

1. 哪些因素可对实验产生影响？
2. 还有哪些造模方法？各种造模方法的优缺点是什么？

Experiment 4 Antidepressant effect of Huang Qin Tang and baicalin on mice model of behavioral despair

【Purpose】To study the method of establishing mice model of behavior despair. To observe the antidepressant effect of Huang Qin Tang and baicalin.

【Principles】When mice are hung upside down by tail suspension, their activities are restricted, and thus exerting despaired hebavious similar to that in immobility. Forced swimming in animal was forced in a cylindrical container to prevent the escape At the beginning, mice struggled hard to escape but cannot escape, then stop the escape attempt, keep immobility, and the immobility state reflects a desperate state of animal. Vast majority of antidepressants may reduce the immobility time in mice behavioral despair model which can be used as antidepressant screening and evaluation. Huang Qin Tang and baicalin can significantly reduce the immobility time of the mice suspend test and forced swimming test suggest that they have antidepressant effect.

【Equipments】Gavage needle, Mice open field tester, Tail suspension device, Mouse Forced Swimming device, Timer.

【Reagents】Baicalin solution, Huang Qin Tang (Scutellaria : prepared Radix glycyrrhizae : radices paeoniae alba : Fructus Ziziphi Jujubae=3 : 2 : 2 : 16), Fluoxetine, saline.

【Animals】Male mice, weighing 18~22 g.

【Methods】

1. Grouping and administration The mice were randomly divided into 4 groups (n=10): control group, positive group (fluoxetine hydrochloride: 20 mg/kg, ig.), baicalin group (40 mg/kg, ig.), Huang Qin Tang group (15.2 g/kg, ig.). The agents were given by gavage (0.2 mL/10g,) once daily for consecutive 7 d before testing.

2. Open field test The experiment is taken 1 h after the last administration. The mice were placed in the middle of the open field tester, recording the last 4 min after spontaneous activity within 6 min. Observe in a quite environment. Observed indicators: the number of crossing (number of walking through the bottom of the grid) and the number of rearing (times of the two forelimbs off the ground more than 1 cm). The open field tester should be thoroughly cleaned between two experiments to avoid the next animal influenced by the smell left. Each animal was tested once.

3. Tail suspend test The experiment is taken 1 h after the last administration. The mice were hung upside down, 1cm from the tip of the tail with adhesive tape attached at

the tail suspension device, keeping the head 15 cm from table. Mice were separated by baffle so that without eye contact to avoid interfering with each other and then record the immobility time of the last 4 min in 6 min (mice stop struggling, or only a small limb movements).

4. Forced swimming test The experiment is taken 1h after the last administration. The mice were placed in forced swimming device [10 cm deep, (25 ± 1) ℃], and separated by baffle so that without eye contact to avoid interfering with each other, and then record the immobility time of the last 4 min in 6 min (mice stop struggling, floating remain motionless in the water, or only move slightly to keep the head floating in the water).

【Results】Write down your data in the table 7-4, table 7-5, table 7-6.

Table 7-4 Effects of HQT and baicalin on the open field test in mice ($\bar{x} \pm SD$)

Group	dose	Animal number	Crossing	Rearing
Control	—			
Positive	20 mg/kg			
Baicalin	40 mg/kg			
HQT	15.2 g/kg			

Table 7-5 Effects of HQT and baicalin on the tail suspend test in mice ($\bar{x} \pm SD$)

Group	dose	Animal number	Immobility time (s)
Control	—		
Positive	20 mg/kg		
Baicalin	40 mg/kg		
HQT	15.2 g/kg		

Table 7-6 Effects of HQT and baicalin on the forced swimming test in mice ($\bar{x} \pm SD$)

Group	dose	Animal number	Immobility time (s)
Control	—		
Positive	20 mg/kg		
Baicalin	40 mg/kg		
HQT	15.2 g/kg		

【Notes】

1. Environment should be quite so as not to interfere with the experiment;

2. Keep the temperature around 25 ℃ in forced swimming test.

【Questions】

1. What are the factors that can affect the experiment?

2. Do you know any other method for establishing depression model? What are the advantages and disadvantages of those methods?

第八章　泻下药实验

凡能通利大便的药物称泻下药。根据泻下作用强弱的不同，可分为润下药、攻下药和峻下逐水药三类，以后者作用最强，攻下次之，润下药性缓和。现代医学按泻下作用机理，将它们分为刺激性泻药、容积性泻药（机械刺激性泻药）和润滑性泻药。泻下药主要研究药物的功效和导泻机理（作用方式）以及致泻作用成分。实验动物，多采用小鼠，大鼠，亦可采用家兔或豚鼠。一般不宜用猫和狗，因猫易发生呕吐，狗对泻药反应迟钝。泻下药研究方法主要有以下几方面，可根据需要选用。泻下药主要药理作用为泻下、利尿、抗感染等。其研究方法主要有以下几方面：

1. 在体实验法

（1）炭末排出时间测定法和排便频度实验：实验多用小鼠，以炭末作为指示剂，灌胃给药，观察泻下药起效时间（即排出含指示剂粪便的时间）、粪便性状、排便数量，并与对照组相互比较，判断泻下药的药效。

（2）肠推进运动实验：以色素为标志，用含有色素（炭末或墨汁）的泻下药给动物灌服或结肠给药，观察色素在肠道推进的距离，反映泻下药对肠道运动的影响判断其对小肠和大肠的作用。常用方法有：小肠推进实验、大肠推进实验和酚红排空定量测定实验。

（3）在体肠道平滑肌实验：记录整体动物不同部位肠管运动情况，观察泻下药对其运动的影响。通常有肠管悬吊法、肠内压测定法、压敏传感器贴壁法和肠生物电测定法。

2. 离体肠管法　记录肠平滑肌活动情况，观察泻下药对肠肌的作用。实验常采用豚鼠、大鼠、家兔的离体肠管作材料，其中，十二指肠兴奋性、自律性较高，对药物反应比较敏感；回肠（特别是豚鼠回肠）自发活动少，易获得稳定的基线。

选择离体肠管法将泻下药与肾上腺素类、胆碱类、组胺类、前列腺素类的拟似药和拮抗药以及氯化钡等药物对肠肌的作用比较研究，可以进一步分析泻下药增强肠运动的机理。

Chapter 8 Experiments on the cathartics

All the drugs used to empty the bowels are cathartic. It can be classified as the drugs for purgation, the drugs for catharis and the drugs for fluid-purging according to their eliminate strength. The drugs for fluid-purging is the strongest, the drugs for catharis is weaker than the drugs for fluid-purging, and the drugs for purgation is the weakest. Modern medical science classifies them as amyctic cathartic, volumetric cathartic and lubricant cathartic, according to their mechanism of action. We mainly study the effectiveness and the action mechanism and the constituent for cathartic in mice and rats as well as rabbits and cavia cobaya. Generally, dogs and cats are not recommended, because cats may vomit, and dogs are insensitive to the cathartic. The main pharmacological actions of cathartic are alvi profluvium, diuresis, anti-infection. The research methods are as follows and they can be adopted when we need:

1. Endosomatic experimental method

(1) The experiment of measuring egesting time of anthracitic suspension and the periodicity of defecation: The anthracitic suspension as the indicator administrated orally by mouse is observed the oneset time (the time of egesting the dejecta containing the indicator), the character of dejecta, the frequency of defecation compared to the control group in order to evaluate the effect of the cathartic.

(2) The experiment of intestinal propelling movements: We give the cathartic containing colorant (the anthracitic suspension or the ink) as the marker to animals, oral administration or at colon. We can judge the pharmacodynamic action to the intestine tracing the movement of the colorant which can reflect the effect of the cathartic to the intestine's enterocinesia. The methods are as follows: the experiment of small intestinal propelling movements, the experiment of large intestinal propelling movements and the experiment of quantified determining phenolsulfonphthalein evacuation.

(3) The experiment of the intestinal smooth muscle: We can observe the effect of the cathartic by recording the enterocinesia of different section through the methods such as:

method of intestinal canal suspending, method of measuring the intestinal pressure, method of pressure-sensitivity sensor, and method of determing the bioelectricity.

2. The experiment of isolated intestinal canal Activity of the intestinal smooth muscle and the cathartic's effect on the muscle are recorded during the experiment. We always use the isolated intestinal canal of guinea pigs, rats, and rabbits among which the duodenum shows higher excitability, autorhythmicity and sensibility to the drugs. Locomotor activity of the ileum (especially the ileum of guinea pig) is minor so that it is easy to get the stabile base line.

We can further analyses the mechanism of the cathartic on strengthening the intestinal enterocinesia by comparing the effect of cathartic on the muscle to the simillimum and antagonist of adnephrin、bilineurin、ergamine、prostaglandin.

实验一　生大黄、芒硝对小鼠小肠运动的影响（炭末法）

【目的】学习用炭末推进法测定动物小肠运动的实验方法。观察泻下药生大黄、芒硝对小肠运动的影响。

【原理】消化道内容物的移动速度与胃排出时间、小肠的运动及消化管内容物的流动性有关。小肠的运动受肠神经及外来神经的控制，当机械和化学的刺激作用于肠壁感受器时，可通过局部的壁内反射而引起小肠蠕动增加，而副交感神经兴奋时可增强小肠运动，交感神经兴奋则产生抑制作用。利用口服炭末在肠道不被吸收的原理，以炭末作为指示剂，测定在一定时间内炭末在肠道的推进距离，可观察泻下药对小肠推进的作用。

【器材】手术剪；眼科镊；直尺；注射器；灌胃针。

【试剂】用含有 2% 阿拉伯胶的水溶液制成 12% 活性炭末混悬液；生理盐水；100% 芒硝水溶液；生大黄水溶液（1 g/mL）。

【动物】小鼠，体重 18~22 g。

【方法】取禁食不禁水 20 h 的小鼠，随机分组，称重，编号。各给药组动物分别灌胃给予 100% 芒硝水溶液（0.2 mL/10 g），生大黄水溶液（0.2 mL/10 g），空白对照组给予等容积蒸馏水。20 min 后各组均灌胃给予 10% 的炭末混悬液 0.6 mL/ 只。20 min 后脱颈椎处死动物，剖开腹腔，分离肠系膜，剪取上端至幽门，下端至回盲部的肠管，轻轻将小肠拉直，准确量取小鼠幽门至炭末推进前沿的长度以及小鼠小肠总长。按下式计算推进百分率：

炭末推进百分率＝（炭末从幽门部到推进前沿的移动距离 / 小鼠小肠总长）× 100%

实验结束后数据作全班统计，计算各组炭末推进百分率的平均数（$\bar{x}$）和标准差（SD），以 t 检验统计法进行组间比较。

【结果】将结果填入表 8-1 中。

表 8-1　生大黄、芒硝对小鼠小肠运动作用的影响

组别	剂量（g/kg）	动物数	炭末移动距离	小肠全长	炭末推进率（%）
空白对照组					
生大黄组					
芒硝组					

【注意事项】

1. 生大黄制剂的制备　取生大黄 100 g，砸成小块后以水浸没。冷浸 24 h 后，过滤，40 ℃水浴浓缩至 1 g/mL。

2. 给药至处死动物的间隔以及处死至取出肠管的时间必须一致。

3. 剪取肠系膜、肠管以及拉直肠管时动作轻柔，不可用力牵拉。

【思考题】

1. 中药泻下药根据泻下作用机制可分为几类？大黄、芒硝分别属于哪一类？

2. 大黄致泻的主要成分及作用机理是什么？临床应用大黄致泻应注意什么？

Experiment 1　The effect of Radix et rhizoma rhei、natrii sulfas on mouse small intestinal propelling movements (anthracitic suspension drived in intestine)

【Purpose】To study the method of anthracitic suspension drived in intestine to determine the small intestinal enterocinesia. To observe the the effect of Radix et rhizama rhei, natrii sulfas on the small intestinal enterocinesia.

【Principles】The speed of alimentary tube contents is related to the time of stomach emptying, small intestinal enterocinesia and the fluidity of the contents. Small intestinal enterocinesia is controlled by the intestinal nerves and other nerves out of the intestine. When the mechanical and chemical stimulus act on the intestinal wall susceptor, small intestinal enterocinesia is increased by local reflex. The parasympathetic nervous system stimulates small intestinal enterocinesia, but the sympathetic nervous system acts to opposite the actions of the parasympathetic nervous system. Take anthracitic suspension as the indicator because it can not be absorbed in the intestine, we measure the distance of anthracitic suspension propelled in the intestine to observe the cathartic action on the small intestinal propelling movements.

【Equipments】scissors, forceps, ruler, syringe, infusion syringe needle for mice.

【Reagents】anthracitic suspension, 12% solution w/v (contended with Acacia, 2% solution w/v), Saline, 100% natrii sulfas solution, Radix et rhizama rhei solution (1 g/mL).

【Animals】Mice, weighing 18~22 g.

【Methods】Mark and weigh the mice fasted for 20 h and divide them into different groups. All the mice are treated by oral administration. Group A: 100% natrii sulfas solution (0.2 mL/10 g), group B: Radix et rhizama rhei solution (0.2 mL/10 g), group C: distilled water 0.2 mL/10 g. 20 minutes later every mouse is given anthracitic suspension 10% solution (0.1 mL/mouse) by oral administration. Kill the animals by vertebrate dislocation 20 minutes after oral administration of anthracitic and then open their abdominal cavities. Free the whole digestive tract from cardia to the end of rectal tube and pave it nicely without traction. Detect the whole length of the distance from the front edge of anthracitic to cardia and compute the percentage of the distance that the anthracitic moved corresponding to the whole length of gastrointestinal tract. Calculate it according to the following formula:

The percentage of anthracitic's moving distance to whole length of GI tract = anthracitic moving distance / whole length of GI tract × 100%

Collect the results of the whole class. Get the mean ($\bar{x}$) and standard deviation (SD), compare the result among the groups by student's t-test.

【Results】 Write down your data in the table 8-1.

Table 8-1 The effect of Radix et rhizoma rhei、natrii sulfas on mouse small intestinal enterocinesia

Groups	Dosage (g/kg)	Animals number	Anthractitic moving distance	Whole length of GI tract	The percentage of anthracitic moving distance (%)
Control group					
Radix et rhizoma thei					
Natrii sulfas					

【Notes】

1. Prepare the solution of Radix et rhizoma rhei comminute radix (100 g) to small pieces, then soak it in the cold water. 24 h later, filter it and concentrate it till 1 g/mL with 40 ℃ water bath.

2. To keep the treat time in control with accuracy, or else it will influence the experimental results dramatically.

3. Avoid traction when cutting the stomach tract, or else the accuracy of detection will be affected much.

【Questions】

1. How many kinds of cathartic are there according to the diarrhea mechanism? Which kind do Radix et rhizoma rhei、natrii sulfas respectively belong to?

2. What are the main constituents and mechanism of Radix et rhizoma rhei leading to diarrhea? What do we have to pay attention to when we use rhei in clinical?

第九章　祛风湿药实验

祛风湿药是一类以祛除风湿，解除痹痛为主要功效的药物。本类药物均能祛风散寒除湿，部分能舒筋活络、止痛、强筋骨，临床主要用于痹证的治疗。现代药理学研究表明，这类药物主要具有抗炎、镇痛、抑制免疫功能，其中少部分成分对免疫功能有促进作用。实验研究祛风湿药时，一般主要根据其抗炎作用来设计，选择的指标主要有肿胀度、毛细血管通透性、肉芽增生等。本章以肿胀和毛细血管通透性为指标，观察中药的抗炎作用。

Chapter 9　Experiments on drugs for dispelling and eliminating dampness

Primary efficacy of drugs for Dispelling and eliminating is concerned with dispelling wind and eliminating dampness, relieving pain induced by impediment. All the drugs can dispel wind, dissipate cold and eliminate dampness, and some of them can soothe sinew, quicken the network vessels, alleviate pain, and strengthen sinew and bone. The drugs are mostly used to treat impediment symptom in clinic. Modern pharmacological study suggests the drugs mostly possess the effects of anti-inflammation, alleviating pain, and immunodepression. Hereinto a few ingredients can enhance immunity. At present, drugs for dispelling and eliminating dampness are mainly researched according to their anti-inflammatory effect. The factors should be objectively and easily chosen by the statistics from the magnitude of swelling, capillary permeability, leucocyte transmigration and granulation formation etc. In this chapter, anti-inflammatory effect of TCM is investigated by detecting edema and capillary permeability.

实验一　复方羌活汤对佐剂关节炎大鼠足肿胀的影响

【目的】学习采用弗氏（Freund's）完全佐剂诱发大鼠多发性关节肿胀的方法，并观察复方羌活汤对弗氏完全佐剂诱导的大鼠足跖肿胀的影响。

【原理】弗氏完全佐剂诱导的大鼠关节炎模型与人的类风湿性关节炎类似，常用于祛风湿药物的筛选。一般大鼠在弗氏完全佐剂注射后的最初 3 天，足跖肿胀明显，随后逐渐减轻。13 天左右再度显著肿胀，出现耳和尾部红斑及炎性小结，22 天左右开始消退。

【器材】天平；足跖容积测量仪；注射器；大鼠灌胃针头。

【试剂】弗氏完全佐剂；复方羌活汤水煎液 2.28 g/mL（金银花、蒲公英、白花蛇舌草、土茯苓、薏苡仁各 30 g；赤芍、紫花地丁各 18 g；贝母、黄柏各 12 g；苍术、羌活各 9 g）；生理盐水；0.4 mg/mL 醋酸泼尼松；苦味酸。

【动物】大鼠，180~220 g，雌雄不限。

【方法】

1. 弗氏完全佐剂的制备方法　将无水羊毛脂与液体石蜡按 4 : 6（V/V，夏天）或 3 : 5（冬天）的比例混匀后，高压灭菌，制备弗氏不完全佐剂。随后，加入适当浓度的灭活乳酸分枝杆菌（终浓度约 5 mg/mL）即成弗氏完全佐剂。

2. 性别相同，体重相近的大鼠 3 只，苦味酸标记，采用足跖容积测量仪测定每只大鼠双侧后肢正常足跖容积。测定时，将鼠后肢拉直放入测量仪玻璃筒内，记录筒内液体水平线与鼠足横线标记处重叠时的足趾容积数值（mL），测定 3 次，其平均值即为大鼠的正常足跖容积。

3. 在第 0 天，于大鼠右后足跖皮内注射弗氏完全佐剂 0.1 mL。甲鼠灌胃给予复方羌活水煎液 1.5 mL/100 g，乙鼠灌胃给予生理盐水 1.5 mL/100 g，丙鼠灌胃给予醋酸泼尼松 1 mg/1.5 mL/100 g。每天 1 次，连续 28 天。于第 0、3、5、7、11、15、19、23、28 天分别测定每只大鼠右后侧足跖容积。于第 11、15、19、23、28 天分别测定每只大鼠左后侧足跖容积。以其与造模前足趾容积的差值表示肿胀度（Δ mL）。

【结果】将数据填入表 9-1 和表 9-2 中。

表 9–1　复方羌活汤对佐剂关节炎大鼠右后侧足跖原发性肿胀的影响

组别	剂量（g/kg）	动物数	右后侧足跖肿胀度（Δ mL）								
			0 d	3 d	5 d	7 d	11 d	15 d	19 d	23 d	28 d
模型组											
复方羌活汤组											
醋酸泼尼松组											

表 9-2　复方羌活汤对佐剂关节炎大鼠左后侧足跖继发性肿胀的影响

组别	剂量（g/kg）	动物数	左后侧足跖肿胀度（Δ mL）				
			11 d	15 d	19 d	23 d	28 d
模型组							
复方羌活汤组							
醋酸泼尼松组							

【注意事项】

1. 不宜选用大于 9 个月或小于 21 天龄的大鼠。
2. 乳化剂的优劣将影响免疫反应的强度。
3. 极少数因不能耐受弗氏完全佐剂而明显影响大鼠一般状态者，应剔除。

【思考题】试述复方羌活汤的抗炎作用机制及临床意义。

Experiment 1 Effect of complex prescription of notopterygii rhizoma decoction on paw edema induced by Freund's adjuvant in rats

【Purpose】

(1) To study the experimental method of multiple arthrocele in rat induced by complete Freund's adjuvant.

(2) To observe the effects of complex prescription of notopterygii rhizome decoction on paw edema induced by complete Freund's adjuvant in rats.

【Principles】This model is similar to rheumatoid arthritis in human and it can be used to screen the anti-arthritis medicines. The edema of hind paw treated with adjuvant significantly increase on day 3 after the adjuvant treatment, and then gradually reduce. On day 13, the paw edema repeatedly elevates, and erythema in ear and tail as well as inflammatory nodules are observed, but such symptom alleviates on days 22 after the adjuvant treatment.

【Equipments】Balance, equipment to measure the volume of paw, syringe, pinheads to gavage rats.

【Reagents】Complete Freund's adjuvant, aqueous extract of complex prescription of notopterygii rhizome decoction 2.28 g/mL (Lonicerae Flos 30 g, Taraxacum mongolicum Hand.-mazz. 30 g, Oldenlandia diffusa (wild) Roxb 30 g, Smilacis Glabrae Rhizoma 30 g, CoicisSemen 30 g, Paeoniae Radix Rubra 18 g, Viola yedoensis Makino 18 g , Fritillariae Bulbus 12 g, PhellodendriCortex 12 g, Atractylodis Rhizoma 9 g and Rhizomza Seu Radix Notopterygii 9 g), normal saline, prednisone suspension 0.4 mg/mL, 2,4,6-trinitrophenol (picric acid).

【Animals】Rats, 180~220 g, male or female.

【Methods】

1. Preparation of complete Freund's adjuvant The ratio between anhydrous lanolin and liquid paraffin is 4/6 (v/v, in summer) or 3/5 (v/v, in winter). The lanolin is heated to melt and mixed with liquid paraffin uniformly, sterilized on the high pressure to get incomplete Freund's adjuvant. Proper concentration of dead Mycobacterium tuberculosis with the final concentration no less than 5 mg/mL is added to incomplete Freund's adjuvant to make complete Freund's adjuvant.

2. Rats of same sex are weighed, marked with picric acid, and randomly divided into three groups. The volumes of hind paws are measured twice by equipment. The average volume of hind paw is taken as the normal value of pre-administration.

3. All rats are orally administered for 28 days.

Rat A is orally administered with the aqueous extract of complex prescription of notopterygii rhizome decoction 15 mL/kg/day.

Rat B is orally administered with normal saline 15 mL/kg/day.

Rat C is orally administered with prednisone 10 mg/15 mL/kg/day.

One hour later following the first oral administration, Complete Freund's adjuvant 0.1 mL is subcutaneously injected into the rat's right hind paw around anklebone. The volume of rat's right hind paw is respectively measured by equipment on day 0, 3, 5, 7, 11, 15, 19, 23 and 28. The volume of rat's left hind paw is respectively measured on days 11, 15, 19, 23 and 28. The swollen degree is calculated as the difference of the hind paw volume after inflammation and that before inflammation.

【Results】The experimental data are filled into the table 9-1、table 9-2.

Table 9–1 the Effect of complex prescription of notopterygii rhizome decoction on the primary paw swelling induced by Freund's adjuvant in rats

Groups	Dose (g/kg)	No. of rats	The right hind paw swelling (Δ mL)								
			0 d	3 d	5 d	7 d	11 d	15 d	19 d	23 d	28 d
Control											
Complex prescription of notopterygii rhizome decoction											
Prednisone											

Table 9–2 the effect of complex prescription of notopterygii rhizome decoction on the secondary paw swelling induced by Freund's adjuvant in rats

Groups	Dose (g/kg)	No. of rats	The left hind paw swelling (Δ mL)				
			11 d	15 d	19 d	23 d	28 d
Control							
Complex prescription of notopterygii rhizome decoction							
Prednisone							

【Notes】

1. The age of rat should be limited between 21 days and 9 monthes.

2. The intensity of immune reaction is influenced by the quality of emulsion.

3. Rats that can not tolerate complete Freund's adjuvant or have abnormal clinical symptom should be discarded from the experiment.

【Questions】

1. What is the mechanism of the anti-inflammatory effect of the complex prescription of notopterygii rhizome decoction?

2. What clinical significance do they have?

实验二　五加皮对小鼠腹腔毛细血管通透性的影响

【目的】观察五加皮对小鼠腹腔毛细血管通透性的影响。

【原理】采用低浓度醋酸为致炎因子，引起急性炎症反应。小鼠静脉注射染料伊文思蓝，再腹腔注射醋酸，通过比色法测定腹腔液染料渗出量，代表炎性渗出的多少。五加皮具有抗炎、镇痛、镇静、免疫抑制等作用，可减少腹腔液染料的渗出量。

【器材】721 型分光光度计；离心机；小鼠固定器；注射器；针头；小鼠灌胃针头；试管；离心试管；剪刀；镊子。

【试剂】五加皮醇提浸膏；0.5% 伊文思蓝溶液（生理盐水配制）；0.6% 醋酸；生理盐水。

【动物】小鼠，18~22 g，雌雄不限。

【方法】

1. 小鼠按体重随机分成两组，其中一组皮下注射五加皮醇提取物（200 mg/kg），另一组为对照组，皮下注射等体积生理盐水。

2. 给药后 1 h，两组小鼠均尾静脉注射 0.5% 伊文思蓝溶液 0.1 mL/10 g，随后立即腹腔注射 0.6% 醋酸溶液 0.2 mL/ 只。

3. 20 min 后，断头放血处死小鼠，剪开腹腔。

4. 用 5 mL 生理盐水冲洗腹腔数次，合并洗涤液，于 2 000 rpm/min 离心 5 min。

5. 取上清，721 型分光光度计 590 nm 处测定吸光度（OD 值）。

6. 以对照组小鼠染料的渗出量为 100%，计算给药组小鼠腹腔渗出的抑制率。

【结果】将实验数据填入表 9-3 内，并按下式计算抑制率。

$$抑制率 = (对照组渗出量 - 用药组渗出量) / 对照组渗出量 \times 100\%$$

表 9-3　五加皮对小鼠毛细血管通透性的影响（$\bar{x} \pm SD$）

组别	剂量（g/kg）	动物数	染料渗出量的光密度值（OD 值）	抑制率
对照组				
五加皮组				

【注意事项】

1. 腹腔注射醋酸溶液的部位力求一致，注射醋酸至处死动物的时间必须严格掌握。

2. 打开腹腔时避免损伤血管，若腹腔内有出血，样本应弃去不用。

【思考题】五加皮抗炎作用的特点和机制是什么？

Experiment 2 Effect of Acanthopanacis Radicis Cortex on abdominal capillary permeability in mice

【**Purpose**】To observe the effect of Acanthopanacis Radicis Cortex on abdominal capillary permeability in mice.

【**Principles**】Low concentration of acetic acid are used as phlegmasia agent to induce acute inflammatory reaction. Even's blue dye is intravenously injected to mice, and then acetic acid is intraperitoneally injected to mice. The absorbance of the liquid from abdominal cavities reflects capillary permeability. Acanthopanacis Radicis Cortex, wich has the effects of anti-inflammation, alleviating pain, sedation and immunodepression, can reduce the dye permeability.

【**Equipments**】spectrophotometer 721, centrifuge, mouse fixing cylinder, syringe (1 mL and 5 mL), injection needle, pinhead to gavage mice, test tubes, centrifuging tubes, scissor, forceps.

【**Animals**】Mice, 18~22 g, male or female.

【**Reagents**】Ethanol extract of Acanthopanacis Radicis Cortex, 0.5% Even's blue dye (dissolved in normal saline), 0.6% acetic acid, normal saline

【**Methods**】

1. The mice are weighed and randomly divided into two groups (control and treatment group). The dry ethanol extract of Acanthopanacis Radicis Cortex (200 mg/kg) is subcutaneously injected in the mice of treatment group and the an equal volume of the normal saline for the control group.

2. One hour later, 0.5% Even's blue dye (0.1 mL/10 g) is intravenously injected into the tails of the mice, and then 0.6% solution of acetic acid per mice (0.2 mL) is intraperitoneally injected to the mice of both groups.

3. 20 min later, The mice were sacrificed by cervical dislocation t and the the peritoneal cavity was opened.

4. The abdominal cavitiy is repeatedly washed by 5 mL saline and the washing liquid is collected and centrifuged at 2,000 rpm for 5 min.

5. The absorbance of extract of the supernatant liquid is measured at the maximum of 590 nm.

6. The average absorbance of each group is calculated and t-test is used to statistically evaluation. The dye permeability of the control group is presumed as one hundred percent and

the inhibitory rate of the exudates in the treating group is calculated.

【Results】 The inhibition rate is calculated according to the subsequent equation and the experimental data are filled into the table 9-3.

Inhibition rate =（dye permeability of the control group−dye permeability of the treating group）

Table 9–3 Effect of Acanthopanacis radicis cortex on capillary permeability in mice（$\bar{x}\pm SD$）

Groups	Dose（g/kg）	No. of mice	The absorbance of the liquid from abdominal cavities	Inhibition rate（%）
Control group				
Acanthopanacis Radicis Cortex group				

【Notes】

1. The injection sites of acetic acid in the peritoneal cavity should be located in the same area and the time for killing mice killed should be strictly controlled.

2. When the mouse peritoneal cavity is opened, the hemorrhage resulted from the lesion of blood vessels should be avoided. If the hemorrhage resulted from blood vessels in the peritoneal cavity is observed, the washing liquid eluent should be discarded.

【Questions】 What are the characteristics and mechanism of the anti-inflammatory action of Acanthopanacis Radicis Cortex?

实验三　秦艽对小鼠巴豆油耳肿胀的影响

【目的】观察秦艽对小鼠巴豆油耳肿胀的影响。

【原理】秦艽味辛、苦、平，具有祛风湿、清湿热、止痹痛之功效。本实验考察秦艽对小鼠抗炎、镇痛药理作用的影响。

【器材】8 mm 打孔器；天平。

【试剂】秦艽水煎液（1 g / 200 mL）；1% CMC-Na 混悬液；2% 巴豆油合剂（含 2% 巴豆油；20% 无水乙醇；73% 乙醚和 5% 蒸馏水）。

【动物】小鼠，体重 18~22 g，雌雄不限。

【方法】

1. 取小鼠 4 只，称重，随机分为 2 组。甲组灌胃给予秦艽水煎液（0.2 mL/10 g），乙组注射适量 1% CMC-Na（0.1 mL/ 10 g）。
2. 半小时后，两组小鼠右耳廓两侧用微量进样器均匀涂布 2% 巴豆油合剂（0.05 mL）致炎，左耳廓作对照。
3. 致炎后 30 min，将小鼠处死，沿耳廓基线取下两耳，用打孔器于同一部位各取一个耳片称重。致炎侧耳片重量减去对照侧耳片重量即为肿胀度。

【结果】根据要求，汇集各组结果进行统计处理。

表 9-4　秦艽对小鼠巴豆油耳肿胀的影响（$\bar{x} \pm SD$）

组别	剂量（g/kg）	动物数	致炎侧耳片重量（g）	对照侧耳片重量（g）	肿胀值
对照组					
秦艽组					

【注意事项】

1. 取材力求部位一致。
2. 打孔器应锋利。

【思考题】秦艽的药理作用及特点有哪些？

Experiment 3 Effect of Largeleaf Gentian Root on auricular tumescence induced by croton oil in mice

【Objective】To observe the effect of Largeleaf Gentian Root on auricular tumescence induced by croton oil in mice

【Principle】Largeleaf Gentian Root is bitter and flat, which can clear rheumatism and heat, and relive arthralgia. This study is to detect the anti-inflammatory and analgesic effect of Largeleaf Gentian Root in mice.

【Equipments】8 mm pin-hole plotter, balance.

【Reagents】water solution of Largeleaf Gentian Root（1 g/200 mL）, 1% CMC-Na, 2% croton oil mixture（2% croton oil, 2% anhydrous ethanol, 73% ethyl ether and 5% distilled water）

【Animals】Mice, 18~22 g, male or female.

【Methods】

1. Four mice are weighted and randomly divided into two groups（control and treatment group）. Give 0.5% indomethacin（0.5 mg/ mL）for the control group by intraperitoneal injection and the an equal volume of 1% CMC-Na（0.1 mL/ 10 g）for the treating group.

2. 30 minutes later, inflammation is evoked at the bilateral of the auricle of the right ears by the steady application of 2% croton oil mixture 0.05 mL with microsyringe, let the left ears be control.

3. 30 minutes later, kill the mice and take the ears along the auricled basic line. Take a piece of ear from the same location of each ear respectively by the pin-hole plotter and weigh them.

The magnitude of ear tumescence is defined as that the difference of the weight of the control side and that of the inflamed side.

【Results】According to the requirements, collect the data of each group to take statistics.

Table 9-4 Effect of Largeleaf Gentian Root on croton oil-induced auricular tumescence（$\bar{x} \pm SD$）

Groups	Dose（g/kg）	No. of mice	The weight of ear at the inflamed side	The weight of ear at the un-inflamed side	Values of swelling
Control group					
Largeleaf Gentian Root group					

【Note】

1. Draw the piece of the ear from the same location.

2. The hole-digger should be sharp.

【Questions】What are the pharmaco-characteristics of Largeleaf Gentian Root?

实验四　淫羊藿苷对脂多糖诱导的巨噬细胞 NO 释放的影响

【目的】观察淫羊藿苷对脂多糖（LPS）诱导的 RAW264.7 细胞中 NO 释放的影响。

【原理】淫羊藿苷是淫羊藿的主要活性成分，属黄酮苷类化合物。研究表明，淫羊藿苷具有显著的抗炎活性。本实验采用格里斯氏（Griess）法考察淫羊藿苷对 LPS 诱导的 RAW264.7 细胞中 NO 释放的影响。

【器材】微孔板读数仪；移液器。

【试剂】胎牛血清；DMEM 培养基；1% 磺胺；0.1% 萘乙烯二胺；$NaNO_2$（0, 20, 40, 60, 80, 100 μmol/L）。

【细胞株】小鼠巨噬细胞系细胞 RAW264.7。

【方法】

1. 分别测定 $NaNO_2$（0, 20, 40, 60, 80, 100 μmol/L）在 540 nm 出吸光度值，制作标准曲线。

2. 将 1% 磺胺，0.1% 萘乙烯二胺按照体积 1 : 1 的比例配制成 Griess 试剂。

3. 将 RAW264.7 细胞接种于 96 孔板（1×10^5 个 / 孔，每孔 100 μL），每组 3 个复孔，37 ℃，5%CO_2 条件下培养 12 h 至完全贴壁。随后，用 LPS（10 μg/mL）和淫羊藿苷（1, 10, 100 μg/mL）处理细胞 24 h。取细胞上清液 100 μL，加入等体积 Griess 试剂，550 nm 测定吸光度值。按照标准曲线，计算出 NO 的量。

【结果】汇集各组结果进行统计处理。

表 9–5　淫羊藿苷对 LPS 诱导的 RAW264.7 中 NO 释放的影响（$\bar{x} \pm SD$）

组别	浓度	NO（μmol/L）
对照组		
淫羊藿苷	1 μg/mL	
	10 μg/mL	
	100 μg/mL	

【注意事项】

1. 每次加标本应更换吸，以免发生交叉污染。

2. 洗涤是最主要的关键步骤，应严格按要求洗涤。

【思考题】淫羊藿的药理作用特点有哪些？

Experiment 4 Effect of Icariin NO production in activated macrophages

[Objective] To observe the effect of Icariin on the production of NO from -stimulated RAW264.7 cells subjected tolipopolysaccharide (LPS) challenge.

[Principle] Icariin is the main active ingredient of epimedium and belongs to flavonoid glycoside. The data shows that it has significant anti-inflammation effect. This experiment is carried out to detect the effect of icariin on the production of NO from LPS-stimulated RAW264.7 cells using Griess method.

[Equipments] Microplate Reader, transferpettor.

[Reagents] Fetal bovine serum (FBS), Dulbecco's Modified Eagle Media (DMEM), 1% sulfanilamide, 0.1% naphthylethylenediamine, $NaNO_2$ (0, 20, 40, 60, 80, 100 μmol/L).

[Cell] RAW264.7 cells, a cell line derived from mice macrophages

[Methods]

1. Detect the absorptive value of $NaNO_2$ (0, 20, 40, 60, 80, 100 μmol/L) at 540 nm and calculate the standard curve.

2. The Griess reagent is prepared with 1% sulfanilamide and 0.1% naphthylethylenediamine, which are mixed to the volume ratio of 1: 1.

3. The RAW264.7 cells were plated at the density of 1×10^5 cells/well and cultured at 37 ℃ and 5% CO_2 for 12 h. Subsequently, the cells were treated with LPS (10 μg/mL) and icariin (1, 10, 100 μg/mL). 100 μL culture media of every well was collected and detected using Microplate Reader at 540 nm. Calculating the concentration of NO according to the standard curve.

[Results] To collect the data of each group and take statistics.

Table 9–5 Effect of icariin on the production of NO from lipopolysaccharide (LPS)-induced RAW264.7 cells ($\bar{x} \pm SD$)

Groups	concentration	NO (μmol/L)
Control group		
Icariin group	1 μg/mL	
	10 μg/mL	
	100 μg/mL	

[Note]

1. The suction nozzle should be changed for every time, and avoiding pollution.

2. Scrubbing is the main procedure, the operation must be strict.

[Questions] What are the pharmaco-characteristics of Largeleaf Gentian Root ?

第十章　利水渗湿药实验

凡能通利水道，渗除水湿的药物称为利水渗湿药。利水渗湿药具有利水消肿，利尿通淋，利湿退黄等功效，主要用于治疗水肿、湿热、淋浊等病症。现代药理研究表明，这类药物主要具有利尿，抗病原微生物，保肝利胆，抗肿瘤，增强免疫功能作用。利水渗湿药实验以利尿通淋为重点，观察药物是否有利尿作用。利尿药筛选的实验中常用的动物为大鼠和狗，其次为家兔和小鼠。

利尿药的动物实验方法分为：（1）急性实验，如直接自输尿管或膀胱收集尿液，适用于较大的动物如兔或狗等。该实验在较短的时间内完成，受外界的影响也较少，然而实验是在麻醉下进行，麻醉药可能对尿液的形成有一定的影响。（2）慢性实验，如代谢笼收集尿液，适用于大鼠或小鼠。为减少尿液蒸发和粪便污染，可使用特殊的集尿装置或用滤纸吸附尿液进行称重。应注意实验环境的影响如气温或湿度等，室温在 20 ℃左右为好。本章主要用尿导管法观察利水渗湿药的利尿作用。

Chapter 10 Experiments of drugs for disinhibiting water and percolating dampness

Primary efficacy of drugs for disinhibiting water and percolating dampness is concerned with freeing waterway, percolating water-damp. The drugs which possess disinhibiting water, detumescence, diuresis, freeing strangury, disinhibiting dampness and abating jaundice, etc are used to treat edema, damp-heat and strangury-turbidity. Modern pharmacological studies suggest that the drugs mostly have the effects on diuretic, anti pathogenic microorganism, hepatoprotection, cholagogue, anti-tumor and immunological enhancing function. Experimental methods for disinhibiting water and percolating dampness emphasize on diuresis and freeing strangury by observing the diuretic effect. Rat and dog are commonly used in screening experiments of diuretics. Rabbit and mice are second to them.

Experimental methods of diuretics in animals usually contain two classes: (1) Acute experiments, for example, directly collecting urine from ureters or bladder, are suitable for larger animals such as rabbit or dog etc. The experiment is completed in a relatively short period of time and less affected by the outside circumstance. Experiment is conducted in anesthesia, however, that anesthetics may have a certain effect on the formation of urine. (2) Chronic experiments, for example, collecting urine by the metabolism cage device, are suitable for rat or mouse. In order to reduce urine evaporation and prevent urine pollution of excrement, urine can be collected by special urine collection device or weighed by the filter paper adsorption. The experiment can be affected by outer environment such as temperature or humidity, and the suitable room temperature is 20 ℃ or so. In this chapter, diuretic effect of drugs for disinhibiting water and percolating dampness is investigated by observing urine volume using urethral catheter method.

实验一 金钱草对家兔的利尿作用(导尿管法)

【目的】了解急性利尿的实验方法,观察金钱草对家兔的利尿作用。

【原理】金钱草有利尿通淋,利湿退黄,清热消肿等功效。现代研究表明,其具有利尿、利胆以及治疗结石症等作用。

【器材】兔固定箱;兔手术台;兔开口器;导尿管(灌胃用);电子称;量筒;烧杯;注射器;聚乙烯管;胶布。

【试剂】金钱草水煎液 2 g/mL;5% 葡萄糖盐水;液体石蜡。

【动物】雄性家兔 2 只,体重 2.2 ~ 2.5 kg。

【方法】

1. 给水负荷 2 只家兔,称重后均置于兔箱中,耳缘静脉注入 5% 葡萄糖盐水 10 mL/kg。

2. 导尿 导尿管尖端先用液体石蜡润滑,再自尿道轻而慢插入至膀胱内,即有尿液滴出,再插入 1~2 cm 即可,最后用胶布将导尿管与家兔固定。

3. 给药 给水负荷后 30 min 给药,给药前先轻压下腹部排空膀胱。甲兔通过灌胃管灌入金钱草水煎液 10 mL/kg,乙兔灌入蒸馏水 10 mL/kg。

4. 收集尿液 给药完毕,记录时间,开始收集尿液,每隔 30 min 测定各兔排泄的尿量 1 次,直至给药后 120 min。

【结果】收集全班数据,计算单位时间内尿量的均数和标准差,并用 t 检验法进行组间显著性检验,将结果填入表 10-1。

表 10-1 金钱草对家兔尿量的影响

组别	剂量(g/kg)	给药后不同时间的尿量(mL)			
		0~30 min	30~60 min	60~90 min	90~120 min
对照组					
金钱草					

【注意事项】

1. 通常选用雄性动物,因为选用雌性动物易误插到子宫腔内而导致实验失败。

2. 每次收集尿液前,需用手轻压下腹部,以排空膀胱的余尿。

3. 插入总深度视动物大小而定,一般家兔约在 8~12cm。

4. 灌胃时,导尿管切勿插入气管,检验方法为:将导尿管外端置于盛水的烧杯中,如有气泡溢出,则为插入气管,应拔出重插。

【思考题】金钱草的利尿作用机制是什么?

Experiment 1 Effects of Christina Loosestrife on urine volume in rabbit (urethral catheter method)

【Purpose】 Study the acute animal test for diuretic action and observe the diuretic effect of Christina Loosestrife in rabbits.

【Principles】 The primary actions of Christina Loosestrife are concerned with diuresis, freeing strangury, disinhibiting dampness and abating jaundice, clearing heat and detumescence. Modern studies show that the Christina loosestrife has diuresis, cholagogue effects and is used for the treatment for lithiasis. So, effect of Christina loosestrife on urine volume in rabbit is observed.

【Equipments】 Rabbit box, operating table for rabbit, mouth-gag for rabbit, urethral catheter, electronic scale, cylinder, beaker, syringe, polyethylene tube, rubberized fabrics

【Reagents】 aqueous extract of Christina Loosestrife 2 g/mL, 5% glucose saline, liquid paraffin.

【Animals】 2 male rabbits, 2.2~2.5 kg.

【Methods】

1. Give water load Two rabbits are weighed and fixed in rabbit box. 5% glucose saline with 10 mL/kg body weight is injected intravenously via the marginal vein of the ear.

2. Urethral catheter method The top of urethral catheter is lubricated by liquid paraffin. Urethral catheter is inserted into urethra slowly and lightly. The urine will flow out along the urethral catheter after urethral catheter is inserted into bladder. Urethral catheter is put further to 1~2 cm again. Finally, the urethral catheter is fixed to the rabbit with some rubberized fabrics.

3. Administration 30 minutes after water load, lower abdomen of the rabbit is pressed by hands to empty the bladder. Aqueous extract of Christina loosestrife (20 g/10 mL/kg) is given to the rabbit by oral administration for the test, while distilled water (10 mL/kg) is given to another rabbit by oral administration for the control.

4. Urine collection After administration, time is recorded and urine is begun to collect. Collect the urine and record the volume every 30 min until 120 min.

【Results】 The data of the whole class is collected. The mean ($\bar{X}$) and the standard difference (SD) of urine volume of two groups in unit time. The significance test among groups by *t*-test should be done. Fill the results into the following table.

Table 10–1　Effect of Christina Loosestrife on urine volume in rabbit ($\bar{X}\pm SD$)

Groups	Dose (g/kg)	Urinary volume in different time after administration (mL)			
		0~30 min	30~60 min	60~90 min	90~120 min
Control					
Treating group					

[Notes]

1. Male animals are usually chosen, because urethral catheter can be easily inserted into the uterine cavity of female animals to induce the failure of the experiment.

2. Lower abdomen of the rabbits is pressed by hands to empty the bladder before urine collection.

3. Inserting total depth of urethral catheter is determined by the size of the animal. Usually, it is about 8~12 cm for rabbit.

4. Urethral catheter should not be inserted into trachea with oral administration. The way to check whether or not the urethral catheter is inserted into trachea is to observe whether or not the air bubble goes out if put the other end of urethral catheter into the water. If urethral catheter is inserted into trachea, the operation should do again.

[Questions] What is the mechanism of the diuretic action of Christina Loosestrife?

第十一章　温里药实验

凡以温里祛寒为主要作用，治疗里寒证的药物称为温里药，又称祛寒药。温里药具有辛散温通、散寒止痛、补火助阳等功效，主要用于寒邪内盛，心肾阳衰所致的各种里寒证。现代药理研究表明，这类药物主要药理作用为：①对心血管系统的影响：强心，扩张血管，抗心律失常，抗心肌缺血，抗休克。②对消化系统的影响：调节胃肠功能，促消化，利胆，止吐，抗溃疡等。③对肾上腺皮质系统功能的影响：附子、肉桂、干姜对垂体-肾上腺皮质系统有兴奋作用，而肉桂能使幼鼠的胸腺萎缩。④对神经系统的影响：镇静，局部麻醉，改善物质代谢，产生热量。⑤抗炎、镇痛。温里药对循环系统的实验分为四类：对离体和在体动物心脏的作用、对血管的作用、对血流动力学的影响和抗休克作用。本章主要介绍温里药对离体蛙心的作用，对狗血流动力学的影响和对缺氧-复氧心肌细胞损伤的保护作用。

Chapter 11　Experiments of drugs for warm interior

Primary efficacy of drugs for warm interior are concerned with warm interior and dispelling cold. The drugs can treat internal cold, so they can be called drugs for dispelling internal cold. The drugs possess the effects on pungent in flavor scattered, eliminating cold and relieving pain, supplementing fire and assisting yang. They are mainly used to cure various interior cold signs induced by cold evil internal exuberance, heart-kidney yang debilitation. Modern pharmacology studies suggest that the drugs have following pharmacological actions. ① Effects on cardiovascular system: cardiotonic effect, vascular dilatation, anti-arrhythmia, anti-myocardial ischemia and anti-shock. ② Effects on digestive system: regulating gastrointestinal function, promoting digestion, cholagogue, anti-vomit, anti-ulcer etc. ③ Effects on adrenocortical system: Radix Aconiti Lateralis Preparata, Cinnamomi Cortex and Zingiberis Rhizoma Exsiccatum can excite adrenocortical system, but Cinnamomi Cortex can make thymus gland atrophy in young mice. ④ Effects on nervous system: sedation, local anesthesia, improving substance metabolism and heat production. ⑤ Anti-inflammation and alleviating pain. Experimental methods of drugs for warm interior in animals usually contain four classes including effects on heart in vitro and in vivo, blood vessels, haemodynamics and shock. In this chapter, drugs for warm interior are investigated by observing effects on the isolated heart of toad, hemodynamic changes in anaesthetized open-chest dogs and ischemia reoxygenation myocardial cells.

实验一　生附子和制附子对离体蛙心的作用（八木氏法）

【目的】学习八木 -Hartung 离体蛙心灌流法。观察生附子、制附子对离体蛙心收缩幅度、频率、节律和心输出量的影响。

【原理】附子中含有多种生物碱，其中以乌头碱、中乌头碱、次乌头碱为主。乌头碱毒性大，使离体蛙心出现短暂的强心作用，随即转入抑制，心收缩力减弱，心律紊乱，最后心跳停止。乌头碱水解产物乌头原碱的毒性仅为乌头碱的 1/2 000~1/4 000，无明显强心作用。生附子浸出液含有大量乌头碱，故对心肌产生明显的毒副作用。附子经长期煎煮后，因乌头碱水解为乌头原碱，毒性大减，而强心成分虽经煎煮、炮制而不被破坏，仍呈现明显的强心作用。

【器材】BL-420 生物技能系统；张力换能器；八木氏蛙心插管；毁髓针；蛙板；蛙心夹；烧杯；移液管；试管夹；铁架台；双凹夹；大剪刀；眼科剪；眼科镊；注射器；缝线。

【药品和试剂】任氏液；低钙任氏液（钙离子含量为正常任氏液的 1/4）；生附子水煎液 0.125 g/mL；制附子水煎液 0.125 g/mL。

【动物】蛙或蟾蜍，体重 70 g 以上，雌雄不限。

【方法】

1. 取蛙或蟾蜍 1 只，用毁髓针捣毁脑和脊髓后，仰位固定于蛙板上。依次剪开胸前区皮肤、胸骨和心包膜，暴露心脏。按下列顺序进行操作：

（1）于左右主动脉下各穿一线备用，然后将心尖翻向头侧；暴露出静脉窦和后腔静脉。

（2）在后腔静脉下穿一线，在穿线处的下方剪一小口，将盛有任氏液的静脉插管由此口插入，用线结扎固定，立即用任氏液从静脉插管冲洗心脏，洗净余血。

（3）翻正心脏，右主动脉结扎。在左主动脉远端剪口，向心脏方向插入动脉插管，如灌流液从动脉流出通畅，则可扎紧动脉插管。

（4）用剪刀将心脏从周围组织中游离出来，调整好方向、角度，将动静脉插管固定在一起。用主动脉下用一丝线结扎除主动脉和后腔静脉以外的所有血管，制成蛙心标本。

2. 用任氏液反复冲洗心脏，直至动脉流出液无色为止。调整静脉插管液面 1.5~2 cm 左右，在整个实验过程中液面高度应保持不变。用蛙心夹夹住心尖，连接好记录装置。

3. 描记一段正常心肌收缩曲线，记录每分钟心跳次数、输出量（滴 / 分）及振幅。然后按下列顺序进行操作：

（1）换入低钙任氏液，待收缩明显减弱趋于恒定时，描记曲线，观察记录上述指标。

（2）向静脉管内加入 0.125 g/mL 的制附子 0.05~0.1 mL，作用明显后，观察记录上述指标。

（3）用滴管移去静脉插管内的全部液体，以任氏液换洗 2~3 次，至心跳恢复正常。描记一段正常心肌收缩曲线，观察记录上述指标。

（4）再换入低钙任氏液，待收缩明显减弱趋于恒定时描记曲线，观察记录上述指标。

（5）向静脉管内加入 0.125 g/mL 的生附子 0.05~0.1 mL，作用明显后，观察记录上述指标。

4. 比较给药前后心脏收缩强度、频率、节律以及从动脉管中博出液体的流速（滴 / 分）。

【结果】

1. 剪贴或复制心脏收缩曲线，并作注明。

2. 计算出用药前后心输出量。

【注意事项】

1. 在后腔静脉插管时，应谨防撕破血管或误插在血管外的薄膜夹层中。

2. 在手术和实验过程中不要损伤静脉窦，心脏离体时要避免扎住静脉窦，并要防止标本漏液。

3. 每次换药前后，静脉插管中液面高度应尽可能保持一致。

4. 生附子和制附子的原植物科、属、种均需一致，否则会影响实验结果。

5. 离体心脏要经常保持湿润。

【思考题】根据用药后的心率、心输出量、心肌收缩力的变化情况，对生附子和制附子的药理作用进行讨论。

Experiment 1　Effects of the Raw Aconite Root and Radix Aconiti Lateralis Preparata on the isolated toad hearts

【Purpose】 Study Yatsuki-Hartung's perfusion method of isolated heart of toad; Observe the effects of the Raw Aconite Root and Radix Aconiti Lateralis Preparata on contractile force, frequency, rhythm and cardiac output in the isolated heart of toad.

【Principles】 The Raw Aconite Root containes many alkaloids chiefly including aconitine, mesaconitine, hypaconitine. Aconitine with strongpoison can reinforce heart transitorily, then turn to inhibit the contraction force of heart and disturb heart rate, finally, leading to the heartbeat stop. The hydrolysis product of aconitine is aconine. Toxicity of aconine with no reinforcing heart effect is only 1/2,000 to 1/4,000 of aconitine's. For lixivium from the Raw Aconite root contains aconitine, thelixivium and can significantly cause heart toxicity. After long time heating in the water, the noxious property of aconitine decreases because aconitine decomposes to aconine. The ingredients of reinforcing hearts will not be destroyed after processing, so it still appears reinforcing heart effect evidently.

【Equipments】 BL-420 biological function system, tension transducer, toad heart cannula of Yatsuki-Hartung's, probe, frog board, toad heart clip, beaker, pipette, tube clip, iron stand, biconcave clamp, shears, ophthalmology scissors, eye forceps, syringes, silk thread.

【Drugs and reagents】 Ringer's solution, Ringer's solution containing Ca^{2+} (0.03 g/L), aqueous extract of the Raw Aconite Root 0.125 g/mL, aqueous extract of Radix Aconiti Lateralis Preparata 0.125 g/mL.

【Animals】 frogs or toads, >70 g, male or female.

【Methods】

1. A toad or frog is taken and its brain and spinal cord are destroyed with a pin. The frog or toad is fixed on the frog board, then, the thoracic cavity is opened and the pericardium is cut to make the heart exposed sufficiently. The experiment operates according to the following orders:

(1) Turn up the heart and make the venous sinus and postcaval vein exposed. Two pieces of thread are put under the left and right aorta respectively.

(2) A piece of thread is put under the postcaval vein. Make an incision beneath the site where the thread is placed. The venous cannula is inserted into the postcaval vein through the incision and fastened cannula is inserted into the postcaval vein through the incision and

fastens by thread to fix. Ringer's solution is used to wash the heart from the venous cannula and the remaining blood is removed.

（3）Turn the heart back. The right aorta is fastened by a thread. Make an incision on the distal edge of the left aorta. Insert the arterial cannula towards the heart. If the perfusion solution flows out fluently from the arterial cannula, fasten the cannula by a piece of thread placed before hand.

（4）The heart is separated from the peripheral tissues. Adjust the direction and angle to fix the arterial cannula and the venous one together. All the blood vessels are ligated except the aorta and postcaval vein with the other piece of thread. The specimen of the frog's heart is made.

2. Ringer's solution is used to wash the heart repeatedly until the effluent solution from theartrial cannula is colorless. Adjust the height of liquid in the venous cannula to 1.5~2 cm and keep the height constant during the whole experiment. Clip the cardiac apex and link the recording equipment.

3. Depict a segment of normal curve. The cardiac contraction force, heart rate, cardiac output（drops/min）are observed and recorded. Then, the experiment is conducted according to the following orders:

（1）Ringer's solution containing low calcium is changed to solution. Depict the curve after the cardiac contraction force weakens obviously. The aforementioned indices are observed and recorded.

（2）Add 0.05~0.1 mL aqueous extract of Radix Aconiti Lateralis Preparata（0.125 g/mL）into the venous cannula, and observe and record the above indices when it acts obviously.

（3）Solution in the venous cannula is removed by pipette. Ringer's solution is used to wash the heart 2 to 3 times until the cardiac contraction force reverts to the normal. Depict a segment of normal curve. The aforementioned indices are observed and recorded.

（4）Ringer's solution containing low calcium is changed to solution again. Depict the curve after the cardiac contraction force weakens obviously. The aforementioned indices are observed and recorded.

（5）Add 0.05~0.1 mL aqueous extract of the Raw Aconite Root（0.125 g/mL）into the venous cannula, and observe and record the above indices when it acts obviously.

The cardiac contraction force, heart rate, rhythm and the cardiac output（drops/min）of the effluent solution from the arterial cannula before and after administration are recorded.

【Results】

1. Copy the curve of heart contraction and mark administered drug and dosage.

2. Record the cardiac output pre-administration and post-administration respectively.

【Notes】

1. The venous cannula is inserted into the postcaval vein, but the postcaval vein should not be cut off. In addition, the venous cannula should not be inserted into the outer membrane

of postcaval vein.

2. During the course of surgery and experiment, be careful not to harm the venous sinus. When all the blood vessels are ligated except the aorta and postcaval vein, be careful not to delegate the venous sinus. In addition, the specimen of the toad's heart should not leak.

3. During experiment, the height of the liquid in the venous cannula should be unchanged.

4. If the Raw Aconite Root is not consistence with Radix Aconiti Lateralis Preparata in family, genus and species, they will affect the experimental results.

5. Keep the isolated heart usually moist.

【Questions】According to changes of the cardiac contraction force, heart rate and cardiac output after administration, discuss the pharmacological action of the Raw Aconite root and Radix Aconiti Lateralis Preparata.

实验二　附子对麻醉犬心脏血流动力学的影响

【目的】学习心脏血流动力学的实验方法,观察附子对麻醉犬心脏血流动力学的作用。

【原理】附子有回阳救逆的功效,具有强心、升压、改善微循环、抗休克等作用。本实验利用血流动力学指标来观察附子对心脏功能及外周阻力的影响。

【器材】MFV-3200 电磁流量计(日本, Nihon Kohden); BL-420 生物机能试验系统; 压力换能器; HX-300 动物呼吸机(成都泰盟科技有限责任公司); 手术剪; 手术刀; 持针钳; 止血钳; 眼科剪; 眼科镊; 三通开关; 针状电极; 气管插管; 动脉插管; 静脉插管; 动脉夹。

【动物】犬,体重 12 kg 以上,雌雄不限。

【试剂】附子注射液 3 g/mL; 去甲乌药碱溶液 0.05 mg/mL; 生理盐水; 肝素钠溶液 500 U/mL; 戊巴比妥钠溶液 3 g/dL。

【方法】

1. 麻醉　犬称重后,前肢皮下头静脉注射戊巴比妥钠 30 mg/kg,使之麻醉,仰卧位固定于手术台上。将心电图电极插入四肢皮下,以标准Ⅱ导联监测动物心电图。

2. 手术

(1) 剪去颈部被毛,正中切开颈部皮肤,分离气管,在气管上做一倒 “T” 形切口,插入气管插管,连接呼吸机(潮气量 130~160 mL,频率 20 次 /min)以保持呼吸通畅。用止血钳拉开气管上方皮肤肌肉,即可在气管两侧见到与气管平行的左右颈总动脉。分离左侧颈总动脉,插入动脉插管(内充满 500 U/mL 的肝素生理盐水),通过压力换能器与 BL-420 生物机能试验系统连接,记录颈总动脉收缩压(SAP)、舒张压(DAP)、平均动脉压(MAP,舒张压 +1/3 脉压差)。分离右侧颈总动脉,插导管进入左心室,与压力换能器相连,通过 BL-420 生物机能试验系统测定左心室收缩压(LVSP),左心室舒张末期压(LVEDP)、左室内压上升及下降最大变化速率($\pm dp/dt_{max}$)。

(2) 剪去胸部被毛,在左肋第 4 肋间切开皮肤,分离肋间肌,打开胸腔,暴露心脏,切开心包膜,做心包摇篮。分离升主动脉根部和左冠状动脉前降支,放置适宜内径的电磁血流量计探头(内径 12 mm, 2 mm),连接于电磁血流量计上测量心输出量(CO)和冠脉流量(CBF)。

(3) 在一侧的腹股沟部位,用手触得股动脉搏动处,剪去该部位的被毛,用手术刀纵切皮肤 3~4 cm,用止血钳分离皮下结缔组织,暴露神经血管束,分离股静脉,结扎远心端,插入静脉插管,并由此注入肝素钠 500 U/(mL · kg)抗凝。

3. 各项指标的测定

(1) 术毕,心电稳定 30 分钟后,测量心率(HR)、SAP、DAP、MAP、LVSP、LVEDP、

$\pm dp/dt_{max}$、心输出量和冠脉流量，作为给药前的各项指标。

（2）分别股静脉注射附子注射液 2 g/kg，去甲乌药碱 5 μg/kg，观察两只犬上述指标的变化。

【结果】

1. 依据公式计算心脏指数（CI）、总外周血管阻力（TPVR）。

$$体表面积 =（BSA,\ m^2）= 体重（kg）^{2/3} \times 0.11$$
$$心脏指数[CI, L/（min \cdot m^2）]=CO/BSA$$
$$总外周血管阻力[TPVR,（kPa \cdot s）/L]=MAP（kPa）\times 60/CO$$

2. 将实验数据填入下列表格，汇集全班数据进行比较。

表 11–1　附子和去甲乌药碱对麻醉犬血流动力学的影响

项目	附子		去甲乌药碱	
	给药前	给药后	给药前	给药后
HR（bpm）				
SAP（kPa）				
DAP（kPa）				
MAP（kPa）				
CO（L/min）				
CBF（L/min）				
LVSP（kPa）				
LVEDP（kPa）				
$+dp/dt_{max}$（kPa/s）				
$-dp/dt_{max}$（kPa/s）				
CI[L/（min · m^2）]				
TPVR[（kPa · s）/L]				

【注意事项】

1. 动脉插管必充满肝素钠溶液，以防凝血。手术过程中见有出血点应结扎小血管，因为肝素化后易引起出血，影响结果。

2. 电磁流量计探头必须大小合适，与血管紧密接触，故实验前需测量血管外颈，以选用合适的探头。实验一般选用比血管外径小 5%~10% 的探头。

3. 记录压力的管道系统内空气必须排尽，微小气泡的存在都将影响血压及室内压波。

4. 为保证探头有良好的传导性，应用前应将探头浸泡在生理盐水中至少 30 min，新探头必须浸泡 2 h。

5. 左室插管在主动脉瓣口不易进入心室（此时从插管可感到心脏跳动），可将插管稍退出，改变角度和方向或抖动插管向前推进，这样往往可顺利插入左心室。

【思考题】通过附子对麻醉犬心脏血流动力学的影响，说明附子的“回阳救逆”功效及治疗“亡阳证”的依据。

Experiment 2 Effects of Radix Aconiti Lateralis Preparata on hemodynamic changes in anaesthetized open-chest dogs in vivo

【**Purpose**】Study the hemodynamic method of heart and observe the effects of Radix Aconiti Lateralis Preparata on hemodynamic changes in anaesthetized open-chest dogs in vivo.

【**Principles**】Radix Aconiti Lateralis Preparata has the effect of restoring yang and rescuing collapse. It has the effect on strengthening heart, boosting pressure, improving microcirculation and anti-shock. Effects of Radix Aconiti Lateralis Preparata on cardiac function and peripheral resistance are observed through hemodynamics indices in experiment.

【**Equipments**】MFV-3000 electromagnetic flow meter (Japan Nihon Kohden), BL-420 biological function experimental system and Pressure transducer and HX-300 ventilator (Chengdu Taimeng technology limited liability company), surgical scissors, surgical scalpel, homeostatic forceps, eye scissors, ophthalmology forceps, three-channel switch of plastic, needle electrode, trachea cannula, arterial cannula, venous cannula, clip, syringe.

【**reagents**】Radix Aconiti Lateralis Preparata injection 3 g/mL, demethylcoclaurine 0.05 mg/mL, normal saline, heparin solution 500 U/mL, pentobarbital sodium solution 3 g/dL.

【**Animals**】dog, >12 kg, sexuality not limited

【**Methods**】

1. Anesthesia The dog is weighed, 3% pentobarbital sodium (30 mg/1 mL/kg) is intravenously injected into the vein in the forelimb to anesthetize animal. Then it is fixed on back position on the operation table. Subsequently, needle electrodes are inserted into four limb hypodermically of the dog. The electrocardiogram (Ⅱ lead) is recorded to determine the heart rate (HR).

2. The procedure of operation

(1) Cut off the fur on the front of the neck and open the skin along the midline of cervical. The trachea is isolated and a trachea cannula is inserted into the trachea, then, connected with HX-300 ventilator (Tidal volume 130~160 mL, frequency 20 /min). Pull apart the skin and muscles above the trachea with homeostatic forceps, then, the left and right common carotid artery paralleling with the trachea can be seen on the both sides of the trachea. The left common carotid is separated and is inserted by arterial cannula full of heparin saline (500 U/mL) The arterial cannula is connected with pressure transducer linking

BL-420 biological function experimental system. Systolic pressure (SAP), diastolic pressure (DAP) and mean arterial blood pressure (MAP, diastolic pressure adds one third of pulse pressure) of common carotid are recorded. The right common carotid is separated, then, the right arterial cannula is inserted into the left ventricle. The right arterial cannula is connected with pressure transducer linking BL-420 biological function experimental system. The left ventricular systolic pressure (LVSP), left ventricular end-diastolic pressure (LVEDP), left ventricular pressure maximal rate of rise and fall (LV$dp/dt_{max}$) are recorded.

(2) Skin is cut off on the left side of the forth rib. Intercostal muscles are separated and then chest is opened. The heart is exposed and cardiac pericardium is opened to make a bassinet of arculacordis. The root of ascending aorta and the left descending coronary artery are separated. Appropriate detectors of MFV-3000 electromagnetic flow meter with internal diameter at 12 mm or 2 mm are set respectively, and then the cardiac output (CO) and coronary blood flow (CBF) are determined.

(3) One side of groin, find the pulse position of femoral artery with fingers and cut off the fur on that position. A longitudinal incision of 3~4 cm is made by surgical scalpel. Subcutaneous tissue is separated with homeostatic forceps. The neurovascular bundle encysted can be exposed. Femoral vein is isolated, A vein cannula is inserted. 500 U/(mL · kg) heparin sodium is injected into femoral vein for anticoagulation.

3. Measurement of each index

(1) After the surgery, stability for 30 min, then, the indexes including HR, SAP, DAP, MAP, LVSP, LVEDP, $\pm dp/dt_{max}$, CO and CBF are determined.

(2) Radix Aconiti Lateralis Preparata injection 2 g/kg and demethylcoclaurine 5 μg/kg are injected into femoral vein, respectively. Then, the above indicators of two dogs are observed.

【Results】

1. The cardiac index (CI) and total peripheral vascular resistance (TPVR) are calculated according to the following equation.

$$\text{Body surface area (BSA, m}^2\text{)} = 0.11 \times (\text{weight, kg})^{2/3}$$

$$\text{Total peripheral vascular resistance [TPVR, (kPa·s) /L]} = \text{MAP (kPa)} \times 60/\text{CO}$$

2. The experimental data are collected and filled into the following table.

Table 11-1　Effects of Radix Aconiti Lateralis Preparata and demethylcoclaurine on hemodynamic changes in anaesthetized dogs *in vivo*.

index	Radix Aconiti Lateralis Preparata		Demethylcoclaurine	
	Pre-administration	Post-administration	Pre-administration	Post-administration
HR (bpm)				
SAP (kPa)				
DAP (kPa)				

(Continued)

index	Radix Aconiti Lateralis Preparata		Demethylcoclaurine	
	Pre-administration	Post-administration	Pre-administration	Post-administration
MAP (kPa)				
CO (L/min)				
CBF (L/min)				
LVSP (kPa)				
LVEDP (kPa)				
$+dp/dt_{max}$ (kPa/s)				
$-dp/dt_{max}$ (kPa/s)				
CI [L/(min · m^2)]				
TPVR [(kPa · s)/L]				

【Notes】

1. Arterial cannula should be filled with heparin sodium solution for anticoagulation. If bleeding blot can be seen, the little blood vessel should be ligated during experiment. Otherwise, experimental result will be affected by bleeding induced by heparinization.

2. Electromagnetic flow meter detector should be suitable and tough blood vessel tightly. External diameter of blood vessel should be determined in order to choose appropriate detector. The detector is used whose external diameter is 10%~15% little than blood vessel.

3. The tubing system for pressure record should not have any bubble, for the wave form of blood pressure and left ventricular pressure can be influenced by little air bubble.

4. Electromagnetic flow meter detector dip in normal saline for at least 30 min but new detector dip in normal saline for 2 h. Then, such detectors have good conductibility.

5. When the left ventricular cannula is difficult to enter left ventriculus at the entrance of aortic valves, we can drop out the cannula slightly, change angle and direction, or twitter the cannula and propel it toward to fluently insert the cannula into left ventricle.

【Questions】How to explain the effect of Radix Aconiti Lateralis Preparata on restoring yang and rescuing collapse and the treatment of yang collapse and yang deficiency syndromes according to its effect on hemodynamic changes in anaesthetized open-chest dogs in vivo?

实验三　附子多糖对缺氧-复氧心肌细胞的保护作用

【目的】学习细胞培养和采用MTT法测定细胞活力方法，观察附子多糖对缺氧-复氧心肌细胞的保护作用。

【原理】原有缺血部位恢复血流后，组织损伤反而加重，即缺血再灌注损伤。缺血再灌注造成心肌细胞损伤并导致疾病发生。建立体外缺氧/复氧模型，以模拟在体心肌细胞缺血再灌注损伤。活细胞线粒体中的琥珀酸脱氢酶能使外源性MTT形成蓝紫色结晶甲瓒，二甲基亚砜能溶解甲瓒，在490 nm处测定吸光值能反映细胞活力。附子多糖具有一个半缩醛羟基，能清除自由基，对处于氧化应激状态的细胞具有保护作用。本实验利用MTT法测定附子多糖对缺氧-复氧心肌细胞活力的影响。

【器材】移液枪；无菌超净台；细胞培养箱；全波长酶标仪；96孔板；75 cm^2 细胞瓶。

【试剂】附子多糖；0.25%胰蛋白酶；DMEM培养基；胎牛血清；青霉素；链霉素；3-(4，5-二甲基噻唑-2)-2，5-二苯基四氮唑溴盐(MTT)；振荡器。

【细胞】大鼠心肌细胞株H9C2。

【方法】

1. 细胞贴壁长成致密单层后，吸除培养液。向瓶内加入2 mL的0.25%胰蛋白酶，于显微镜下观察，发现细胞皱缩变圆，轻轻摇动培养瓶，直到细胞脱落，再加2 mL含10%胎牛血清的DMEM以终止胰酶反应。1 000 rpm离心5 min后重悬细胞，细胞悬液接种于96孔板(1×10^4 cell/well)中预培养24 h。

2. 实验分组　正常组在含10%胎牛血清的DMEM培养基中于5% CO_2，95%空气的培养箱中静置培养。模型组在无血清DMEM培养基中，置于37 ℃三气培养箱中低氧(5% CO_2, 2% O_2, 93% N_2)培养。附子多糖组处理同模型组，但提前0.5 h加入0.1 g/L、1 g/L、10 g/L的附子多糖。

3. 模型组和附子多糖组低氧培养4 h后，置于37 ℃，含5% CO_2，95%空气的培养箱中静置培养4 h，以完成缺氧/复氧损伤。然后各组加入0.02 mL MTT(5 mg/mL)，37 ℃下继续孵育4 h后，弃上清，加入DMSO，选择490 nm波长，在酶标仪上测定各孔光吸收值(OD值)。

【结果】将结果填入表11-2中。

表 11-2　附子多糖对缺氧 - 复氧心肌细胞的保护作用

分组	浓度(g/L)	OD_{490} 值
正常组		
模型组		
附子多糖组	0.1	
	1	
	10	

【注意事项】

1. 接板时注意控制好胰酶消化时间。
2. 接板后注意摇匀细胞,以防分布不均。
3. MTT 的配制和保存注意避光。

【思考题】

1. MTT 法测定细胞活力的原理是什么?
2. 附子多糖保护缺血再灌注心肌细胞的机制是什么?

Experiment 3　Protective effect of monkshood polysaccharide on myocardial cells against hypoxia-reoxygenation-induced injury

【**Purpose**】To learn the methods of cell culture and determination with cell viability by MTT method; Study the protective effect of monkshood polysaccharide on hypoxia-reoxygenation -induced myocardial cells injury.

【**Principles**】When original ischemia part restore blood flow, tissue damage become heavier, which is called ischemia-reperfusion injury. Ischemia-reperfusion injury may cause many diseases. Myocardial cell model of hypoxia-reoxygenation injury was established to simulate myocardial ischemia-reperfusion injury in vivo. Mitochondria of living cells can exogenous succinate dehydrogenase to make MTT form crystal violet formazan. Dimethyl sulfoxidecan can dissolve formazan and the dissolved formazan is measured at 490 nm. The absorbance values reflect the cell viability. Monkshood polysaccharide with a hemiacetal hydroxyl can remove free radicals and play a protective effect on the oxidative stress in cells. Effects of monkshood polysaccharide on hypoxia-reoxygenation-induced myocardial cells injury are observed by MTT method.

【**Equipment**】pipettes, aseptic clean bench, incubator, Thermo Scientific Varioskan Flash, 96-well plates, 75 cm^2 flasks.

【**Reagents**】monkshood polysaccharide, 0.25%trypsin, DMEM medium, fetal bovine serum, penicillin, streptomycin, 3-(4,5-dimethyl-2)-2,5-diphenyltetrazolium bromide, oscillator.

【**Cell**】rat cardiomyoblasts line H9C2.

【**Methods**】

1. Discard the old medium when cells grow into a dense monolayer. Added 2 mL of 0.25% trypsin and observe the flask under microscope. When cell shrinkage round, and the flask is gently shaken until desquamated cells is observed. Then, add DMEM 2 mL containing 10% fetal bovine serum to terminate the pancreatic enzyme reaction. The cells are collected after centrifugated at 1,000 rpm for 5 min, seeded in 96-well plate (1×10^4 cell / well) and cultured for 24 h.

2. Experiment groups　Normal group in DMEM medium containing 10% fetal bovine serum is cultured in incubator (5% CO_2, 95% air). Model group in serum-free DMEM medium is cultured in incubator (5% CO_2, 2% O_2, 93% N_2). To monkshood polysaccharide group, cells are incubated with monkshood polysaccharide (0.1, 1, 10 g/ L) for 0.5 h, then,

they are treated as the model group.

3. After 4 h treatment, model group and monkshood polysaccharide group are incubated in 37 ℃, 5% CO_2, 95% air incubator for another 4 h treatment. Then, all groups are added 0.02 mL MTT (5 mg/mL) and incubated at 37 ℃ for 4 h. The supernatant is removed, and DMSO is added to dissolve the formazan crystals. The optical absorbance was measured at 490 nm.

【Result】

Table 11-2 Protective effect of monkshood polysaccharide on hypoxia-reoxygenation-induced myocardial cells injury

Groups	Concentration (g/L)	OD_{490}
Normal		
Control		
monkshood polysaccharide	0.1	
	1	
	10	

【Notes】

1. Take attention to the trypsin digestion time when seeding.
2. Shake the plate to assure equidistribution.
3. Prepare MTT solution in the dark.

【Questions】

1. What is the mechanism of MTT cell viability assay?
2. What is the mechanism of protective effect of monkshood polysaccharide on hypoxia-reoxygenation-induced myocardial cells injury?

第十二章　理气药实验

理气药是一类具有疏通气机，调整脏腑功能，消除气滞、气逆为主要作用的药物。理气药具有行气止痛、疏肝、降逆平喘等功效，主要用于气滞和气逆证。现代药理学研究表明，这类药物主要药理作用为：①对消化系统的影响：调节胃肠运动，调节消化液分泌、利胆。②对支气管平滑肌的影响：多数理气药具有松弛支气管平滑肌作用。③调节子宫平滑肌作用。④对心血管系统的作用：枳实注射液能明显升高麻醉犬的血压；青皮对多种实验性休克有治疗作用，使休克状态的低血压迅速回升；枳实、枳壳等具有强心作用。以上作用在灌胃给药时均不能呈现。

理气药调节胃肠运动的常用实验方法为：离体标本实验法、在体实验法及胃肠推进运动实验法。

（1）离体标本实验法：一般选用家兔、豚鼠及大鼠的肠管、胃、胆囊等器官进行，用换能器记录平滑肌的舒缩运动和张力变化。

（2）在体实验法：一般用麻醉犬或家兔，打开腹腔直接观察肠管，胆囊及子宫的舒缩活动。

（3）胃肠推进运动实验法：一般用小鼠，灌胃给药后，观察炭末（或墨汁）在小肠的推进率。

本章主要介绍理气药对离体肠管、胆汁分泌、实验性胃溃疡、疼痛、失血性休克低血压的影响。

Chapter 12 Experiments of drugs for rectifying Qi

Drugs for rectifying qi have the effect of dredging qi dynamic, regulating bowels and viscera, eliminating Qi stagnation and counter flow. These drugs possess the effects on moving Qi to alleviate pain, regulating the liver, down bearing Qi and calming panting etc. They are mostly used to treat Qi stagnation and counter flow. Modern pharmacological studies suggest that the drugs have following pharmacological actions: ① Effects on digestive system, including regulating gastrointestinal function and digestive juice secretion as well as cholagogue. ② Most of the drugs can loosen tracheal smooth muscle. ③ Regulating uterus smooth muscles. ④ Effects on cardiovascular system: Fructus Aurantii Immaturus injection can significantly increase blood pressure in anaesthetized dog. Pericarpium Citri Reticulatae Viridie can prevent experimental shock and increase blood pressure in shock model. Fructus Aurantii Immaturus and Fructus Aurantii possess cardiotonic effect. However, cardiovascular effect of those drugs can't be observed by oral administration.

There are many methods applied to measure the effects of drugs for rectifying qi on the function of the gastrointestinal smooth muscles such as experimental methods of isolated specimens, in vivo experimentation and gastrointestinal propulsive motility experiment.

(1) Experimental methods of isolated specimens are usually researched in organs such as intestinal canal, stomach and gallbladder of rabbit, guinea pig and rat. Movement and tension of smooth muscle are recorded by transducer.

(2) Experimental methods in vivo are usually researched in anaesthetized dog or rabbit, whose abdominal cavity is opened and movements of intestines, gallbladder and uterus are observed.

(3) Mice are given traditional Chinese medicine (TCM) by oral administration, then the propelling rates of the charcoal powder in the small intestine are determined to observe the effect of TCM on gastrointestinal movements.

In this chapter, TCM are investigated by observing the effects on the isolated intestine, bile secretion, experimental gastric ulcer, pain and hypotension induced by hemorrhage shock.

实验一　青皮、枳壳、四逆散对豚鼠离体肠平滑肌的影响

【目的】学习温血动物离体器官的实验方法；观察青皮、枳壳和四逆散对离体平滑肌的影响。

【原理】动物的离体消化道平滑肌在接近于在体情况的适宜环境下，具有自发性运动机能。化学物质 Ach 和组胺均可引起平滑肌收缩。青皮有疏肝破气，消积化滞之功；枳壳有理气宽中行气消胀之力；四逆散能疏肝理气，调和肝脾。三者对肠平滑肌均有明显的解痉作用，均能拮抗 Ach 和组胺所致的平滑肌收缩。

【器材】BL-420 生物机能实验系统；HW-400S 恒温平滑肌槽；张力换能器；氧气发生器；哺乳动物手术器械；注射器（1 mL）；烧杯；移液枪；表面皿；缝针；棉线。

【试剂】青皮水煎液 1 g/mL；枳壳水煎液 1 g/mL；四逆散水煎液 1 g/mL（枳实、芍药、柴胡、炙甘草各 5 g，共煎成 20 mL）；pH 均为 6 左右。10^{-4} 乙酰胆碱溶液（g/mL）；10^{-4} 组胺溶液（g/mL）；台氏液等。

【动物】豚鼠 1 只，体重 200~300 g，雌雄不限，空腹 6 小时以上。

【方法】

1. 调节恒温平滑肌槽，浴槽内的台氏液保持 37.0 ± 0.5 ℃。

2. 取豚鼠一只，猛击头部使其昏迷后，立即剖开腹腔，找到盲肠与回肠交界处，结扎，取回肠，置于室温、已饱和的冷台氏液中，沿肠壁分离肠系膜，用台氏液将肠内容物冲洗干净，将肠管剪成约 1.5~2 cm 的肠段，肠管两端从里向外各穿 1 线，将肠段固定于恒温平滑肌槽中，上端接肌张力换能器，负荷约 2 g。恒温平滑肌槽中加入 20 mL 的预温的台氏液，氧气调节流速为每秒出现 1~2 个气泡。用 BL-420 生物机能实验系统记录肠肌张力变化。一般经平衡 15 min 以上，待基线平稳后，即可进行下列实验：

（1）在浴槽中加入青皮水煎液 0.2 mL，观察 10 min，并记录其作用曲线。

（2）更换浴槽中台氏液 3 次，待基线稳定后，加入 10^{-4} 乙酰胆碱溶液 0.1 mL，当肠肌收缩显著时，即加入青皮水煎液 0.1~0.2 mL，观察 10 min，并记录其作用曲线。

（3）更换浴槽中台氏液 3 次，待基线稳定后，加入 10^{-4} 组胺溶液 0.1 mL，当肠肌收缩显著时，即加入青皮水煎液 0.1~0.2 mL，观察 10 min，并记录其作用曲线。

（4）取另一肠段，按以上（1）~（3）顺序，观察枳壳及四逆散水煎液对离体肠肌的作用。

【结果】复制青皮、枳壳及四逆散水煎液对离体肠平滑肌的作用曲线，注明药物和剂量。

【注意事项】

1. 回肠位于小肠末端，平滑肌层较薄，自律性较低，越靠近回盲部自律性越低，基线越平稳。

2. 剪取肠管及冲洗，固定肠管等操作必须轻柔，尽可能不用金属及手指触及。
3. 肠管两端穿线时切勿将肠腔扎闭，否则会影响药物的作用强度。
4. 加药前必须准备好更换用的 37 ℃台氏液。
5. 实验中始终要通入 O_2，气泡量不要太多，以每秒 1~2 个为宜。

【思考题】

1. 通过青皮、枳壳及四逆散对离体小肠平滑肌的影响，分析中药的理气作用。
2. 为何选择豚鼠进行离体肠肌实验？

Experiment 1 Effects of Pericarpium Citri Reticulatae Viride, Fructus Aurantii and Si-Ni-San on isolated intestinal smooth muscle of Guinea pig

【Purpose】

1. To learn the experiment methods of organ of warm-blood animal in vitro.

2. To observe effects of Pericarpium Citri Reticulatae Viride, Fructus Aurantii and Si-Ni-San on isolated ileum of Guinea pig.

【Principles】 Under the suitable conditions, isolated intestinal smooth muscles of many animals can keep the spontaneous moving functions. The contractile response of intestinal smooth muscles is induced by acetylchloride and histamine respectively. Citri reticulatae Pericarpium viride has the effects on coursing the liver and breaking qi, dispersing food and transforming stagnation. Fructus Aurantii has the effects on rectifying qi and loosening the center, moving qi and dispersing distention. Si-Ni-San has the actions on coursing the liver and rectifying qi, harmonizing spleen-stomach. The three drugs possess the evident spasmolytic effect and they all could inhibit the contraction induced by acetylchloride and histamine.

【Equipments】 BL-420 biological function system, HW-400S constant temperature smooth muscle trough, tension transducer, oxygen generator, operating instruments of mammalian, syringe（1 mL）, beaker, pipette, bath dish, needle, silk thread.

【Reagents】 Aqueous extract of Pericarpium Citri Reticulatae Viride 1 g/mL, aqueous extract of Fructus Aurantii 1 g/mL, aqueous extract of Si-Ni-San 1 g/mL（Fructus Aurantii Immaturus 5 g, Paeoniae Radix 5 g, Bupleuri Radix 5 g, and Honey-Fried Licorice 5 g are decocted together into 20 mL.）, The pH of above aqueous extracts are around 6. acetylcholine solution 10^{-4} g/mL, histamine solution 10^{-4} g/mL, Tyrode's solution.

【Animals】 Guinea pig, 200~300 g, male or female, fasting for more than 6 h.

【Methods】

1. Constant temperature smooth muscle trough is adjusted to make the temperature of Tyrode's solution at 37.0 ± 0.5 ℃.

2. Beat the head with a mallet to make Guinea pig coma, then the abdominal cavity is opened. The end of ileum is ligated with a thread between cecum and ileum. Ileum is taken and put into Tyrode's solution saturated with O_2 in room temperature. Ileum is isolated along mesenterium and washed with Tyrode's solution to get rid of intestinal materials. The length

of ileum piece should be 1.5~2 cm. Attach a thread to each end by inserting a needle from inside to outside. Inferior thread is fixed in the bottom of the organ bath and superior thread is connected with the tension transducer with load about 2 g. 20 mL Tyrode's solution preheated is added to the bath tube. O_2 can be controlled at 1~2 bubbles per second. The tension and contraction of the ileum are recorded by BL-420 biological function system. A length of base line is recorded until the base line becomes steady. The procedure usually needs more than 15 minutes. Then the following orders are conducted.

(1) Add 0.2 mL aqueous extract of Pericarpium Citri Reticulatae Viride to the bath. The tension and contraction of the ileum piece are recorded for 10 min.

(2) Tyrode's solution is changed 3 times. Then, 0.1 mL acetylcholine solution is added to the bath when the base line becomes steady. When the ileum piece contracts obviously, 0.1 mL water extract of Pericarpium Citri Reticulatae Viride is added to the bath. The tension and contraction of the ileum piece are recorded for 10 min.

(3) Tyrode's solution is changed 3 times. Then, 0.1 mL histamine solution is added to the bath when the base line becomes steady. When the ileum piece contracts obviously, 0.1 mL aqueous extract of Pericarpium Citri Reticulatae Viride is added to the bath. The tension and contraction of the ileum piece are recorded for 10 min.

(4) Effects of Fructus Aurantii and Si-Ni-San on isolated ileum of Guinea pig are observed respectively by another piece of the ileum according to the above procedure.

【Results】Trace and copy the curve of Pericarpium Citri Reticulatae Viride, Fructus Aurantii and Si-Ni-San on isolated ileum of Guinea pig. Those should be indicated the drug and dosage.

【Notes】

1. The ileum is located in the distal end of intestine. Smooth muscular layer of the ileum is thin. It has relatively low autorhytmicity. The closer it approaches the ileocecal position, the lower its autorhythmicity is, and the steadier the base line is.

2. The ileum should be cut, washed and fixed lightly and should not be touched with metal or the finger.

3. Don't seal the ileum lumen when its both sides are ligated. Otherwise, the effect of the drugs will be influenced.

4. Tyrode's solution with 37 ℃ should be prepared for exchange before adding drugs.

5. O_2 should be added during the whole experiment and be controlled at 1~2 bubbles per second.

【Questions】

1. How to explain the effect of rectifying qi on TCM according to the effect of Pericarpium Citri Reticulatae Viride, Fructus Aurantii and Si-Ni-San on isolated ileum of Guinea pig?

2. Why choose Guinea pig in the isolated intestinal muscle experiment in vitro?

实验二　茵陈蒿汤对大鼠胆汁分泌的影响

【目的】学习测定大鼠胆汁分泌量的实验方法；观察茵陈蒿汤对大鼠胆汁分泌的影响。

【原理】胆汁由肝细胞分泌后储存于胆囊中，经胆总管流入十二指肠。胆汁的分泌排泄与消化功能以及黄疸的形成有密切关系。茵陈蒿汤是治疗湿热黄胆证的经典方剂，其作用机制与促进胆汁的排泄功能有关。大鼠为无胆囊动物，对大鼠进行胆管插管，可以动态观察茵陈蒿汤对胆汁分泌的影响。

【器材】注射器；细塑料管（直径为 1~2 mm）；手术剪；眼科镊；止血钳；手术刀；大鼠手术台；移液枪；离心管（2 mL）；缝线；眼科剪。

【试剂】茵陈蒿汤水煎剂 2 g/mL（茵陈 18 g，栀子 12 g，大黄 6 g）；3% 去氢胆酸；3% 戊巴比妥钠溶液。

【动物】大鼠 3 只，体重 300 g 左右，雌雄不限。

【方法】

1. 大鼠禁食、不禁水 12 h，称重后分为三组。

2. 实验前每组大鼠腹腔注射戊巴比妥钠液 30 mg/kg，麻醉后仰位固定，沿腹正中线切开约 2 cm，打开腹腔，以胃幽门为标准，翻转引出十二指肠，从乳头部追踪胆总管。在乳头部上方 3~5 mm 处，用镊子将覆盖在上面的被膜连续剥离 5~10 mm，暴露胆总管。

3. 在胆总管的乳头侧及其上方，穿过 2 根细线备用。将靠近乳头部的细线牢固结扎，用眼科剪在胆管上向肝脏方向作 V 形切口，插入细塑料管，即可见有淡黄色胆汁流出，结扎固定细塑料管，用塑料离心管收集胆汁，手术后用止血钳夹闭腹壁。

4. 待稳定 20 min 后，先收集 30 min 胆汁，作为给药前胆汁分泌的正常值。

5. 甲组大鼠由十二指肠注入茵陈蒿汤水煎剂 0.5 mL/100 g，乙组由十二指肠注入等体积的生理盐水，丙组由十二指肠注入去氢胆酸液 0.5 mL/100 g。给药后每隔 30 min 收集胆汁一次，共 4 次，分别记录胆汁流量，与给药前作自身对照，并按下列公式计算胆汁分泌百分率。

$$\text{胆汁分泌百分率}=\frac{\text{给药后胆汁分泌量（mL/30 min）}}{\text{给药前胆汁分泌量（mL/30 min）}}\times 100\%$$

【结果】将实验数据填入表 12-1、表 12-2 中，汇集全班数据进行比较。

表 12–1　茵陈蒿汤对大鼠胆汁分泌的影响

组别	剂量（g/kg）	胆汁流量（μL）				
		给药前 30 min	给药后（min）			
			0~30	30~60	60~90	90~120
生理盐水						
茵陈蒿汤						
去氢胆酸						

表 12–2　茵陈蒿汤对大鼠胆汁分泌的影响

组别	剂量（g/kg）	给药后胆汁分泌百分率（%）			
		0~30 min	30~60 min	60~90 min	90~120 min
生理盐水					
茵陈蒿汤					
去氢胆酸					

【注意】

1. 手术时，创口要小并切勿损伤肝脏及十二指肠。
2. V 形切口时，勿将胆管切断，并应保持插管通畅。
3. 动物要注意保温，尤其在冬季更应注意。
4. 药物要预热到 38 ℃才可给药。

【思考题】

1. 通过茵陈蒿汤对胆汁分泌的影响，分析中药的理气作用和利湿退黄作用。
2. 为何选择大鼠进行利胆实验？

Experiment 2 Effects of Capillaris decoction on the bile excretion in rats

【**Purpose**】1. To learn the method of detecting quantity of the excreted bile of rat. 2. To investigate the cholagogic effect of Capillaris decoction.

【**Principles**】The bile is secreted by the hepatocyte and stored in the cholecyst. The bile passes through general bile duct and then runs into the dodecadactylon. The excretion of bile has close relation with digestive function and aurigo formation. Capillaris decoction is classical prescription to cure the syndrome of damp-heat and aurigo. Such effect is related to promoting the secretion of bile. Rats have no cholecyst. Effects of Capillaris decoction on the excretion of bile can be observed dynamically by the intubation of bile duct in the rat.

【**Equipments**】syringes, slim plastic tube (diameter 1~2 mm), surgical scissors, eye forceps, homeostatic forceps, surgery knife, operating table of rat, pipe (1 mL), centrifugal tubes (2 mL), silk thread and ophthalmology scissors.

【**Reagents**】aqueous extract of Capillaris decoction 2 g/mL (Artemisiae Capillaries Herba 18 g, Gardeniae Fructus 12 g, Rhei Rhizoma 6 g), 3%dehydrocholic acid. 3% pentobarbital sodium, normal saline.

【**Animals**】Rats, weight about 300 g, male or female.

【**Methods**】

1. 12 h-fasted rats are weighed and divided into three groups randomly.

2. The rats are anesthetized by intraperitoneal injection of 3% pentobarbital sodium with dosage of 30 mg/kg, then, they were fixed supinely. Cut off the fur along the midline on the abdomen and incise the skin and peritoneum about 2 cm. The pylorus are taken as standard, the duodenum are turned over, and the papilla of dodecadactylon will be seen so that the general bile duct can be tracked from the papilla. About 3~5 mm above the papilla, strip the capsule covering on the papilla with the forceps for about 5~10 mm continuously to expose the common bile duct completely.

3. 2 silk threads were put through the end of the bile duct near the papilla and the above. The thread was knotted firmly near papilla. A reversed "V" shaped incision is sheared with ophthalmology scissor on the bile, the polyethylene plastic tube is inserted from the notch to the liver and the tube is fixed with the thread prepared. The bile flow out from the tube and the centrifugal tubes are used to collect bile. At last, abdominal cavity is temporarily closed with hemostatic forceps.

4. The bile flow out 20 min, then it was collected for 30 min, the volume was calculated and taken as the basal secretion of bile before administration.

5. Aqueous extract of Capillaris decoction (1 mL/100 g) was given to each rat in group1 from duodenum, saline (1 mL/100 g) was given to each rat in group2 from duodenum, 3% dehydrocholic acid (1 mL/100 g) was given to each rat in group3 from duodenum. The bile is collected four times every 30 min, then, the data post-administration is compared with that pre-administration.

Percentage of bile secretion = bile excretion in 30min post-administration/bile excretion in 30min pre-administration × 100%

【Results】 The bile secretion percentage according to the above equation is calculated and the experimental data of all the class are collected and filled into the table 12-1 and table 12-2.

Table 12–1 Effects of Capillaris decoction on the bile excretion in the rat

Groups	Dose (g/kg)	Bile excretion (μL/30 min)				
		Pre-administration	Post-administration (min)			
		30 min	0~30	30~60	60~90	90~120
Normal saline						
Capillaris decoction						
Dehydrocholic acid						

Table 12–2 Effects of Capillaris decoction on the bile excretion in the rat

Groups	Dose (g/kg)	Percentage of bile secretion after administration (%)			
		0~30 min	30~60 min	60~90 min	90~120 min
Normal saline					
Capillaris Decoction					
Dehydrocholic acid					

【Notes】

1. The wound should be as small as possible and be careful not to damage liver and duodenum in the operation.

2. "V" shaped incision is sheared on the bile, but the bile should not be cut off. Furthermore, it should not be jammed.

3. Keep the animals warm, especially in winter.

4. The drug should not be used until it is warmed to 38 ℃.

【Questions】

1. How to explain the effect of rectifying Qi, disinhibiting dampness and abating jaundice on Traditional Chinese medicine according to the effect of Capillaris decoction on bile excretion in rat?

2. Why choose rats in the cholagogic experiment?

实验三 延胡索抗大鼠实验性胃溃疡的作用(应激反应法)

【目的】学习应激性胃溃疡的实验方法;观察延胡索总碱抗大鼠应激性胃溃疡的作用。

【原理】大鼠受到应激刺激后,交感神经系统兴奋性升高,血管收缩,引起黏膜缺血、缺氧、抵抗力下降。副交感神经 - 垂体 - 肾上腺系统兴奋性升高,胃酸、胃蛋白酶和胃泌素分泌增加,从而引起应激性溃疡。延胡索所含生物碱具有镇静,扩张血管,促进血液循环,提高机体对缺氧的耐受能力;同时,能降低胃酸酸度,抑制胃蛋白酶活性等作用。因此,延胡索具有抗大鼠应激性胃溃疡的效能。

【器材】恒温水浴装置;大鼠手术台;天平;手术剪;大镊子;注射器;烧杯;透明尺;钟罩;眼科镊。

【试剂】延胡索总碱溶液 8 mg/mL;乙醚;1% 甲醛溶液(V/V)。

【动物】大鼠 150~180 g, 雌雄不限。

【方法】

1. 取 2 只大鼠,禁食、不禁水,24 h 后用乙醚轻度麻醉,四肢仰卧位固定在大鼠手术台上。

2. 甲鼠肌注延胡索总碱 80 mg/kg,乙鼠肌注生理盐水 10 mL/kg。于给药后 30 min 将固定好的大鼠直立浸于 20 ℃的恒温水槽内,水面以齐剑突为宜。

3. 水浸应激 18 h 后,颈椎脱臼法处死大鼠,打开腹腔。结扎幽门及贲门后取胃,每胃由腺胃部注入 6 mL 生理盐水,将其放入 1% 甲醛溶液中固定 10 min 后,沿胃大弯剪开,检查溃疡病变。应激性溃疡在腺胃部沿血管走行分布,表面覆盖凝血。擦去凝血,可见深褐色条索状溃疡。以溃疡长度总和的毫米数作为胃溃疡指数,并计算溃疡抑制率。

$$\text{溃疡抑制率}=\frac{\text{对照组溃疡长度总和}-\text{实验组溃疡长度总和}}{\text{对照组溃疡长度总和}}\times 100\%$$

【结果】将实验数据填入表 12-3,汇集全班数据进行统计学比较。

表 12-3 延胡索总碱对大鼠应激性溃疡的作用

组别	剂量(mg/kg)	动物数	溃疡指数(mm)	抑制率(%)
生理盐水				
延胡索总碱	80			

【思考题】

1. 延胡索所含生物碱有哪些药理作用?

2. 延胡索总碱抗应激性胃溃疡的作用机制是什么?

Experiment 3 Effects of Corydalis on experimental gastric ulcer in rat (stress ulcer)

【Purpose】Study the method of stress ulcer in stomach induced by water immersion-restraint stress; Observe the effect of Corydalis on preventing stress ulcer.

【Principles】When the rats are received stress stimulation, excitability of sympathetic nervous system increases and blood vessel contracts, then the gastric mucosa is short of blood and oxygen, resistibility decreases. Excitability of parasympathetic nerve-hypophysis-adrenal gland system increases, then the volume of gastric juice, the acidity of gastric juice, and the pepsin activity increase which result in stress ulcer. Corydalis contains alkaloids which not only have the effect on sedation, dilatation of blood vessels, facilitating blood circulation and increasing the endurable ability to oxygen deficiency, but also demonstrates the ability to attenuate the acidity of gastric juice and the activity of pepsin. So Corydalis can be sued for the prevention and treatment of gastric ulcer.

【Equipments】homeothermic water bath, steel fixing board of rats, operating table of rat, balance, operating scissor, forceps, syringe（1 mL）, beaker, transparent ruler, bell glass, ophthalmology forceps.

【Reagents】total alkaloids from Corydalis 8 mg/mL, ether, normal saline, 1% formaldehyde solution（V/V）.

【Animals】rats, weight 150~180 g, male or female.

【Methods】

1. After fasting rat for 24 h, the rats are weighed and divided into two groups randomly. The rats are nartcotizednarcotized superficially with diethyl ether and fixed on the steel fixing board.

2. All rats are administered by intramuscular injection. Rat A was given total alkaloids from corydalis 80 mg/kg. Rat B was given saline 10 mL/kg. 30 min later, the rats fixed firmly are dipped in homeothermic water bath in 20 ℃. The water surface flushing with xiphoid is suitable.

3. 18 h later, the rats are killed with dislocation of cervical vertebra and their peritoneal cavity is opened. When pylorus and cardiacardio are ligated, then, stomach is taken out. 6 mL saline is injected into stomachus glandularis. Cut stomach along the big curvature and gastric ulcer is observed. Stress ulceration is distributed along the vascellum in stomachus glandularis, and the surface is coved by blood clotting. Erasing blood clotting, ulcer with puce

stria will be observed. The total length of ulcer is taken as ulcer index of gastric mucosa, and moreover, the inhibition of gastric ulcer is calculated according to the following formula.

$$\text{Inhibition rate} = (\text{total ulcer length of control group} - \text{total ulcer length of treating group}) / \text{total ulcer length of control group} \times 100\%$$

【Results】 The experimental data are collected and filled into the following table. The significance test among groups by *t*- test should be done.

Table 12–3 Effects of corydalis on gastric stress ulcer in rat.

Groups	Dose（mg/kg）	No. of mice	Ulcer index（mm）	Inhibition rate（%）
Normal saline				
Corydalis	80			

【Questions】

1. What are the pharmacological effects of total alkaloids from Corydalis?
2. What is the mechanism of anti-stress ulcer action of s total alkaloids from Corydalis?

实验四　延胡索对小鼠的镇痛作用(热板法)

【目的】了解用热板法筛选镇痛药的实验方法,观察延胡索的镇痛作用。

【原理】各种伤害如热刺激引起的疼痛性刺激通过感觉纤维传入脊髓,最后到达大脑皮层感觉区而引起疼痛。热板法是筛选镇痛药的经典方法:小鼠的足部受到刺激而产生疼痛时,就发生舔足的疼痛反应,以接触热板到舔足所需的时间作为痛阈值。延胡索能活血行气止痛,本实验以此为观测指标,观察延胡索对小鼠的镇痛作用。

【器材】热板测痛仪 GJ-8402 型;烧杯;秒表;天平;注射器(1 mL);针头;鼠笼。

【试剂】派替啶注射液 1 mg/mL;生理盐水;苦味酸;胡索水煎醇沉液 4 g/mL。

【动物】雌性小鼠 3~4 只,体重 18~22 g。

【方法】

1. 动物选择　调节热板温度至 55 ± 0.5 ℃,小鼠置于热板上。测定自放在热板上至出现舔后足或抬后足并回头的时间(s),作为该小鼠的正常痛阈值。每只小鼠测定 2 次,每次间隔 5 min,以平均值不超过 30 s 为合格,共选出 3 只小鼠。

2. 给药　取预选合格的小鼠 3 只,分别编号。甲鼠腹腔注射延胡索水煎醇沉液 0.2 mL/10 g,乙鼠腹腔注射派替啶注射液 0.2 mL/10 g,丙鼠腹腔注射生理盐水 0.2 mL/10 g。

3. 给药后的 15、30、45、60、90 min 分别测定各小鼠的痛阈值。若小鼠在热板上 60 s 无痛觉反应,应取出,按 60 s 计。将结果记入表内。

4. 按下列公式计算用药后不同时间点的痛阈提高百分率。

$$痛阈提高百分率=\frac{给药后痛阈值-给药前痛阈值}{给药前痛阈值}\times 100\%$$

(如用药后痛阈值减去用药前痛阈值为负数,则痛阈提高百分率以零计算)

【结果】将实验数据填入表 12-4,汇集全班数据进行比较。

表 12-4　延胡索对小白鼠的镇痛作用

组别	给药前痛阈值(s)	给药后痛阈值				痛阈提高百分率			
		15 min	30 min	45 min	60 min	15 min	30 min	45 min	60 min
生理盐水									
延胡索									
哌替啶									

【注意事项】

1. 室温以 15~20 ℃为宜，过低则小鼠反应迟钝，过高则过于敏感，而引起跳跃，影响实验的准确性。

2. 正常小鼠一般放在受热平板上 10~15 s 内出现不安、举前肢、舔前足、踢后肢、跳跃等现象，这些动作均不作为疼痛指标。

3. 一般不选用雄鼠，因雄鼠阴囊可触及热板，易呈现敏感反应，影响结果。

【思考题】

1. 试述延胡索的镇痛作用机制。

2. 热板法和小鼠甩尾法在对药物的敏感性与反应性质方面有何异同？

Experiment 4 Analgesic effect of Corydalis (the hot plate method)

【Purpose】To learn the hot plate method of screening analgesic drugs and observe the analgesic effect of corydalis.

【Principles】Various injuries such as ached stimulation caused by heat transmit into spinal cord through sensory nerve fiber, and then reach sensory area of cerebral cortex to produce pain. Hot plate method is canonical method of screening analgesic drugs. If the paws of mouse are stimulated with heating, the mouse immediately licks its hindpawshind paws as a response. The duration from touching the hot plate to licking hindpawshind paws is considered as the latent period of the pain threshold. Corydalis has the effect of quickening the blood, moving Qi and alleviating pain. In this experiment, analgesic effect of corydalis is observed by hot plate method.

【Equipments】electric hot plate (GJ-8402), beaker, stopwatch, balance, syringes (1 mL), pinhead, mouse cage.

【Reagents】pethidine injection 1 mg/mL, normal saline, picric acid, decoction of Corydalis refined by alcohol sedimentation 4 g/mL.

【Animals】3~4 female mice, 18~22 g.

【Methods】

1. Place the mouse on the hot plate heated to constant temperature of 55 ± 0.5 ℃ . Mouse is removed from the hot plate until it licks hindpawshind paws or raises hindpawshind paws and turns the head. The duration is the latent period of the pain threshold. Each mouse will be measured twice at an interval of 5 minutes. Select three mice each of whose mean threshold of the pain is shorter than 30 seconds.

2. All mice are administered by intraperitoneal injection.

Mouse A was given Corydalis decoction 0.2 mL/10 g.

Mouse B was given pethidine injection 0.2 mL/10 g.

Mouse C was given saline 0.2 mL/10 g.

3. Pain threshold is measured respectively at 15, 30, 45, 60 and 90 min post-administration according to the above method. The mice should be taken away from the hot plate immediately if they have no pain reaction after 60 s, and the pain threshold is recorded as 60 s.

4. The increased percent of pain threshold post-administration should be calculated according to the following equation.

The increment percentage of pain threshold=(post-treating pain threshold−pre-treating pain threshold)/ pre-treating pain threshold × 100%

(If post-treating pain threshold less than pre-treating pain threshold, the increased percent of pain threshold is recorded as zero.)

【Results】The experimental data are collected and filled into the following table.

Table 12–4 Effect of corydalis on the pain induced by hot plate in mice

Groups	pre-treating pain threshold(s)	post-treating pain threshold				the increment percentage of pain threshold			
		15 min	30 min	45 min	60 min	15 min	30 min	45 min	60 min
Normal saline									
corydalis liquor									
pethidine									

【Notes】

1. The room temperature will influence this experiment to some degree. The appropriate temperature is 15~20 ℃ . Mouse acts slowly at too low temperature. If the temperature is too high, mice get sensitively to jump. The accuracy of the result will be affected by the change of temperature.

2. Normal mice will show the activities of restlessness, raising forelimb, lamping forefoot, kicking hindlimb, jumping, within 10~15s after putting on the hot plate. Such reactions are not taken into consideration as pain reaction.

3. Male mouse is not suitable for this experiment, because the scrotum will droop when heated and the skin of scrotum is sensitive to pain, and thus influence the results.

【Questions】

1. How to expound the mechanism of analgesic effect of corydalis?

2. What are the similarities and differences between hot-plate test and the tail-flick in the evaluation of drug efficiency?

实验五　青皮、枳实对家兔血压的升压作用

【目的】观察青皮、枳实对家兔低血压状态的影响。

【原理】青皮可以兴奋α受体，枳实可以通过兴奋α，β受体而产生升高血压的作用。本实验以麻醉家兔的低血压状态为模型，观察青皮、枳实对家兔的升压作用。

【器材】BL-420生物机能系统；压力换能器；手术台；手术剪；眼科剪；眼科镊；止血钳；聚乙烯管（内径1 mm）；动脉插管；气管插管；注射器。

【试剂】1%戊巴比妥钠溶液；肝素钠注射液6 250 U/mL；生理盐水；青皮注射液（含生药4g/mL）；枳实注射液（含生药4 g/mL）。

【动物】家兔3只，2.2~2. 5 kg，雌雄不限。

【方法】

1. 麻醉　家兔3只称重后，分别耳缘静脉缓慢注射1%戊巴比妥钠溶液3 mL/kg，使之麻醉，待动物角膜反射消失后，将仰卧位固定于手术台上，打开手术台底面电灯保温。

2. 手术

（1）颈部：剪去颈部被毛，正中切开颈部皮肤5~7 cm，分离皮下组织，暴露胸骨舌骨肌，再用止血钳于正中线分开肌肉，分离气管，在气管上做一倒"T"形切口，插入气管插管，结扎固定。用止血钳拉开气管上方皮肤肌肉，即可在气管两侧见到与气管平行的左右颈总动脉。分离右侧颈总动脉，插入动脉插管（内充满肝素化生理盐水），以三通活塞连接BL-420生物机能系统上的压力换能器。

（2）腹股沟：在两侧的腹股沟部位，用手触得股动脉搏动处，剪去该部位的被毛，用手术刀纵切皮肤3~4 cm，用止血钳分离皮下结缔组织，再将耻骨和缝匠肌的焦点处分离，并将缝匠肌后部向外拉开，其下方可见筋膜包绕的神经血管束。分离一侧的股静脉，结扎远心端，向近心端插入静脉插管，用于注入500 U/（mL · kg）肝素以防止血液凝固。另一侧分离出股动脉，插入一根聚乙烯管用于放血。

3. 描记一段正常颈动脉血压曲线后，股动脉放血，使颈动脉血压持续稳定在6.67 kPa，持续30分钟。

4. 甲兔耳缘静脉注射生理盐水，乙兔耳缘静脉青皮注射液，丙兔耳缘静脉注射枳实注射液。观察给药后15、30、45、60 min血压的变化。

【结果】将实验数据填入下列表格，汇集全班数据进行比较。

表 12-5 青皮枳实对家兔低血压状态的影响

组别	给药后颈动脉收缩压(kPa)			
	15 min	30 min	45 min	60 min
生理盐水				
青皮				
枳实				

【注意事项】

1. 麻醉不可过深，以免血压过度降低。

2. 股动脉放血的速度不宜过快，如血压低于 6.67 kPa，可由股静脉缓慢回输少量血液，使血压稳定在 6.67 kPa 左右。血压不宜放得过低，否则易引起失血性休克并死亡。

3. 注意动脉插管和静脉头皮针内不要凝血。

4. 压力换能器的高度与心脏在同一水平为准。

5. 在实验过程中，需保持动脉插管与颈动脉平行，以免刺破动脉。

【思考题】试述青皮、枳实升压的药理学机制。

Experiment 5 Effects of Pericarpium Citri Reticulatae Viride and Fructus Aurantii Immaturus on hypotension induced by hemorrhage in rabbits

【Purpose】Effects of Pericarpium Citri Reticulatae Viride and Fructus Aurantii Immaturus on hypotension induced by hemorrhage in rabbits are observed

【Principles】Pericarpium Citri Reticulatae Viride can excite α adrenergic receptor. Fructus Aurantii Immaturus can excite α and β adrenergic receptor. So they can increase the blood pressure. Effects of Pericarpium Citri Reticulatae Viride and Fructus Aurantii Immaturus on hypotension induced by bloodletting in rabbits are observed.

【Equipments】BL-420 Biological function system, pressure transducer, operating table of rabbit, surgical scalpel, surgical scissors, eye scissors, ophthalmology forceps, homeostatic forceps, polyethylene tube (inner diameter 1mm), arterial cannula, trachea cannula, syringe (1 mL)

【Reagents】1% pentobarbital sodium solution, heparin sodium injection 6,250 U/mL normal saline, Pericarpium Citri Reticulatae Viride injection 0.15 g/mL, Fructus Aurantii Immaturus injection 0.15 g/mL.

【Animals】rabbit, 2.2~2.5 kg, sexuality not limited.

【Methods】

1. Anesthesia The rabbit is taken and weighed. 1% pentobarbital sodium (30 mg/kg) is slowly intravenously injected into ear vein for anesthetization. After confirming the disappearance of the corneal reflex, the animal is fixed its back on the operating table.

2. Operation

(1) Cut off the fur on the front of the neck and open the skin along the midline of cervical under the inferior border of larynx. Separate subcutaneous tissue with homeostatic forceps and expose the sternohyoid muscle. Separate the muscle in midline with homeostatic forceps, then expose trachea. The trachea is isolated and a trachea cannula is inserted into the trachea as well as tied firmly. Pull apart the skin and muscle above the trachea with homeostatic forceps, then, the left and right common carotid artery paralleling with the trachea can be seen on the both sides of the trachea. Right common carotid artery is isolated and an arterial cannula filled with 0.5% heparin saline is inserted. The arterial cannula is connected with pressure transducer linking BL-420 Biological function system.

(2) Groin: Both sides of groin, find the pulse position of femoral artery with fingers and

cut off the fur on that position. A longitudinal incision of 3~4 cm is made by surgical scalpel. Subcutaneous tissue is separated with homeostatic forceps. Secondly, Sartorius muscle and pectineus at their point of intersection are separated. Then the back of sartorius muscle is pulled outward, below which the neurovascular bundle encysted can be seen. Femoral vein is isolated in the one side of groin. A vein cannula is inserted. 500 U/(mL · kg) heparin sodium is injected into femoral vein for anticoagulation Femoral artery is isolated in another side of groin. A polyethylene tube is inserted into femoral artery for bloodletting.

3. Depict a segment of normal curve on blood pressure. After bloodletting from femoral artery, the blood pressure on carotid artery is constantly at 6.67 kpa.for 30 min.

4. Rabbit A is intravenously injected l saline 10 mL/kg. Rabbit B is intravenously injected Pericarpium Citri Reticulatae Viride injection 1.5 g/kg and 10 mL/kg. Rabbit C is intravenously injected Fructus Aurantii Immaturus injection 1.5 g/kg and 10 mL/kg. The blood pressure is observed four times every 15 min after administration.

【Results】The experimental data are collected and filled into the following table.

Table12-5 Effect of Pericarpium Citri Reticulatae Viride and Fructus Aurantii Immaturus on hypotension induced by hemorrhage in rabbits

Groups	Systolic pressure on carotid artery after administration (kPa)			
	15 min	30 min	45 min	60 min
Normal saline				
Pericarpium Citri Reticulatae Viride				
Fructus Aurantii Immaturus				

【Notes】

1. Do not anesthetize the rabbit too deep otherwise the blood pressure will decline excessively.

2. The speed of bloodletting from femoral artery should not be quickly. If blood pressure is under 6.67 kPa, some blood is slowly intravenously injected into the femoral vein to keep blood pressure stabilization. Blood pressure should not decline excessively by bloodletting, otherwise the animal will get hemorrhagic shock and die.

3. Pay attention to the arterial catheter and scalp needle, and do not let blood coagulate in them.

4. The height of the pressure transducer should be set at the same level with the rabbit heart.

5. The arterial cannula and the common carotid artery are kept in parallelism to avoid artery being cut in experiment.

【Questions】What is the mechanism of increasing blood pressure effect of Pericarpium Citri Reticulatae Viride and Fructus Aurantii Immaturus?

第十三章　活血化瘀药实验

活血化瘀药药理作用广泛，对机体的血液循环、免疫及神经系统等都有明显影响，相应的研究方法也很多。目前常采用血液流变学、血流动力学和微循环观察等方法研究活血化瘀药。

血液流变学是研究血液的流动性、凝固性、黏聚性和变形性的学科。它主要取决于血液的黏度，而影响血液黏滞性的重要因素是红细胞压积、红细胞黏附和聚集的程度、红细胞变形能力、血浆黏度、血管壁内面光滑度、管壁弹性、血液温度以及 pH 值等，其中红细胞的形态、容积对血液黏滞性有明显影响。血浆黏度是由所含的高分子量蛋白、脂蛋白和糖类决定的。所以在活血化瘀药的研究中，常通过测定全血黏度、血细胞压积、红细胞聚集、红细胞电泳时间、血细胞变形能力及黏度、血凝块与血栓弹性或表观黏度、血小板聚集、毛细管流动中逆转现象及临界半径、前列腺环素和血栓素比值等指标，观察活血化瘀药对血液流变学、血小板和血液凝固过程的影响。

心脏功能及血流动力学是研究循环药理的基本手段，也是活血化瘀药研究的重要部分。它主要包括对心率、血压、冠状动脉流量、心肌营养血流量、冠脉阻力及总外周阻力、左心室做功、肺动脉压、心输出量及心搏出量、左心室压与左室收缩性、心脏指数及心搏指数的测定。研究血流动力学的实验方法大致分为两种，即创伤性和非创伤性测定方法。创伤性测定方法是指对实验动物有创伤的实验方法，包括直接的血压测定、左室内压的测定、主动脉流量的测定、心肌营养血量的测定、心肌梗死面积的测定等。冠脉流量是研究活血化瘀药防治冠心病的重要指标。但增加冠脉流量的药物不一定都有抗心肌缺血作用，应以多种指标综合分析，才能获得较准确的结论。冠脉流量测定分两种，即整体冠脉流量测定和离体冠脉流量测定。心肌营养血流量测定通常利用同位素 86 铷（86Rb）测定小鼠心肌营养血流量，现已广泛用于心肌缺血药的初筛。另外用超声心动图、心音图、心电图、颈动脉及心尖搏动图等进行无创伤性心功能测定，从不同角度研究活血化瘀药对心脏功能状态及血流动力学的影响，亦已广为应用。心脏泵血功能由前负荷、后负荷和收缩性能三个变数决定，搏出量主要决定于心肌产生的张力和缩短的程度，因而受负荷状态影响明显。只能在特定条件下，如前、后负荷不变，或即使改变但泵功能变化的方向与负荷改变的原定影响方向相反时，才可根据泵功能指标粗略判断收缩性能的急性改变。可见，血流动力学指标对评定心肌收缩性能的价值也有局限。

微循环是指微动脉与微静脉之间的微细循环，它分布在全身的各个脏器和组织中。研究微循环的方法很多，主要是显微镜直接观察法。一般分为两大类：体表观察法和内脏微循环观察法。体表观察在临床上主要有甲襞、眼球视网膜、齿龈、唇黏膜、耳鼓膜及舌尖等部位的微循环；动物实验有家兔球结膜和眼睑微循环、家兔舌尖微循环、兔耳微循环等。内脏微循环主要用动物的肠系膜、心肌和肝脏等脏器来观察活血化瘀药对微循环的影响，常用大白鼠、家兔、豚鼠、小白鼠的肠系膜进行观；也可利用脏器“开窗”手术做慢性实验。

活血化瘀药主要治疗血瘀证。目前采用的血瘀证模型主要可分为三类：(1) 病因模型：根据中医药理论，采用物理、化学及自然衰老方法模拟血瘀证致病因素造模，部分模型可以活血化瘀药进行反证。(2) 病理生理模型：根据西医血管病理生理学，多采用手术方法引起血管阻塞、内皮损伤或微循环障碍造模。(3) 生物表征模型：以物理、化学及手术等方法模拟中医血瘀证临床表现造模。其中的病因模型多采用大鼠、小鼠和兔为实验对象，主要方法为：①气虚血瘀模型：如动物强迫游泳方法。②血虚血瘀证模型：如动脉放血法。③阴虚血瘀证模型：如应用糖皮质激素和肾上腺素致阴虚火旺造模。④阳虚血瘀证模型：采用低温冷冻法。⑤外伤血瘀证模型：如以杠杆压挤法造模。⑥寒凝血瘀模型：采用冰冷冻法。⑦热毒血瘀模型：采用内毒素或细菌注射法。⑧痰浊血瘀证模型：以高脂饮食造模。⑨气滞血瘀证模型：如采用电针刺激。⑩自然衰老血瘀证模型等。

Chapter 13 Experiments concerned with drugs for invigorating blood circulation and eliminating stasis

Drugs for invigorating blood circulation and eliminating stasis have extensive pharmacological actions and obviously affect the functions of blood circulation system, immune system and nervous system. There are many experimental methods for the investigation of these drugs, and those relevant to hemorheology, hemodynamics and microcirculation are frequently adopted in recent years.

Hemorheology is a subject dealing with blood fluidity, coagulability, viscosity and deformability. The rheological properties of blood mainly depend on its viscosity which is influenced by the volume of packed red cells, degrees of adhesion and aggregation of erythrocytes, erythrocyte deformability, plasma viscosity, smoothness of inner surface of vessel wall, vessel wall elasticity, blood temperature, pH et al. Among these factors, the shape and volume of erythrocyte affect blood glutinousness significantly. Plasma consistency is depended on the contents of high-molecular-weight protein, lipoprotein and carbohydrate in it. So in most relevant experiments, the following indexes are measured for studying the effects of drugs for invigorating blood circulation and eliminating stasis on the hemorheology and the coagulation process of platelet or blood. These indexes include whole blood viscosity, packed cell volume, erythrocyte aggregation, erythrocyte electrophoretic time, deformation capability and viscosity of hematocyte, blood clot and thrombus elasticity or apparent viscosity, platelet aggregation, the retroconversion phenomenon and transition radius when blood flowing in capillary, ratio of prostacyclin to thromboxane.

Cardiac function and hemodynamics, the basic ingredients of pharmacological research related to circulation system, are the important parts in studies of the drugs for invigorating blood circulation and eliminating stasis. The indexes measured include heart rate, blood pressure, blood flow of coronary artery, nutritional blood flow in myocardium, coronary artery resistance, total peripheral resistance, left ventricular work, pulmonary artery pressure, cardiac output, stroke volume, left ventricular pressure, left ventricular contractibility, cardiac index, stroke index. In general, there are two types of experimental methods for studying hemodynamics:traumatic and non-traumatic assay methods. Traumatic assay methods are those traumatic to the experimental animals, including direct assays of blood pressure, left intraventricular pressure, blood flow of aorta, nutritional blood flow in myocardium, infarct size of myocardium. Blood flow of coronary artery is an important index in the evaluation of the prevention and cure of coronary heart disease with drugs for invigorating blood circulation and eliminating stasis. Because not every drug with the function of increasing blood flow of coronary artery could improve myocardial ischemia, more precise conclusion should be drawn on the basis of analyzing various indexes. The methods for detecting blood flow of coronary artery are divided into two types: in vivo and in vitro assay. Myocardium nutritional blood flow is obtained by using isotope 86Rb, which is generally applied in preliminary screening of anti-myocardial ischemia drugs. In addition, non-traumatic assays such as ultrasonic cardiogram, phonocardiogram, electrocardiogram, carotic pulse graph and apexcardiogram are widely applied to investigate the effects of drugs for invigorating blood circulation and eliminating stasis on cardiac function and hemodynamics from different points of view. Blood-pumping function of heart is depended on three variable indexes:preload, afterload and contractibility. Stroke volume, determined by the tension and the decurtation degree of the cardiac muscle, is obviously affected by loading conditions. Only under the definite conditions such as invariable preload or afterload, or the direction of changing pumping function just opposite to that of the load changes, the probable decision of acute changes in contractibility could be made on the basis of pumping functions. So, evaluation of cardiac contractility from hemodynamic indexes is remained to be defined.

Microcirculation, distributing in every organ and tissue all over the body, is the minicirculation between arterioles and veinules. Many methods can be adopted to investigate microcirculation, among which direct observation with microscope is frequently applied. Universally, there are two types of approaches:body-surface observation and internal-organ observation. Clinically, body-surface observation includes observing the microcirculation in nail walls, retina, gum, lip mucosa, ear drum and tip of the tongue. In animal experiments, circulations in bulbar conjunctiva, eyelid, tip of the tongue of rabbit can be observed. Internal-organ microcirculations in animal mesentery, myocardium and liver are usually adopted in the evaluation of drugs for invigorating blood circulation and eliminating stasis. Mesentery of rat, rabbit, guinea pig or mouse is commonly used. In chronic experiments, opening window operation can be adopted.

Drugs for invigorating blood circulation and eliminating stasis mainly aim at curing the syndrome of blood stasis. At present, the models of syndrome of blood stasis include three types. The first is the model of etiological factor. According to the theory of Chinese medicine science, physical or chemical methods, or natural senility are used to mimic etiological factor of syndrome of blood stasis, and a part of these models could be demonstrate by successful treatment with drugs for invigorating blood circulation and eliminating stasis. The second is the pathophysiological model. According to the theory of vascular pathophysiology in western medicine, models can be established by surgical angiemphraxis, endothelium injury or microcirculation disturbance. The third is the biological exosyndrome model, which is made by mimicing the clinical manifestations in the syndrome of blood stasis with physical, chemical or surgical methods. In the first model, experimental animals can be rats, mice or rabbits, and the main methods are described below: ① Deficiency-of-vital-energy-induced blood stasis model. For example, by forcing animals to swim for some time; ② Blood-deficiency-induced blood stasis model by artery depletion method; ③ Blood stasis model induced by Yin asthenia. The model induced by glucocorticosteroid or epinephrine-induced asthenic Yin causing excessive pyrexia is an example; ④ Yang- asthenia-induced blood stasis model by treatment at low temperature; ⑤ Blood stasis model by surgical trauma of hand with spike extruding; ⑥ Blood stasis model of cold coagulation by cryoapplication; ⑦ Model resulted from toxic heat by injection of endotoxin or bacterium; ⑧ Phlegm-induced model by high fat diet; ⑨ Qi-stagnancy-induced blood stasis model by electro-acupuncture stimulation; ⑩ Natural-senile-induced model.

实验一 丹参、川芎和复方丹参对离体豚鼠心脏冠脉流量的影响

【目的】掌握离体心脏冠脉流量的测定方法；观察丹参、川芎和复方丹参对离体心脏冠脉流量、心率及心肌收缩力的影响；了解抗心肌缺血药的作用原理。

【原理】心肌的血液及氧由主动脉根部发出的左右两支冠状动脉供应，血液经毛细血管由冠状静脉窦回到右心房。离体心脏则经主动脉插管，将充氧、恒温、恒压的洛氏液通过冠状动脉灌流心肌。

心肌供血、供氧和需氧之间不平衡可引发心绞痛发作。活血化瘀药丹参、川芎及复方丹参能扩张冠脉，增加冠脉流量；垂体后叶素收缩冠脉，减少冠脉流量；异丙肾上腺素虽增加冠脉流量，但加快心率，增强心肌收缩力，使心肌需氧量增加。

【器材】灌流装置；记录装置；超级恒温器；玻璃主动脉插管；量杯；培养皿；1 mL 注射器；剪刀；小镊子；烧杯；弹簧夹；充氧的橡皮球胆；秒表。

【动物】豚鼠。

【试剂】丹参注射液 0.75 g/mL；川芎注射液 1.25 g/mL；复方丹参注射液 3 g/mL（丹参、降香各 1.5 g）；硫酸异丙肾上腺素 10 μg/mL；脑垂体后叶素 1 U/mL；洛氏液。

【方法】调节超级恒温器使恒定在（37 ± 1）℃。泵出的水打入冷凝管，使灌流液保持恒温。冷凝管下端经橡皮管与主动脉插管相连，冷凝管上端连灌流瓶。A 灌流瓶中进气管之下端水平面即控制灌流液面之高度。调节灌流液面高度距离主动脉根部 50 cm 左右。B 灌流瓶不断通入恒定的氧气，使瓶内洛氏液被氧气饱和。当全部管道内充满已充氧气的洛氏液后用弹簧夹夹住。

取约 300 g 的豚鼠，用锤子击后脑致死，颈动脉放血。剪开胸腔和心包膜，轻轻提起心脏。剪断与心脏连接的血管，取出心脏，立即放入低温（4 ℃左右）洛氏液中并轻轻挤压，排出余血。在升主动脉与肺动脉间穿过一根丝线，在升主动脉最高处剪开一小切口，插入主动脉插管，结扎固定。打开弹簧夹，使洛氏液由冠脉经心肌而入右心房，从腔静脉和肺动脉的断端流出。用蛙心夹夹住心尖，其连线连接于记录装置杠杆（或肌力换能器），描记心脏搏动曲线，用秒表记录心率；在心脏下方置一量筒以测定冠脉流量。

使心脏适应和恢复 10~15 min 后，冠脉流量、心率及心搏幅度基本稳定。连续测量 3 min 的每分钟流量，若数量相近，以其平均值作为给药前的正常流量。豚鼠以 10~15 mL/min 为宜，可根据心脏大小适当调节灌流压而加以控制。从主动脉插管上端的橡皮管（或主动脉插管之侧管）注入下述各药，测定给药后 1~10 min 内每分钟流量、心率及心搏幅度，找出其极值，算出给药后流量之最大增减值。每给药 1 次，需待其恢复正常流量后再作第 2 次给药。

（1）丹参注射液 0.2 mL；（2）复方丹参注射液 0.2 mL；（3）川芎注射液 0.2 mL；

（4）硫酸异丙肾上腺素溶液 0.2 mL。

【结果】丹参、复方丹参和川芎能增加离体豚鼠心脏冠脉流量。异丙肾上腺素虽增加冠脉流量，但明显地增加心率和心肌收缩力。结果记入表 13-1。

表 13-1 丹参、复方丹参及川芎对离体豚鼠心脏冠脉流量、心率及心搏幅度的影响

药物	浓度	冠脉流量（mL/min）			心率（次/min）			心搏幅度（mm）		
		给药前	给药后	增减率%	给药前	给药后	增减率%	给药前	给药后	增减率%
空白										
丹参										
复方丹参										
川芎										
异丙肾上腺素										

注：增减率 =[（给药后均值 – 给药前均值）/ 给药前均值］× 100%

【注意事项】

1. 本实验也可采用大白鼠或兔心脏。

2. 洛氏液必须用新鲜蒸馏水配制。

3. 制备离体心脏时注意保护心房，勿伤及窦房结；主动脉插管不能过深，以免堵塞冠脉，更不能插入左心室。整个手术和插管过程操作应迅速。

4. 为了保持冠脉流量、心率和心搏幅度正常稳定，实验必须在恒温、恒压和充氧下进行。

5. 市售的丹参、复方丹参及川芎注射液由于公司或批号不同，会影响实验结果，应先预试验。

【思考题】

1. 丹参、川芎及复方丹参为什么可以用于治疗冠心病心绞痛，而异丙肾上腺素则禁用于冠心病心绞痛？

2. 为什么不能单纯以增加心脏冠脉流量作为筛选抗心绞痛药的指标？

Experiment 1　Effects of Danshen Root, Chuanxiong and Complex Prescription of Danshen on blood flow of coronary artery of Guinea pig heart in vitro

【Purpose】To master the assay method of the blood flow of coronary artery in isolated heart and observe the effects of Danshen Root, Chuanxiong and complex prescription of Danshen on blood flow of coronary artery, heart rate and myocardial contractility. Understand the mechanisms of myocardial ischemic antagonist.

【Principles】Blood and oxygen in myocardium are supplied by left and right coronary arteries from aortic root. Blood goes through blood capillary into coronary sinus venosus by which returns to right atrium. In isolated heart, myocardium perfusion is completed by aortic cannula through which Lock's solution with oxygenation. at constant temperature and constant pressure is added and pass through coronary artery to myocardium.

Angina pectoris attack could be initiated by the imbalance between blood and oxygen supply and oxygen requirement. Drugs for invigorating blood circulation and eliminating stasis such as Danshen, Chuanxiong and complex prescription of Danshen can dilate coronary artery, increase the blood flow of coronary artery, while hypophysin decreases the blood flow of coronary artery by inducing coronary contraction. Isoprenaline increases oxygen requirement of myocardium by accelerating heart rate and enhancing myocardial contractility, although it increases the blood flow of coronary artery.

【Equipments】Perfusion device, recording apparatus, ultrathemostat, glass aortic cannula, cylindrical glass, culture dishes, syringes (1 mL), scissors, pincette, beaker, pinch clamp, rubber bulb for oxygenation, seconds-counter.

【Animals】Guinea pigs.

【Agents】Danshen injection (0.75 g/mL), Chuanxiong injection (1.25 g/mL), Danshen complex prescription (3 g/mL, Danshen 1.5 g, Chuanxiong 1.5 g), isoprenaline sulfate (10 μg/mL), pituitrin (1 U/mL) and Lock's solution.

【Methods】Ultrathemostat is adjusted to (37 ± 1)℃. Water pumped out is led in condensation tube to keep the perfusate at a constant temperature. Inferior extremity of condensation tube is connected to aortic cannula, while the superior extremity connected to perfusion bottle. In perfusion bottle A, water level in onlet duct is the controlled height of perfusate which is adjusted to the level 50 cm-distance to the aortic root. Lock's solution in bottle B is constantly oxygenated until saturation and pinch clamp is clamped when the whole tube is filled with oxygenated Lock's solution.

Guinea pig of 300 g body weight is put to death by attack with hammer on hindbrain and blood is let out from carotid artery. Thoracic cavity is shaved and cardiac pericardium is opened. The heart is raised gently and vessels connected to heart are cut off. The isolated heart is put into Lock's solution at about 4 ℃ and squeezed gently to clear the remained blood. A silk suture is put between ascending aorta and pulmonary artery, and a little incision is made at the topmost of ascending aorta for inserting aortic cannula fixed with ligation. Pinch clamp is opened and Lock's solution from coronary artery flows through cardiac muscle to right atrium dextrum, and flows out from the broken ends of caval vein and pulmonary artery. Apex cordis is clamped with frog heart clip which connected to recording apparatus (hand spike or muscle force transducer) by a thread to record the heart beat curve. Heart rate is recorded by seconds-counter and the blood flow of coronary artery is measured with cylindrical glass put under the heart.

After 10~15 min of accommodation and restoration, when the blood flow of coronary artery, heart rate and amplitude of heart beat are at constant states, three continuous minute volumes are measured.If the values are similar, the mean value is looked as the normal flow before drug treatment. Perfusion velocity is controlled by adjusting the perfusion pressure according to the size of heart, for example, 10~15 mL/min is proper for a guinea pig heart. Drugs are added from the rubber tube connected to the superior extremity of aortic cannula (or the canalis lateralis of aortic cannula) and the minute volumes, heart rate together with heart beat amplitude from 1~10 min are recorded. The extremum is used to calculate the maximum increase or decrease value. After the flow volume recovers to the normal level, the next treatment of drug is permitted.

(1) 0.2 mL of Danshen injection. (2) 0.2 mL of Danshen complex prescription injection. (3) 0.2 mL of Chuanxiong injection. (4) 0.2 mL of isoprenaline sulfate injection.

【 Results 】 Danshen, Danshen complex prescription and Chuanxiong can elevate the blood flow of coronary artery in in-vitro guinea pig heart, while isoprenaline increases the blood flow of coronary artery as well as heart rate and myocardial contraction. The data are filled into table 13-1.

Table 13–1 The effects of Danshen, Danshen complex prescription and Chuanxiong on the blood flow of coronary artery, heart rate and myocardial contraction in isolated guinea pig heart

Drug	Concentration	Blood flow of coronary artery (mL/min)			treatment treatment Heart rate (time/min)			treatment treatment Amplitude (mm)		
		before treatment	after treatment	change rate%	before treatment	after treatment	change rate%	before treatment	after treatment	change rate%
Blank										
Danshen										

(Continued)

Drug	Concen-tration	Blood flow of coronary artery (mL/min)			treatment treatment Heart rate (time/min)			treatment treatment Amplitude (mm)		
		before treatment	after treatment	change rate%	before treatment	after treatment	change rate%	before treatment	after treatment	change rate%
Danshen complex										
Chuan xiong										
Isoprenaline										

Note: increase or decrease percentage =[(mean value after drug treatment-mean value before drug treatment)/ mean value before drug treatment] × 100%

【Notes】

1. The heart of rat or rabbit is also adopted in this experiment.

2. Lock's solution is prepared with water recently distilled.

3. Cardiac atrium should be carefully protected in the process of in-vitro heart preparation so as not to injury the sinus node. Aortic cannula should not be inserted too deep in order to avoid obstruction of coronary artery and insertion into left ventricle is specially avoided. The operation and insertion of aortic cannula should be completed quickly.

4. Experiment should be done under the conditions of constant temperature, constant pressure and oxygenation in order to maintain the stable blood flow of coronary artery, heart rate and heart beat amplitude.

5. Experimental results are affected by qualities of danshen, danshen complex prescription and chuanxiong injections sold in market because of the different sources, so preliminary test should be done first.

【Questions】

1. Why danshen, danshen complex prescription and chuanxiong injections could be used to treat coronary artery disease or angina, while isoprenaline is prohibited to be adopted?

2. Why the factor of increasing blood flow of coronary artery should not be regarded as the unique index for screening antianginal drug?

实验二　血府逐瘀汤对大白鼠肠系膜微循环的影响

【目的】通过血府逐瘀汤对微循环影响的实验，揭示该方活血化瘀的部分实质。

【原理】血府逐瘀汤为活血化瘀良方，能改善微循环。本实验借助显微电视录像装置观察大白鼠肠系膜微循环变化（包括血管口径、血流速度变化）以了解组织血流灌注的情况。

【器材】微循环显微彩色录像系统；冷光源；二道生理记录仪；大白鼠肠系膜观察台；超级恒温水浴；5 000 mL 广口瓶；小型水浴槽；手术剪刀；眼科镊；2 mL 注射器；缝合线。

【动物】SD 大鼠。

【试剂】血府逐瘀汤水煎醇沉液 2 g/mL（当归 10 g、生地黄 10 g、桃仁 12 g、红花 10 g、枳壳 6 g、赤芍 6 g、柴胡 3 g、桔梗 5 g、川芎 5 g、牛膝 10 g、甘草 3 g，共煎成 40 mL）；生理盐水；肝素钠注射液；乌拉坦溶液 20 g/100 mL；平衡克氏液（其中含 NaCl 7.7 g、KCl 0.35 g、$CaCl_2 \cdot 2H_2O$ 0.29 g 、$MgSO_4 \cdot 7H_2O$ 0.3 g、$NaCHO_3$ 2 g，蒸馏水加至 1 000 mL，充 95%N_2+5%CO_2 混合气体半小时，以排除平衡克氏液中的氧气）。

【方法】选取空腹 12 h 的大鼠 6 只，体重 180~220 g，用乌拉坦 1.4 g/100 g 肌注麻醉。将手术野毛剪净。分离颈动脉，连接血压换能器，以二道生理记录仪监测血压，按 Chambers 法制备大鼠回肠系膜微循环标本，用 37 ℃恒温平衡克氏液不断向标本上滴注，每分钟 50 ± 5 滴以保持标本的恒温、恒湿、恒 pH 和一定的离子浓度。用 Leitz 镜头（10 T）和 CD-2 型彩色显微电视录像装置观测记录。在监测器屏幕上测定给药前后（小肠给药：血府逐瘀汤水煎醇沉液 0.8 mL/100 g）细动脉（A3）、细静脉（V3）口径的变化，并用二道生理记录仪同步记录血压的变化，判断微循环改善的情况。

【结果】给药后细动脉、细静脉口径不同程度增大，以动脉扩张更为明显。参照表 13-2 记录。

表 13-2 血府逐瘀汤对大白鼠肠系膜血管口径的影响

动物号	A_3 口径(μm)				V_3 口径(μm)			
	给药前	给药后			给药前	给药后		
		10 min 差值	20 min 差值	30 min 差值		10 min 差值	20 min 差值	30 min 差值
1								
2								
3								
4								
5								
6								
差值 $\bar{x}\pm SD$								
P 值								

【注意事项】

1. 保持活体肠系膜标本温度为(37 ± 1)℃。因温度对肠系膜微循环影响较大,很易产生实验结果的偏差。

2. 腹部手术切口在 1.5~2 cm 为宜。切口过大肠管易涌出,影响观察;过小寻找观察部位不便,并会影响血液循环。

3. 实验结果的数据是用 Leitz 镜头和彩色显微录像装置观察测量所得。屏幕上可观察到微循环的动态变化。

【思考题】根据本实验结果讨论血府逐瘀汤活血化瘀作用的实质。

Experiment 2 Effect of Xuefuzhuyutang on the mesentery microcirculation in rats

【**Purpose**】To reveal the mechanisms of Xuefuzhuyutang in invigorating blood circulation and eliminating stasis by observing the effect of this complex prescription on microcirculation.

【**Principles**】Xuefuzhuyutang is an effective prescription for improving microcirculation. In this experimental, micro-video recording system is applied to observe the changes of mesentery microcirculation (including changes in blood vessel caliber and blood flow rate) in rats to get the message of the blood perfusion in tissues.

【**Equipments**】Multicolor micro-video recording system for microcirculation, Cold light source, two channels electrophysiolograph, observation desk for rat mesenary, ultrathemostat, 5,000 mL-volume wide-mouthed bottle, organ bath, surgical scissors, pincette, syringe of 2 mL volume, sutural line.

【**Animals**】Sprague-Dawley (SD) rats.

【**Agents**】Xuefuzhuyutang was extracted with water decoction followed by ethanol precipitation, 2 g/mL (Angelica Root, 10 g, crude Rehmannia Root, 10 g, Peach Seed, 12 g, Carthamus Tinctorius, 10 g, Citri Immaturus Exsiccatus, 6 g, Paeoniae Radix, 6 g, Bupleurum Chinense, 3 g, Platycodon Root, 5 g, Chuanxiong, 5 g, Achyranthis Radix, 10 g, Licorice Root, 3 g, decocted to 40 mL.), saline, heparin sodium injection, ethyl carbamate solution (20 g/100 mL), balanced Kreb's solution (NaCl 7.7 g、KCl 0.35 g、$CaCl_2 \cdot 2H_2O$ 0.29 g 、$MgSO_4 \cdot 7H_2O$ 0.3 g、$NaCHO_3$ 2 g, distilled water is added to 1 000 mL, and 95%N_2+5%CO_2 of mixed gases is filled in to remove the oxygen in Kreb's solution.)

【**Methods**】6 rats weighed 180~220 g, fasted for 12 h, are anesthetized by intramuscular injection of 1.4 g/100 g of urethane. Hair on operating field is cut off. Carotid artery is isolated and connected with blood pressure transducer for blood pressure monitoring by two channels electrophysiolograph. The mesenaric microcirculation sample of rat ileum is made according to the method of Chambers. 50 ± 5 drops per minute of balanced Kreb's solution of constant temperature is dropped onto the sample constantly to keep the sample at a state of constant temperature, humidity, pH and ion concentration. The changes are recorded under Leize lens (10 T) on the CD-2 multicolor Micro-video recording system. The data of caliber and blood flow rate of small artery (A_3) and small vein (V_3) are measured on monitor screen before and after drug treatments (0.8 mL/100 g of extracted solution of

Xuefuzhuyutang is administered by small intestine), and blood pressure is simultaneously recorded by two channels electrophysiolograph, both of which are indexes to evaluate the microcirculation state.

【Results】 Multicolor micro-video recording system for microcirculation, Cold light source, two channels electrophysiolograph, observation desk for rat mesenary, ultrathemostat, 5,000 mL-volume wide-mouthed bottle, organ bath, surgical scissors, pincette, syringe of 2 mL volume, sutural line.

After drug treatment, the diameters of small artery and small vein increase in various degrees, and the change of small artery is prominent. Data are recorded according to table 13-2.

Table 13–2 Effect of Xuefuzhuyutang on the blood vessel diameters of mesentery microcirculation in rats

Animal number	A_3 diameter (μm)				V_3 diameter (μm)			
	before	after treatment			before	after treatment		
		10 min change	20 min change	30 min change		10 min change	20 min change	30 min change
1								
2								
3								
4								
5								
6								
change $\bar{x} \pm SD$								
P value								

【Notes】

1. Keep the temperature of in-vivo mesenary specimen at 37 ± 1 ℃. Temperature affects the mesenary microcirculation stronger, which could produce the deviation of experimental data.

2. Operative incision on abdominal region is properly controlled at 1.5~2 cm. If the incision is too large, intestinal is easy to be squeezed out. On the contrary, too small of incision would interfere blood circulation and make it difficult to search observation site.

3. Experimental data are measured by Leize lens and Multicolor Micro-video recording system, and the dynamic changes of microcirculation would be observed on the screen.

【Questions】 Please discuss the mechanisms concerned with the invigorating-blood-circulation-and- eliminating- stasis action of Xuefuzhuyutang according to the experimental data.

实验三　丹参和川芎对大白鼠"血瘀"证血液流变学的影响

【目的】了解大白鼠急性"血瘀"证模型的复制方法,同时观察活血化瘀药丹参或川芎对急性"血瘀"证的防治作用。

【原理】中医理论认为"大怒致瘀","外寒也可致瘀"。给大白鼠注射大剂量肾上腺素,模拟暴怒时的机体状态;随之以冰水浸泡动物,模拟外寒侵袭。两种因素的综合作用可复制出大白鼠血液流变性呈黏、浓、凝状态的急性"血瘀"证模型。

丹参活血凉血祛瘀,川芎活血行气通经,二者对血液黏、浓、凝状态均有明显改善。据此证明此"模型"的可靠性,同时也说明改善血液流变学是活血化瘀药的作用原理之一。

【器材】剪刀;1 mL 和 2 mL 注射器;20 mL 烧杯;小水桶及冰块;试管;红细胞压积管;滴管;兽用长注射针头;离心机;黏度细胞电泳自动计时仪。

【动物】Wistar 大白鼠。

【试剂】肝素钠粉剂;生理盐水;肾上腺素 1 mg/mL;丹参水煎液(浓缩为 1.5 g/mL);川芎水煎液(浓缩为 1.5 g/mL)。

【方法】将 280~350 g 体重的 Wistar 大白鼠按下列设计分组,每组 8 只。雌雄各半。

1. 空白对照组　每天灌水 10 mL/kg,连续 7 天。

2. "血瘀"模型对照组　每天灌胃水 10 mL/kg,连续 7 天。于第 7 天皮下注射肾上腺素 0.8 mg/ kg,4 h 后再注射 1 次,共 2 次。在第 1 次注射后 2 h,将大白鼠浸入冰水 5 min,然后禁食,于次日清晨进行实验检测。

3. 中药实验组　为丹参或川芎实验组。每天灌胃丹参或川芎水煎液 15 g/kg,连续 7 天。于第 7 天按第(2)项所述方法复制"血瘀"模型,次晨取血检测。

上述各组动物均不麻醉,剪开颈动脉放血。每只动物血样分别置于 2 支离心管内,其中 1 支加入少量肝素钠抗凝,另 1 支不加任何药品,让血液自然凝固(详见后附之"血样准备")。用血黏细胞电泳自动计时仪检测,并计算下列各项血液流变学指标:

(1)全血黏度(比):(ηb),高切变速度(700~600/s)、低切变速度(70~20/s)之全血黏度分别计算:

全血黏度(比 ratio)= 全血流速(s)/ 生理盐水流速(s)　　(式 16-1)

(2)全血还原黏度(比)=(ηb-1)/ H　　(式 16-2)

H 为红细胞压积(除去红细胞压积影响因素)

(3)血清(或血浆)黏度(比)= 血清(或血浆)流速(s)/ 生理盐水流速(s)(式 16-3)

(4)纤维蛋白原黏度(比)= 血浆黏度(比)- 血清黏度(比)　　(式 16-4)

(5)红细胞压积:记录红细胞压积管刻度(白细胞部分不计入)

(6)红细胞电泳率(W):

W = 单位时间移动距离(μm/s)/ 单位电场强度(V/cm) (式 16-5)

附:血样准备

①全血:取抗凝血放置 10 min,用单层纱布过滤除去杂质和小凝块。用前充分混匀。

②血清:直接取血,放置后离心即可。

③血浆:测定全血粘度后,将所余抗凝血离心即可。

④红细胞压积:将抗凝血用带长针头的 2 mL 注射器将全血注入压积管内,以 3 000 rpm 离心 30 min。观察红细胞液面刻度,记下读数。

【结果】丹参、川芎能降低血瘀模型动物增高的全血黏度、血浆黏度、纤维蛋白原黏度及红细胞压积,缩短已延长的红细胞电泳时间。可参照表 13-3 记录数据。

表 13-3 药物对大白鼠急性“血瘀”证血液流变性的影响

分组	动物数	全血黏度		血清黏度(比)	血浆黏度(比)	纤维蛋白原黏度(比)	红细胞电泳时间(s)	红细胞压积(%)
		低切变速度(70~20/s)	高切变速度(700~600/s)					
空白对照								
“血瘀”模型								
丹参								
川芎								

附:血液流变性指标的意义

血液流变性改变是“血瘀”证主要客观诊断指标之一。“血瘀”证的血液流变性特点为:黏、浓、凝、聚。

1. 黏

(1)全血黏度(比):反映血液流变性的总体变化,即包括血液中血细胞有形成分及血浆中可溶性成分的变化。“血瘀”证表现为全血黏度(比)增高。

(2)全血还原黏度(比):低、高切变速度:由于红细胞(RBC)压积是影响全血黏度(比)的主要因素之一,为除去 RBC 压积的影响,故以全血还原黏度(比)表示单位 RBC 压积产生的黏度,有利于压积不同的全血黏度之间的比较。

全血黏度及全血还原黏度(低切变速度)可反映 RBC 聚集性的变化,全血黏度和全血还原黏度(高切变速度)则反映 RBC 变形能力的改变。

(3)血清黏度和血浆黏度:二者反映血中可溶性成分的变化,血浆仅比血清多一个纤维蛋白原因素。影响二者黏度的因素如下:根据可溶性成分产生黏度能力表示(以白蛋白为 1),胆固醇 278,纤维蛋白原 139,甘油三酯 121,β 脂蛋白 3.2,Ig 和 IgA 2.7。

2. 浓 指血液浓度增高。包括 RBC 压积和血浆中血脂及免疫球蛋白等大分子成分的改变。RBC 压积增高,说明全血过浓,有血瘀存在可能性大。

3. 凝　指纤维蛋白原浓度增高，即指血细胞凝固性增大。通常用纤维蛋白原黏度（比）及血液凝固时间来检测。"血瘀"证时，表现为纤维蛋白原增多，血液易凝。

4. 聚　指血细胞聚集程度增高，表现为RBC及血小板的电泳时间增大，反映细胞膜负电荷密度降低，RBC间排斥力小而易聚集。它是"血瘀"证检测指标之一。如RBC电泳速度快，则反映RBC表面负电荷密度大，RBC不易聚集。此外，血沉也反映RBC聚集力，但在正常大白鼠血沉变化无规律，故未选用该指标。

【思考题】

1. "血瘀"证的形成受哪些因素影响？本实验所选两种刺激因素，其产生"血瘀"证的机理如何？

2. 丹参和川芎均为活血化瘀药，但性质和功用尚有不同，请结合实验结果分析两药的作用特点。

Experiment 3 Effects of Danshen and Chuanxiong on the rheological properties of blood in rats with syndrome of Blood Stasis

【Purposes】To understand the preparation method of acute model of syndrome of blood stasis in rats, and observe the preventive and therapeutic effects of Danshen and Chuanxiong, the drugs for invigorating blood circulation and eliminating stasis, on acute syndrome of blood stasis.

【Principles】According to the theory of Chinese medical science, blood stasis could be induced by rage and exogenous cold-evil. Body state in rage is mimiced by high dose of epinephrin exposed to rats, and invasion of exogenous cold-evil is mimiced by soaking the animal into ice water. Acute model of blood stasis in rats, with the blood rheological properties of stickiness, thickness and coagulation, could be prepared by the complex actions of these two factors.

Danshen, with functions of promoting blood flow, cooling the blood and removing blood stasis, and Chuanxiong, impulsing energy and promoting veins and arteries, improve the functions of blood with stickiness, thickness and coagulation properties, which demonstrates the reliability of the model and suggests that improving rheological properties of blood is one of the mechanisms of drugs for invigorating blood circulation and eliminating stasis.

【Animals】Wistar rats.

【Agents】Heparin sodium powder, normal saline, 1 mg/mL of epinephrin, Danshen decoction (condensed to 1.5 g/mL), and Chuanxiong decoction (condensed to 1.5 g/mL).

【Equipments】Shears, syringes (1 mL or 2 mL volume), beaker of 20 mL volume, little bucket, ice cubes, tubes, hematocrits, dropping pipette, centrifuger, automatic chronograph of blood viscosity and cell electrophoresis.

【Methods】Wistar rats weighed 280~350 g are divided into four groups, each group with 8 rats and female and male are equated.

1. Normal control Rats are orally administered with 10 mL/kg of water every day for 7 days.

2. Blood-stasis model control Rats are orally administered with 10 mL/kg of water every day for 7 days. 0.8 mg/kg of epinephrin is subcontanously injected on day 7 for two times with an interval of 4 h. 2 h after the first injection, rats are immersed into ice water for 5 min, and fasted until the next morning for experiment.

3. Groups of tested drugs　Rats are orally administered with 15 g/kg of Danshen or Chuanxiong decoction every day for 7 days. On day 7, rats are treated according to the method in model control.

Rats above are cut at carotid artery for blood letting. The blood sample of each animal is collected in two centrifuge tubes, one is pre-treated with heparin sodium for anticoagulation, the other without any treatment for natural blood coagulation (Please refer to the part blood sample preparation as follow.). Data are recorded by automatic chronograph of blood viscosity and cell electrophoresis, and hemorheological indexes are calculated.

(1) Whole blood viscosity (ratio) (ηb), at high shear velocity (HSV, 700~600/s) or low shear velocity (LSV, 70~20/s):

whole blood viscosity (ratio) = flow rate of whole blood (s) / flow rate of normal saline (s)

(formula 16-1)

(2) Whole blood reduced viscisity (ratio) = (ηb−1) / H (H is the volume of packed red blood cells, in order to eliminte the effect of the volume of packed red blood cells)

(formula 16-2)

(3) Serum (or plasma) viscosity (ratio) = flow rate of serum (or plasma) (s) /flow rate of normal saline (s)

(formula 16-3)

(4) Fibrinogen viscosity (ratio) = plasma viscosity (ratio) – serum viscosity (ratio)

(formula 16-4)

(5) Volume of packed red blood cells. Directly record the volume of red blood cells in the hematocrits.

(6) Erythrocyte electrophoresis rate (w)

w = moving distance in unit time (μm/s) / electric field intensity on unit distance (V/cm)

(formula 16-5)

Annotations: Preparation of blood sample

① Whole blood. Anticoagulated blood is let aside for 10 min, filtered with monolayer gauxe to remove foreign material and little clots. It should be fully mixed before use.

② Serum. Blood is collected, and centrifuged after several minutes.

③ Plasma. The remained anticoagulated blood is centrifuged after the whole blood viscosity is measured.

④ Volume of packed red blood cells. Anticoagulated blood is added into the hematocrits by 2 mL−volume syringe with long pinhead, centrifuged at 3,000 revolutions per minute (rpm) for 30 minutes, and the scale at the level of red blood cells is recorded.

【Results】 Danshen and Chuanxiong can decrease the whole blood viscosity, plasma viscosity, fibrinogen viscosity and the volume of packed red blood cells, and shorten the lengthened erythrocyte electrophoretic time in models of blood stasis. Data are filled in table 13-3.

Table 13–3 Effects of drugs on the rheological properties of blood in rats with syndrome of blood stasis

Group	Animal number	Whole blood viscosity		Serum viscisity (ratio)	Plasma viscosity (ratio)	Fibrinogen (ratio)	Erythrocyte electrophoresis rate (s)	Volume of packed RBC (%)
		LSV (70~20/s)	HSV (700~600/s)					
Blank								
Model								
Dan shen								
Chuan xiong								

Appendix: Significance of the rheological properties of blood

The change in the rheological properties of blood is one of the objective diadynamic criterias in the syndrome of blood stasis. The characters of the rheological properties of blood in syndrome of blood stasis are: stickiness, thickness, coagulation and aggregation.

1. Stickiness.

(1) Whole blood viscosity (ratio) reflects the overall changes in the rheological properties of blood, which includes the changes of the formed element of blood and the soluble components in plasma. In syndrome of blood stasis, this index increases.

(2) Whole blood reduced viscosity (ratio) at high or low shear velocity. The volume of packed red blood cells is one of the main factors which influence the whole blood viscosity (ratio), so the whole blood reduced viscosity, indicating the viscosity of unit volume of packed red blood cells, is introduced, which is helpful for comparison between the viscosities of different packed volumes.

In general, whole blood viscosity and whole blood reduced viscosity in low shear velocity reflect the aggregation properties of RBC, while the ones in high shear velocity reflect the changes of deforming ability.

(3) Serum viscosity and plasma viscosity. Both of them reflect the changes of soluble components, and the latter contains one more factor of fibrinogen. The factors affecting these two viscosities are described as below according their contributions to viscosity——albumen 1, cholesterol 278, fibrinogen 13, triglyceride 121, β lipoprotein 3.2, immunoglobulin and Ig A 2.7.

2. Thickness. It reflects the increase of haemoconcentration, including the changes of the volume of packed RBC and the macromolecular components in plasma such as blood fat and immunoglobulins. If the volume of packed RBC increases, the whole blood is thicker, the possibility of blood stasis is more than usual.

3. Coagulation refers to the increase of fibrinogen, which suggests that the coagulability of blood cells increase. In general, fibrinogen viscosity and clotting time of blood are the indexes

to be measured. In the syndrome of blood stasis, content of fibrinogen increases and the blood tends to coagulate.

4. Aggregation refers to the degree of cell gathering, with the appearances of the increased electrophoretic times of RBC and platelet. It suggests that negative charge on cell membrane decrease, resulting in RBCs aggregation by lowering the repelling force between RBCs. It is one of the indexes to be measured in syndrome of blood stasis. The faster electrophoresis rate of RBC indicates the more negative charge on cell membrane and RBC is uneasy to aggregate. Furthermore, blood sedimentation rate also reflects the aggregation ability. This index is not adopted here because of its irregularity even in normal rats.

【Questions】

1. What factors affect the formation of syndrome of blood stasis? Why these two factors adopted in this experiment could result in blood stasis?

2. Danshen and Chuanxiong are drugs for invigorating blood circulation and eliminating stasis with some differences in their peculiarity and functions. Please analyze their characters of action.

实验四　当归抗大白鼠血栓形成的作用

【目的】掌握大鼠体外颈总动脉 - 颈外静脉血流旁路形成血栓的方法；观察当归抗血栓形成的作用。

【原理】本实验利用大鼠体外颈总动脉颈外静脉旁路法形成血小板血栓。当动脉血流中的血小板接触丝线的粗糙面时黏附于线上，血小板聚集物便环绕线的表面形成血小板血栓。血小板的黏附聚集功能受到抑制时，形成血栓的重量就较轻。因此，从血栓重量可测知血小板的黏附聚集功能。当归为活血药物，其有效成分阿魏酸钠对血小板聚集功能有抑制作用，可抑制大鼠血栓的形成。

【器材】手术剪；手术钳；丝线（4 号、7 号）；聚乙烯管（内径 1~2 mm）；动脉夹；注射器（5 mL、0.25 mL）；分析天平；称量瓶。

【动物】大白鼠。

【试剂】当归水煎乙醇沉淀液 1 g/mL；肝素钠注射液 12 500 U/mL；戊巴比妥钠 3 g/dL；阿司匹林；生理盐水。

【方法】取 350 g 雄性大白鼠 20 只，称重后随机分为两组。每鼠经腹腔注射戊巴比妥钠 0.05 g/kg 麻醉。气管内插入聚乙烯管以清除分泌物。分离右颈总动脉和左颈外静脉。动脉插管由连接在一起的 3 段聚乙烯管组成，两端的长约 3 cm，中段长 6 cm。在其中段（约 6 cm）放入一根长 5 cm 的 4 号手术丝线，将肝素钠生理盐水溶液（50 U/mL）充满聚乙烯管。当管的一端插入左颈外静脉后，从聚乙烯管注入肝素钠 50 U/kg。夹住管壁，插管的另一端插入右颈总动脉。手术完成后立即静脉注射药物（给药组）或生理盐水（空白对照组）。5 min 后开放血流，则血液从右颈总动脉流经聚乙烯管，返回左颈外静脉。开放血流 15 min 后中断血流，迅速取出丝线称重。总重量减去丝线重即血栓湿重。按下列公式计算抑制率：

$$血栓形成抑制率 = [(对照组血栓重 - 给药组血栓重) / 对照组血栓重] \times 100\%$$

【结果】当归给药组大鼠血栓湿重明显降低。参照表 13-4 记录。

表 13-4　当归对大鼠血栓形成的影响

分组	剂量（g/kg）	动物数（只）	血栓湿重（mg）	血栓形成抑制率（%）
对照组				
当归组				

【注意事项】

1. 手术过程要求迅速,操作熟练。
2. 注意及时吸出气管分泌物,保持呼吸道通畅。
3. 严格控制并准确给予肝素钠的剂量,否则影响血栓的形成。

【思考题】通过本实验,试讨论当归抗血栓形成的作用和机理。

Experiment 4　Antithrombotic effect of Angelica Root in a rat thrombosis model

【**Purposes**】To master the preparation method of arteriovenous shunt thrombosis model in rats, and observe the thrombosis-preventing effect of Angelica root.

【**Principles**】Platelet thrombus is induced by applying the model of rat arteriovenous shunt thrombosis. The platelets in the blood flow in artery would adhere to the silk thread when they contact the rough surface of the thread, leading to the formation of platelet thrombus with the aggregates surrounding the thread surface. The platelets functions of adherence and aggregation could be speculated by the weigh of the thrombus, because if these functions are downregulated, the weight of the thrombus is lighter. Angelica Root, a hemorheologic agent with the effective component of sodium ferulate, could inhibit the formation of thrombus in rat model.

【**Equipments**】Surgical scissors, surgical clamp, suture silk (No.4 and 7), polyethylene tute (inner diameter 1~2 mm), bulldog clamp, syringe (5 mL, 0.25 mL), analytic balance, weighing bottle.

【**Animals**】Rats.

【**Agents**】Extraction of Angelica Root by water decoction and ethanol precipitation (1 g/mL), heparin sodium injection (12,500 U/mL), sodium pentobarbital (3 g/dL), aspirin and normal saline.

【**Methods**】Male rats weighed about 350 g are divided into 2 groups at random and anesthetized by intraperitoneal injection of 0.05 g/kg of pentobarbital sodium. A polyethylene tubing is inserted into the air tube to clear the secretion, then the right common carotid artery and the left external jugular vein are isolated. The polyethylene tubing (12 cm total long) taken as the arterial cannula is composed of three parts——two cannulaes (about 3 cm long respectively) connected with the central part (6 cm long) which contains a 5 cm silk thread and is filled with heparin saline solution (50 U/mL). After the polyethylene tubing is inserted into the left external jugular vein, 50 U/kg of the heparin saline solution is injected through the polyethylene tubing, then the tubing is clamped and the other end of the polyethylene tubing is inserted into the right common carotid artery. The drug or saline solution is immediately injected intravenously to the rat. After 5 minutes, the clamp is opened and the blood returns to left external jugular vein from right common carotid artery through polyethylene tubing. The central part of the shunt is removed after 15 minutes of blood circulation, and the silk thread carrying the thrombus is pulled out. The wet weight of the thrombus is then determined. The wet weight is the total weight subtracting the silk weight. The inhibition ratio is calculated by the followed formula:

Thrombosis inhibition ratio=[(thrombus weight of control group-thrombus weight of drug-tested group)/ thrombus weight of control group] × 100%

[Results] The wet weight of thrombus in rats treated with Angelica Root decreased significantly. Data are filled in the table 13-4.

Table 13-4 Effect of Angelica Root on thrombus formation in rats

Group	dose (g/kg)	Animal number	Wet weight of thrombus (mg)	Thrombosis inhibition ratio (%)
Control				
Angelica Root				

[Notes]

1. The operation should be done practisedly and quickly.

2. The trachea secretion should be cleared promptly to maitain the respiratory tract easy and smooth.

3. The dose of heparin sodium, which will influence the thrombus formation, should be strictly controlled.

[Questions] Please try to discuss the effects of Angelica Root on thrombus formation and the related mechanisms.

实验五　丹参对垂体后叶素所致急性心肌缺血的影响

【目的】观察丹参对垂体后叶素所致急性心肌缺血心电图的影响。

【原理】垂体后叶素可使包括冠状动脉在内的全身血管收缩。利用垂体后叶素这一作用，静脉注射后可使动物产生急性心肌缺血状态，以心电图 ST 段及 T 波产生的变化为指标，观察给予药物后对其的对抗作用。

【器材】手术器械；电脑及记录装置；头皮静脉注射针头；注射器；大鼠固定台。

【动物】SD 大鼠。

【试剂】20% 乌拉坦溶液；丹参注射液；垂体后叶素；生理盐水。

【方法】取体重 200~300 g 的大鼠一只，20% 乌拉坦溶液（5 mg/kg）腹腔麻醉，仰位固定在大鼠固定台上。

打开电脑，点击桌面上的 BL-420 图标，选择做心电图的实验内容，将之与电脑主机相连的针状电极插入大鼠四肢皮下，做好描记心电图的准备。

在大鼠大腿内侧股动脉波动处剪开皮肤，暴露股静脉，插入与注射器相连的头皮静脉针头，缓缓推注生理盐水，已备给药。

描记一段正常心电图后，股静脉注射垂体后叶素 1 U/kg，10 s 内注射完毕，再推注生理盐水 0.5 mL/100 g，观察并记录心电图的变化，直至 30 min 时停止。

另取一只大鼠，用乌拉坦麻醉，在诱发急性心肌缺血前静脉注丹参注射液 2 mL/100 g，用同法诱发大鼠急性心肌缺血。给垂体后叶素后立即和 5 min 再次静注丹参注射液 1 mL/100 g，观察并记录丹参注射液对急性心肌缺血大鼠的影响。

【结果】描记或绘制两只大鼠心电图（Ⅱ导联）的变化情况及所有药物。

【注意事项】

1. 给垂体后叶素的剂量可依据动物的缺血性心电图的改变作适当调整。

2. 正常实验的动物应筛选垂体后叶素对心电图有明显改变者。

【思考题】丹参注射液对急性心肌缺血模型有何作用？它与祖国医学对丹参的认识有何关系？

Experiment 5 The effects of Salvia miltiorrhiza on acute myocardial ischemia caused by pituitrin

【Purposes】To study the protective effect of Salvia miltiorrhiza on acute myocardial ischemia caused by pituitrin.

【Principles】Pituitrin induces vasoconstriction including coronary vessels, and intravenous injection of pituitrin can induce acute myocardial ischemia in animalos.. As an indicator of change generated by ST segment and T wave in ECG, observe the antagonistic effects of administrated drugs.

【Equipments】Surgical instruments, computers and recording devices, scalp vein needles, syringes, rat fixed units.

【Animals】Rat.

【Agents】20% urethane solution, Salvia injection, pituitrin, saline.

【Methods】Place the rat back on the table, binding its limbs with cotton thread.

Turn on the computer, then click the icon of BL-420 on the desktop and choose the experimental contents about electrocardiogram. The needle electrodes which connect with computer host are inserted into the skin of the rat. Make preparation for recording electrocardiogram.

Cut the skin in the thigh artery fluctuations of rats, to expose femoral vein, inserting scalp intravenous needle which connect with the syringe, then push saline injection slowly for drug delivery.

After recording a period of normal electrocardiogram, inject pituitrin intravenously within 10 seconds. Make another saline injection of 0.5 mg/100 g. Observe and record the changes of electrocardiogram for 30 minutes.

Take another rat, then inject 20% Urethane solution（5 mL/kg）into the abdominal cavity. Inject salvia miltiorrhiza injection 2 mL/100 g intravenously before acute myocardial ischemia is induced. Then induce acute myocardial ischemia in rats by the same methods. After injecting pituitrin for 5 minutes, inject Salvia miltiorrhiza injection of 1 mL/100 g intravenously immediately, then observe and record the influence of Salvia miltiorrhiza injection on acute myocardial ischemia in rats.

【Results】Tracings or draw two rat electrocardiogram（Ⅱ lead）changes in the situation and the use of drugs.

【Notes】

1. The dose of pituitrin can make the appropriate adjustments according to the changes of ischemic ECG.

2. Only use the animals which demonstrate a significant change in ECG in response to pituitrin treatment.

【Questions】

1. What is the role of Salvia injection on acute myocardial ischemia model?

2. To know the implication of Salvia action in Chinese medicine.

第十四章　止咳、化痰、平喘药实验

镇咳、祛痰和平喘药被广泛用于治疗支气管炎症和哮喘。镇咳药分为中枢性镇咳药和末梢性镇咳药两大类。前者直接抑制延脑的咳嗽中枢,后者抑制咳嗽反射弧中的感受器或外周神经的某一环节而产生镇咳作用。引咳物不同,所致咳嗽的类型也不同,最常用的是化学物质刺激、机械刺激和电刺激引咳。祛痰药通过各种方式,使呼吸道的分泌量增多,使黏着于呼吸道黏膜的痰液变稀、液化而易于咳出。筛选祛痰药有直接收集气管分泌液法和测定气管的酚红排泌量法。此外,呼吸道黏膜纤毛运动对于排痰也有重要作用,因此观察纤毛运动也有助于祛痰药的研究和评价。支气管平滑肌痉挛是引起哮喘的直接原因,因此多数平喘药都作用于支气管,使平滑肌松弛。支气管平滑肌对药物反应有明显的种属差异,其中以豚鼠最为敏感,也最常用。实验可以用离体气管,也可以用整体动物。

Chapter 14　Experiments of antitussive, expectorant and antiasthmatic agents

Antitussive, expectorant and antiasthmatic agents are widely used in treating bronchial inflammation and asthma. There are two groups of antitussive agents: the central antitussive and peripheral antitussive. The former directly inhibits the medullar cough center and the latter mainly suppresses the receptor or one point of the coughing reflex arc (coughing reflex arc consists of receptor, afferent nerve, cough center, efferent nerve and effector). The types of cough may be different when different irritants are given. Chemical, mechanical and electric irritation are usually used to trigger coughing. Expectorants are claimed to increase the quantity of excretion of the respiratory tract to make the sputum less viscous, and therefore the sputum is more easily cleared. Collecting tracheal secretory fluid directly and detecting the phenolsulfonphthalein excreted by the trachea are two ways to screen the expectorant. In addition, ciliary movement of respiratory mucosa plays an important role in clearing sputum away, therefore detecting ciliary moment has some benefits to our study and evaluation of the action of expectorant agents. Bronchial spasm is the most direct cause of asthma, so most anti-asthma agents can relax the bronchial smooth muscle. There are obvious species differences in response to the same drugs. The smooth muscle of guinea pigs is sensitive to smooth muscle contraction, and thus widely used in experiments. Both the in-vitro trachea and in-vivo animal models can be used.

实验一　桔梗对小白鼠氨水引咳作用实验

【目的】学习小鼠氨水引咳法；观察桔梗的止咳作用。

【原理】用化学药物引起动物咳嗽，以观察受试药物的止咳作用。氨水是一种具有刺激性的化学物质，小鼠吸入氨水气雾后即可引起咳嗽。通过计算单位时间内小鼠的咳嗽次数可以分析药物的镇咳作用。

【器材】超声雾化器；橡皮管；小鼠固定器；烧杯；1 mL 注射器；针头；灌胃针头；10 mL 量筒；天平；小鼠笼。

【药品和试剂】磷酸可待因；生理盐水；浓氨水；桔梗水煎液 1 g/mL。

【动物】小鼠。

【方法】小鼠按体重随机分三组，第一组灌服桔梗水煎液 20 g/kg（0.2 mL/10 g），第二组给同容积生理盐水，第三组腹腔（或皮下）注射可待因 30 mg/kg（0.1 mL/10 g）。灌服药物和生理盐水 1 h、腹腔注射可待因 0.5 h 开始接受喷雾。喷入浓氨水的气雾 10 秒，2 分钟后喷雾终止，立即取出小鼠，观察 1 min 内咳嗽次数。若 1 min 内出现 3 次以上典型咳嗽动作（腹肌收缩，同时张大嘴，有时可有咳声）者为“有咳嗽”，否则算作“无咳嗽”。按序贯法（上下法）求出引起半数小鼠咳嗽的喷雾时间（EDT50）。计算 R 值，若 R 值大于 130%，说明药物有止咳作用；若 R 值大于 150%，则表明有显著止咳作用。

$$R=\frac{\text{给药组}EDT_{50}}{\text{对照组}EDT_{50}}\times 100\%$$

【结果】结果填入表 14-1。

表 14-1　桔梗水煎液对小鼠的止咳作用（序贯法）

分组	剂量（g/kg）	动物数	EDT_{50}（S）	R 值（%）	1 分钟内咳嗽次数
对照组					
桔梗					
可待因					

【注意事项】天冷季节水密度大，为确保雾化正常，槽内水温以 15~20 ℃为宜。

【思考题】桔梗止咳的机理是什么？

Experiment 1 The antitussive effect of Platycodon Root on ammonia water-induced cough response in mice

【Purpose】

1. Study the method of preparing the mouse model of cough by ammonia water.
2. Observe the antitussive effect of Platycodon Root.

【Principles】 The antitussive activity of tested drugs can be observed in chemicals-induced cough models. The ammonia water is amyctic and can be sprayed well-distributed into a sealed container when link to the air compressor. The mice will show cough response when inhaling irritative ammonia. Therefore, the antitussive effect of drugs will be evaluated by recording the times of cough in a given time range.

【Equipments】 Ultrasonic nebulizer, rubber tube, mice holder, beaker, 1 mL syringe, pinhead, pinhead for intragastric administration, 10 mL cylindrical glass, scale, mouse cage.

【Drugs and reagents】 codeine phosphate, saline, strong ammonia, water extracts of Platycodon Root 1 g/mL.

【Animals】 Mice.

【Methods】 Mice were divided into 3 groups, 9~10 mice per group, and treated orally with water extracts of Platycodon Root（20 g/kg）, an equal volume of saline as the blank control or injected intraperitoneally with codeine phosphate（30 mg/kg）as the positive control. Mice were put into the ultrasonic nebulizer 1 h after saline and Platycodon Root administration or 0.5 h after codeine phosphate treatment before exposure to the sprayed ammonia water for 10 s. The mice were kept in the nebulizer for 2 min. The cough times of each mouse in 1 min was recorded. If the mouse shows the cough response（at least three times typical coughing per min）, the mouse is regarded as a cough-positive mouse, otherwise it is called a negative one. Then the EDT_{50} and R value are calculated according to the formula presented as below.

$$R = (\text{drug treated group } EDT_{50} / \text{control group } EDT_{50}) \times 100\%$$

If $R > 130\%$, the agents can be regarded with antitussive effect, and if $R > 150\%$, it can be said that the effect is significant.

【Results】 Reference values can be seen in Table 14-1.

Table 14–1 The antitussive effect of Platycodon Root in mice (sequential method)

Group	Dose (g/kg)	*n*	EDT_{50} (S)	*R* (%)	Times of cough in 1 min
Control					
Platycodon Root					
Codeine					

【 Notes 】The water temperature should be controlled at 15~20 ℃ in winter, so the ultrasonic nebulizer could work well.

【 Question 】What is the antitussive mechanism of Platycodon Root?

实验二　桔梗对小白鼠的化痰作用

【**目的**】学习酚红从呼吸道排泌的实验方法，观察桔梗对小白鼠气管段酚红排泌的影响。

【**原理**】于小白鼠腹腔注射酚红后，后者可以部分地从气管分泌排出。桔梗能增强呼吸道分泌功能，现时也使黏膜排泌的酚红量增加，将气管放入定量的生理盐水中，加碳酸氢钠使其显色。用分光光度计测出酚红的排泌量，从而得知药物的化痰作用。

【**器材**】1 mL 注射器；试管架；10 mL 试管；小鼠灌胃针头；手术剪；眼科镊；蛙板；大头针；分光光度计及比色杯；天平；约 100 mL 烧杯；细棉线；低速离心机。

【**药品**】桔梗水煎液 1 g/mL；复方甘草合剂；酚红溶液 1 mg/mL 及 5 mg/mL；碳酸氢钠溶液 50 mg/mL。

【**动物**】小白鼠。

【**方法**】小白鼠呼吸道酚红冲洗法：酚红在碱性溶液中显红色，用碳酸氢钠溶液将呼吸道内排泌的酚红洗出后，用比色法测其排泌量，从而定量的反应药物的化痰能力。实验前小白鼠禁食 8~12 h，随机分为对照组和给药组。分别灌胃自来水及药物 0.2 mL/10 g。30 min 后每只小鼠腹腔注射酚红溶液 0.2 mL/10 g。再 30 min 后，脱颈椎处死，仰位固定。颈部拉直，解剖分离出气管。在气管下穿一细棉线，以备固定气管插管用。气管插管从甲状软骨插入气管约 0.3 cm，用备好的棉线结扎固定。用 1 mL 注射器吸取 5 g/dL 碳酸氢钠溶液 0.5 mL，推注入气管内。反复连续推 3 次，灌洗呼吸道。最后用注射器将灌洗液抽出注入试管中，按上述方法操作 4 次，合并洗出液约 2 mL，于 1 000 rpm 离心 5 min，取上清于 546 nm 处比色。用碳酸氢钠溶液灌洗气管时，用量要准确；此外，推抽注射速度宜慢，要使液体尽可能抽出，不要把空气推入气管内。

酚红标准液制备：精密称取酚红 0.5 g，溶解于 0.5 mol/L 碳酸氢钠溶液中，加生理盐水到 1 00 mL，摇匀。

酚红标准液配制：用分析天平准确称取一定量酚红，以 5 g/dL 碳酸氢钠溶解，使 1 mL 含酚红 1 000 μg。然后依次稀释，配成每毫升含 1、2、3、4、5、6、7、8、9、10、15、20 μg 的标准比色管，每管容量 3 mL，密封备用。

【**结果**】填入表 14-2。

表 14-2 桔梗提取液对小鼠气管酚红排泌的影响

分组	剂量(g/kg)	酚红排泌量(μg/mL)
桔梗		
甘草合剂		
空白对照		

【注意事项】

1. 解剖气管时勿损伤甲状腺周围血管,以免将血液带进注射器而影响比色。
2. 气管周围如果有出血,尽快用滤纸吸干。
3. 小鼠应及时处死。

【思考题】根据实验结果,分析中药化痰药物作用的强弱,并与临床使用情况比较,效果是否一致?

Experiment 2　The expectorant effect of Platycodi Radix in mice

【Purpose】

1. Study the method of phenolsulfonphthalein secretion test to screen expectorant agents.

2. Observe the effect of Platycodi Radix on phenolsulfonphthalein secretion from the mice's respiratory tract.

【Principles】After phenolsulfonphthalein indicator is injected into mouse's abdominal cavity, it can be partly secreted by bronchi. Platycodi Radix can increase the secretion in bronchi as well as phenolsulfonphthalein secretion in the mucosa of the respiratory tract. Therefore, the expectorant function of the sample can be indirectly deduced by the effect on phenolsulfonphthalein secretion. Phenolsulfonphthalein appeared red in alkali solution and phenolsulfonphthalein in the respiratory tract can be rinsed out by $NaHCO_3$ solution and quantified by colorimetric method through a spectrophotometer.

【Equipments】syringe（1 mL, 0.25 mL）, test tube rack, 10 mL test tube, mice perfusing stomach implement, operating scissors, ophthalmologic forceps, pins, frog board, spectrophotometer, scales, 100 mL beakers, cotton thread, centrifugal machine.

【Drugs and Reagents】Saline, water extract of Platycodi Radix（1 g/mL）, Mistura Glycyrrhizae Composita , phenolsulfonphthalein（0.5 g/dL）, $NaHCO_3$ 50 mg/mL, saline.

【Animals】Mice, weighing 20~24 g.

【Methods】Mice were divided into 3 groups and were orally given with Platycodi Radix（15 g/kg）and saline respectively. Thirty minutes later, a phenolsulfonphthalein solution（5 mg/0.2 mL/10 g body weight）is injected into the mouse's abdominal cavity. After another 30 minutes, the mice are killed by cervical dislocation. The bronchus is isolated and a tracheal intubation is inserted into bronchus（about 3-mm long）and fixed by thread. 0.5 mL $NaHCO_3$ solution is injected into the tracheal slowly and suction into a tube. The work above is repeated 4 times and the collected fluid would be about 2 mL. The fluid is mixed together, centrifuged at 1,000 rpm for 5 min, then the absorption of the supernatant is detected at 546 nm with a spectrophotometer. The quantity of phenolsulfonphthalein（μg/mL）is counted according to the OD values and the data is compared with that of blank group.

Preparation of standard curve: phenolsulfonphthalein is dissolved in 0.5 mol/L $NaHCO_3$ solution to prepare the primary solution with a concentration of 1 mg/mL. Then, the primary solution is diluted with 0.5 mol/L $NaHCO_3$ one by one to get a series of concentration of 1、2、3、4、5、6、7、8、9、10、15、20 μg/mL, and the related absorptions are determined with a spectrophotometer at 546 nm. At last, the standard curve is fitted according the concentrations and corresponding absorptions by computer.

【Results】Polygala Root can increase the phenolsulfonphthalein secretion in the bronchi in mice.

Table 14–2 The effect of water extract of Polygala Root on phenolsulfonphthalein secretion from mouse's bronchus

Group	Dose (g/kg)	phenolsulfonphthalein secretion (μg/mL)
Polygala Root		
Mistura Glycyrrhizae Composita		
Control		

【Notes】

1. The bronchus should be isolated gently in case of damaging thyroid and blood vessel nearby.

2. The blood adhered to the bronchus should be cleaned by the filter paper as soon as you can.

3. Mice must be killed on time.

【Question】Analyze the expectorant effect of traditional Chinese medicine according to the results of this experiment.

实验三　小青龙汤对豚鼠组胺引喘的平喘作用

【目的】学习用组胺喷雾诱导豚鼠哮喘的方法。观察小青龙汤的平喘作用。

【原理】小青龙汤是治疗老年人的慢性支气管炎、支气管哮喘等的常用方剂。本实验利用磷酸组胺造成哮喘模型，观察小青龙汤的平喘作用。组胺类药物以喷雾法给药，可引起豚鼠支气管痉挛、窒息，使动物抽搐而跌倒。利用这种模型，可观察支气管平滑肌松弛药的平喘作用。

【器材】台秤；注射器；喷雾装置；秒表。

【药品和试剂】0.5 g/mL 小青龙汤醇提液；1 mg/mL 磷酸组胺；生理盐水。

【动物】幼年豚鼠，雌雄兼用。

【方法】实验前一天选体重 150~200 g 幼年豚鼠若干只，分别置喷雾箱内，以 53.3~66.6 kPa（400~500 mmHg）压力喷入 1 mg/mL 磷酸组胺 1 mL，动物在吸入以上药液后经过一定的潜伏期，即产生哮喘反应，动物“哮喘”反应的发生先是呼吸加速，然后呼吸困难，最后抽搐以致跌倒。动物一出现抽搐，即拉开箱门取出动物，必要时辅以人工呼吸，以免动物因窒息而死亡。同时记录引喘潜伏期（从喷雾开始到抽搐跌倒的时间），一般不超过 150 s，超过 150 s 者可认为不敏感，不予选用。

次日将预选过的“哮喘”豚鼠随机分为 2 组，每组 10 只，一组灌胃 0.5 g/mL 小青龙汤 10 g/kg，一组灌胃相同剂量的生理盐水，给药后 15 min 重复给药一次，给药后 30 min，分别放入喷雾装置内按预选时的同样条件分别喷雾磷酸组胺。记录喷雾开始至症状出现的时间（以抽搐、跌倒为准）作为潜伏时间，记录各组动物潜伏期。

【结果】将各组动物的潜伏期填入表 14-3。

表 14-3　小青龙汤的平喘作用

分组	给药剂量（g/kg）	引喘潜伏期（秒）	
		给药前	给药后
生理盐水组			
小青龙汤组			

【注意事项】

1. 每鼠每天只能测定一次引喘潜伏期，同一天多次测定会影响实验结果。
2. 一般观察 360 s，不跌倒者引喘潜伏期以 360 s 计算。
3. 有刺激性的药物，腹腔给药减少动物呼吸，可出现假阳性结果。

【思考题】分析小青龙汤的平喘作用机理。

Experiment 3 The antiasthmatic effect of Xiaoqinglong decoction in guinea pig stimulated with histamine

【Purpose】

1. Study the method of inducing asthma model in Guinea pigs by spraying histamine.

2. Observe the antiasthmatic effect of Xiaoqinglong decoction.

【Principles】Xiaoqinglong decoction is a traditional formula usually used in the treatment of chronic bronchitis and bronchial asthma in aged people. The current experiment aime to to observe the antiasthmatic effect of Xiaoqinglong decoction in the asthmatic model induced by histamine challenge. Histamine spraying induces bronchial spasm and asphyxia in guinea pig, and therefore this model is usually used to investigate the effects of antiasthmatic agents on bronchus relaxation.

【Equipments】Bench scale, spraying assembly, syringe, seconds-counter.

【Drugs and reagents】Ethanol extract of Xiaoqinglong decoction 0.5 g/mL, histamine phosphate 1 mg/mL, saline.

【Animals】Guinea pigs, 150~220 g, male or female.

【Methods】One day before the experiment, young guinea pigs are kept in a spraying assembly and exposed to 1 mL sprayed histamine phosphate at the stable pressure of 53.3~66.6 kPa. Then the response of the animals was observed. In general, the guinea pigs breathe deeper and faster at first, and then they show signs of dyspnoea, tic and stumble. When the guinea pigs stumble, take the animals out of the spraying assembly as soon as possible, or they will die. The latent period of inducing asthma (time from beginning of spray to the appearance of tic and stumble) was recorded. Generally, the latent period is no more than 150 s. If the period exceeds 150 s, the guinea pig is not qualified for the experiment because it is not sensitive to the stimulation.

On the second day, the sensitive guinea pigs are divided into 2 groups, 10 animals per group. Guinea pigs in one group are treated orally with the ethanol extract of Xiaoqinglong decoction (10 g/kg), the other group of animals are orally administrated with saline. Fifteen min later, Xiaoqinglong decoction or saline is given orally again at the same dose. Thirty min later, guinea pigs are put into the spraying assembly according to the above-mentioned protocols. The latent period of each guinea pig is recorded.

【Results】The latent periods of the two different groups of guinea pigs are filled in the Table 14-3.

Table 14-3　The antiasthmatic effect of Xiaoqinglong decoction in guinea pig

Group	Dose (g/kg)	Latent period (s)	
		Before treatment	After treatment
Saline			
Xiaoqinglong decoction			

[Notes]

1. Each guinea pig can only be used one time for the measurement of the latent period in one day because some guinea pigs may be tolerant to histamine if they contact histamine for several times.

2. If the latent period exceeds 360 s, take it as 360 s.

3. Some amyctic drugs might reduce the animal breath and thus induce a false-positive results.

[Question] Analyze the antiasthmatic mechanisms of Xiaoqinglong decoction.

实验四　贝母辛对豚鼠气管条的舒张作用

【**目的**】学习用豚鼠气管条的制备方法。观察贝母辛的气管舒张作用。

【**原理**】贝母辛是从彭泽贝母中分离出的生物碱类成分，具有扩张支气管作用。本实验利用乙酰胆碱体外诱导豚鼠气管条收缩，并观察贝母辛的舒张作用。

【**器材**】BL-420 生物机能实验系统；HV-4 型离体组织器官恒温灌流系统；移液器。

【**药品和试剂**】10 mg/mL 贝母辛（DMSO 溶解后以双蒸水配成混悬液）；氯化乙酰胆碱（或磷酸组胺）；DMSO；克氏液［Krebs solution 组成（mM）：NaCl 118, KCl 4.7, KH_2PO_4 1.18, $MgSO_4$ 1.18, $NaHCO_3$ 25, glucose 5.6, $CaCl_2$ 2.5］。

【**动物**】豚鼠，雌雄兼用。

【**方法**】

1. 气管条的制备　处死豚鼠，迅速取出气管置于冷的通有 95 %O_2 +5 %CO_2 混合气体的克氏液中，剔除周围的软组织。将豚鼠气管剪成螺旋条，宽约 3 mm，长约为 20 mm。悬挂于盛有 5 mL 克氏液的恒温（37 ± 0.5）℃浴槽中，上端接肌肉张力换能器，连接 BL-420 生物机能实验系统，将气管螺旋条初负荷给予 1.5 g。每 15 min 换液 1 次，平衡约 1 h 后开始正式实验。

2. 对乙酰胆碱（ACh）诱导的豚鼠气管平滑肌收缩的影响　待气管螺旋条基线稳定后，以累积法加入 ACh（终浓度为 1×10^{-9}~1×10^{-4}），记录各浓度引起气管收缩张力值（G）。加入 ACh（终浓度为 1×10^{-4}）引起的最大收缩幅度记为 G_{max}，此时的最大收缩率记为 E_{max}（100 %），以 $G/G_{max} \times 100$ % 计算气管条对不同 Ach 浓度产生的收缩率，绘制 Ach 量效关系曲线。以克氏液冲洗气管条 3 次，每 15 min 更换 1 次，待基线恢复到实验前，分别加入终浓度为 0.01、0.05 mmol/L 贝母辛溶液，孵育 20 min 后重复上述 Ach 的加入过程，记录各浓度引起气管收缩幅度（G'），计算收缩率（G'/G_{max}）。同时设置溶剂（DMSO）对照组。

【**结果**】将实验结果填入表 14-4。

表 14-4　贝母辛的气管舒张作用

分组	给药浓度（mol/L）	收缩率（%）											
		给药前						给药后					
		10^{-9}	10^{-8}	10^{-7}	10^{-6}	10^{-5}	10^{-4}	10^{-9}	10^{-8}	10^{-7}	10^{-6}	10^{-5}	10^{-4}
DMSO	—												
贝母辛	0.01												
	0.05												

【**注意事项**】药液避光低温保存，尽快用完。

【**思考题**】分析贝母辛的舒张气管平滑肌作用。

Experiment 4　The Effect of Peimisine on ACh-induced contraction of tracheal strips from guinea pigs

【Purpose】

1. Learn the method of preparing guinea pig tracheal strips.

2. Observe the smooth muscle relaxant effect of peimisine.

【Principles】 Peimisine is an alkaloid isolated from Fritilllaria monantha Migo and is reported with bronchial smooth muscle relaxation activity. In the current study, we will induce the contraction of guinea pig tracheal strips with acetylcholine (ACh) and observe the relaxant effect of peimisine.

【Equipments】 BL-420 biofunctional laboratory system, HV-4 organ bath system, micropipette.

【Drug and reagents】 Peimisine 10 mg/mL, DMSO、Krebs solution. (mM: NaCl 118, KCl 4.7, KH_2PO_4 1.18, $MgSO_4$ 1.18, $NaHCO_3$ 25, glucose 5.6, $CaCl_2$ 2.5.)

【Animals】 Guinea pigs, male or female.

【Methods】

1. Preparation of tracheal spiral strips　guinea pigs are killed and the tracheas are immediately isolated and cleared the adherent connective tissue. Tracheas are cut into 20 × 3 mm spiral strips and suspended in 5 mL organ baths containing Krebs solution. The tissues were maintained at 37 ℃ and continually gassed with 5% CO_2 in O_2. A passive tension of 1.5 g was applied to tracheal preparations. Tension was maintained in Krebs solution (Change the solution every 15 min) for a 60 minute equilibration period until it achieved a steady state.

2. ACh-induced contraction of tracheal spiral strips　After the response of tracheal preparations recover to the baseline, these strips are contracted with ACh (final concentration 1×10^{-9}~1×10^{-4}) (ACh is added into the baths cumulatively), and the contraction (G) is recorded. The contraction induced by the addition of 1×10^{-4} ACh is regarded as the maximal response (G_{max}), and the contraction rate at this point is the maximal contraction rate (E_{max}, 100%). Thus G/Gmax is calculated as the contraction rate in response to various concentrations of ACh in order to prepare the dose-effect curve. The strips are then rinsed three times with Krebs solution at the internal of 15 min. After the baseline recovers to that before the addition of ACh, tissue preparations are pretreated with 0.01 or 0.05 mmol/L (final concentration) peimisine for 20 min prior to exposure to ACh (1×10^{-9}~1×10^{-4}) as mentioned above. The tension is recorded as G', and the contraction rate after treatment of

peimisine is calculated as G'/G_{max}. DMSO is used as a blank control.

【Results】Data are filled into table 14-4.

Table 14-4 The effect of peimisine on ACh-induced contraction of tracheal strips in guinea pigs

Group	Conc. (mol/L)	Contraction rate (%)											
		Before treatment of peimisine						after addition of peimisine					
		10^{-9}	10^{-8}	10^{-7}	10^{-6}	10^{-5}	10^{-4}	10^{-9}	10^{-8}	10^{-7}	10^{-6}	10^{-5}	10^{-4}
DMSO	—												
Peimisine	0.01												
	0.05												

【Note】The reagents and peimisine should be kept in dark at low temperature and used as soon as possible.

【Questions】Analyze the effect of peimisine on tracheal smooth muscle.

第十五章　安神药和平肝息风药实验

凡以镇静安神为主要功效的药物称为安神药。多用于心气虚、心血虚或心火盛以及其他原因所致的心神不宁、烦躁易怒、失眠多梦、头晕目眩等证。现代药理学研究证明，多数安神药具有抑制中枢神经系统的作用，不同的安神药还分别具有明目、解毒、润肠等功效。

凡具有平肝息风或潜阳镇静作用的药物称为平肝息风药。这一类药物主要用于肝阳上亢、肝风内动所致内风诸病，如阳邪热盛所致高热神昏，四肢抽搐之证等。平息肝风药主要具有镇静、抗惊厥、降压等药理作用，另外还有抗炎、镇痛、解热，抗肿瘤，影响机体免疫功能，影响心血管系统功能以及调节消化系统功能等作用。由于平息肝风药可以作用于中枢神经系统及心血管系统，所以在研究这类药物时，一般从降压和对中枢神经系统方面的影响来设计实验动物模型和实验指标。常用的实验方法如下：

1. 降压实验　血压的测定有直接测压法（插管法）和间接测压法（大鼠尾动脉测压法等）。降压药的研究常分为三个步骤：①首先观察药物对正常麻醉动物的急性降压作用：将动物麻醉后，直接测量其颈动脉或股动脉的血压。此法简单，但由于与临床实际有距离，所以仅用于初筛。②慢性实验治疗法：用高血压模型动物来观察药物的治疗作用. 动物的高血压模型有肾型、神经型、内分泌型和遗传性等，血压测定常采用间接测压法。此法接近临床实际情况，主要用于复试。③降压作用机制研究：通过上述实验证明药物有降压作用后，近一步通过对中枢、神经节、递质、受体、血管平滑肌、水盐代谢等方面试验来分析药物的作用环节。

2. 中枢神经抑制实验　包括镇静、催眠、抗惊厥实验以及镇痛和解热实验。一般常在小鼠腹腔或灌胃给药后，观察是否出现安静、活动减少、嗜睡或睡眠等外观行为的改变。可采用光电管法、吊笼法、转轮法观察药物对小鼠自由活动的影响以及与戊巴比妥类药物的协同作用。戊巴比妥类是典型的中枢抑制药，凡是对中枢神经有抑制作用的药物，一般都能增强其中枢抑制作用。对此，常用延长戊巴比妥所致睡眠时间及对戊巴比妥阈下催眠剂量的影响来进行研究。对抗中枢兴奋药的作用，是利用它们能减低兴奋药的过度自发活动来筛选；也可用其对抗中枢兴奋药毒性，以提高半数致死量来衡量；还可以利用其对抗某种兴奋药的效应来确定作用部位。抗惊厥实验，主要是利用电刺激和化学制剂引起动物惊厥发作，观察药物的影响。常用致惊剂有戊四唑、士的宁等。镇痛实验常用化学刺激法、热刺激法、电刺激法、机械刺激法等各种致痛方法引起疼痛，观察药物的镇痛作用。

Chapter 15 Experiments for tranquilizer and Liver-Wind suppressing medicine

It is named as tranquilizer which function is sedative and tranquilized. This kind of drugs are commonly used in syndrome of inquietude, vexation, agitation, irascibility, insomnia, excessive dream and vertigo mainly induced by deficiency of Heart Qi and Blood or exuberance of Heart Fire. Modern pharmacology research has proved that different tranquilizers also have activities of improving vision, resolving toxicity and moistening intestines besides of suppressing central nerve system.

Drugs which can suppress Liver-Wind or subside Yang for sedation belong to the kind of medicine suppressing hyperactive liver for calming endogenous wind in Traditional Chinese Medicine（TCM）.They are mainly applied for Liver-Yang ascending and internal stirring of Liver-Wind, such as syndrome of high fever, dizzy and convulsion limbs induced by excessive Yang. In TCM, it is said they not only have activities of sedation, anti-convulsion, lowering blood pressure, anti-inflammation, analgesic and anti-tumor, but also have functional modulations on immunity, cardiovascular and digestive system. Considering effects on central nerve and cardiovascular system, animal models and related targets which affect blood pressure and CNS are always used. Experiments methods in common use are as following:

1. Experiments for depressing blood pressure（BP） There are two ways to detect BP that is direct（intubatton tests）and indirect measurement（test of rat tail blood pressure, etc.）. Study on antihypertensive medicine is usually disparted into three steps：① Firstly, we should investigate their acute depression on BP in normal and anesthetic animals：Usually, animals are measured BP in carotid and femoral arteries directly. This test is easy but only used in original screening on account of little coincident with clinic practice. ② Chronic treatment tests：It is introduced to study drug action by indirect measurement. Experiment hypertensive model covered are induced by numerous reasons such as renal, nerve, incretion and transmissibility, etc. These methods which are close to clinic truth are mostly used in retrial. ③ Study on mechanism：On

the base of foregoing tests' results we can discover the antihypertensive and then investigate its mechanism further by tests of nerve centre, ganglion, neurotransmitters, accepter, vas smooth muscle and metabolism of water and sodium.

2. Experiments for suppressing centre nerve It concludes sedative-hypnotic and anti-convulsion tests as well as experiments on easing pain and releasing heat. Sedative experiment is mostly used to evaluate drugs function after peritoneal injection or oral administration. We can design photoelectric cell test, activity cage or rota-rod test to assess the locomotion movement in mice. Whether animals appear to be quiet, less of movement, sleepy or sleeping, it is illustrated that the drug has sedative or suppressive property. Furthermore, tests of synergism with pentobarbital are also applied. Any medicines which possess inhibitive effect on CNS usually can enhance the function from pentobarbital, which is the typical suppressor of central nerve. Hence, it is the common experiments to study potentiation of pentobarbital-induced sleep at hypnotic and sub-hypnotic dosage. Besides, antagonize effect against analeptics also can be evaluated by original screening test on locomotion activity which is increased by analeptics and decreased by suppressor of central nerve. Otherwise, half lethal concentration (LD_{50}) is cited in evaluating antagonize effect on analeptics toxicity. These tests can illustrate functional site as well. Furthermore, we can observe drug effect in anticonvulsant experiments which lead the outbreak of convulsion by electricity and chemical stimulation. And chemical stimulation concludes pentylenetetrazol and strychnine belonging to common convulsants. Finally, animals stimulated by chemical, heat, electricity and even machine are test for evaluating abirritation from medicines in Pain Relief Experiment.

一、中枢神经系统实验

实验一　天麻对小白鼠入睡个数的影响

【**目的**】通过天麻对小鼠入睡个数的影响，了解它的镇静作用。

【**原理**】天麻具有息风、平肝、定惊等功效，有镇静和抗惊厥作用。本实验用阈下剂量戊巴比妥钠与天麻合用，观察天麻与戊巴比妥钠的协同作用。如有协同作用，则可使小鼠入睡个数增加。由此来验证天麻对中枢神经系统的抑制作用。

【**器材**】注射器；天平。

【**试剂**】天麻注射液 2 mL/ 支（合原生药 0.5 g）；生理盐水；苦味酸溶液。

【**动物**】小白鼠。

【**方法**】以翻正反射消失 1 min 以上为入睡指标。取健康小鼠，按体重随机分为 2 组，用苦味酸标记。分别腹腔注射天麻注射液 0.2 mL/10 g 及等容量生理盐水。给药 30 min 后每鼠腹腔注射戊巴比妥钠 30 mg/kg，比较给药组与对照组的入睡个数，用卡方检验进行统计分析。

【**结果**】实验结果按表 15-1 记录。

表 15–1　天麻对小鼠入睡个数的影响

组别	动物数	剂量（g/kg）	入睡动物数
对照组			
天麻组			

【**注意事项**】

1. 戊巴比妥钠溶液要新鲜配制。
2. 每次实验前都要预试，找出戊巴比妥钠的阈下剂量。
3. 实验过程中要保持安静。

1 Experiment on CNS

Experiment 1 Effect of Gastrodia Elata on falling asleep in mice

【**Purpose**】For investigating the sedative effect of Gastrodia Elata by observing falling asleep in mice.

【**Principles**】As one of Traditional Chinese medicine, which can pacify the liver, extinguish wind and calm fright, GE has an efficiency on sedation and anti-convulsion. In order to prove the inhibition of GE on CNS, we observe the synergetic effect of GE with sub-hypnotic dosage of pentobarbital sodium in mice, which is indicated by the increased number of mice falling asleep after combination.

【**Experiments**】Injectors, Scale, etc.

【**Reagents**】Injection of Gastrodia Elata 2 mL/vial (crude drug in whole is 0.5 g), saline, picric acid solution.

【**Animals**】Mice.

【**Methods**】Randomize mice into 2 groups according to body weight and mark each with picric acid. Peritoneal injection of Gastrodia Elata (0.2 mL/10 g weight) and saline with equal volume was administered 30 min before the test。 Following injection of pentobarbital sodium (24 mg/kg was used as sub-hypnotic dosage), each mouse was observed for the sleep onset, and the loss of righting reflex over 1 min is considered to be asleep. And then Chi-square test is used to compare the animal numbers of falling asleep.

【**Results**】Note test results according to the table 15-1.

Table15–1 The effect of GE on mice number of falling asleep

Groups	*N*	Dose (g/kg)	Number of falling asleep
Control			
GE Group			

【**Notes**】

1. Solution of pentobarbital sodium need to be made freshly.
2. please titrate the sub-hypnotic dosage of pentobarbital sodium before the true test.
3. Keep quiet during the test.

实验二　酸枣仁对小鼠的镇静作用

【目的】观察酸枣仁对小鼠自发活动的影响。

【原理】自发活动是正常动物的生理特征。自发活动的多少往往能反映中枢兴奋或抑制作用状态。自发活动减少的程度与中枢抑制药的作用强度成正比。

【器材】药理生理多用仪器及附件；注射器；鼠笼。

【试剂】200% 酸枣仁溶液；生理盐水等。

【动物】小白鼠。

【方法】

1. 将药理生理多用仪前面板左中钮开关下拨“计数”，把两端装有中型插头的导线一端插入多用仪后面板“计数输入”插口，另一端插入活动计数盒，再用地线引出线将多用仪后面板“地线”接线柱与附件盒上黑色线柱相连，然后把金属安放入附件盒，圆心放置在突起的尖端上即可进行实验。取活动度相近的小鼠 4 只，称重，标记。分别将小鼠放入自发活动记录装置的盒内，使其适应环境 5 min。然后开始计算时间，观察并记录 5 min 后数码管上显示的数字，作为给药前的对照值。

2. 将小鼠随机分组，每组两只。其中两只灌胃酸枣仁溶液（0.1 mg/10 g，0.05% 溶液 0.2 mL/10 g）；两只腹腔注射生理盐水 0.2 mL/10 g。给药后将小鼠放回盒内，每个 10 min 按上述方法记录活动次数一次，连续观察两次（即至 30 min）。

【结果】实验数据记录于表 15-2 中。

表 15-2　酸枣仁对小鼠的镇静作用

鼠号	体重	药物及剂量	5 min 内活动计数			
			给药前		给药后	
			10~15 min	25~30 min	10~15 min	25~30 min

【注意事项】环境应尽量安静。

【思考题】本方法适用于测定哪些药物？

Experiment 2　Calming effect of Semen in mice

【Purpose】Study about the effects of Semen to spontaneous activity of mice.

【Principles】Spontaneous activity is a normal physiological characteristics of animals. The number of spontaneous activity can often reflect the state of excitability or inhibition. The degree of reduction in spontaneous activity is proportional with potency of central inhibitor.

【Experiments】Pharmacological and physiological multi-instrument accessories, syringes, squirrel.

【Reagents】200% Semen solution, saline and so on.

【Animals】Mice.

【Methods】

1. Twist the switch on the front panel to stir "count" . One end of the plug is inserted into the multipurpose instrument "count input" and another one is inserted into the skill box. Connect the multi-purpose instrument panel "wire" to the column in Annex box on the black terminal with ground pinout. Then the metal box was put into the accessories. The experiment center of the circle can be placed on the tip of the spike. After weighing and tagging, The mouse was placed in a spontaneous activity recording device boxes, which can adapt to the environment for 5 minutes. And then began to calculation time, observe and record 5 minutes after the digital tube display digital, as to the value before the control.

2. The mice were randomly divided into 2 groups:the treatment and the control. 2 rats in each group. Ziziphi Spinosae Semen solution was given by intragastric administration (0.1 mg/10 g, 0.05% solution 0.2 mL/10 g) and mice in the control were given same volvum of salin. , After administration, mice are put back to the box, and spontancous activity was observed for 10 minutes (repeat two times).

【Results】Write down your data in the table 15-2.

Table 15-2 The calming effect of Semen in mice

mouse	weight	drug dosage	Activities count in 5 minutes			
			Before administration		after administration	
			10~15 min	25~30 min	10~15 min	25~30 min

[Note] Experiments should be conducted in a quiet place as much as possible.

[Questions] What drugs are applicable to this method?

实验三　柴胡加龙骨牡蛎汤总皂苷对皮质酮诱导 PC12 细胞损伤的保护作用

【目的】学习皮质酮诱导 PC12 细胞损伤模型的制备方法；观察柴胡加龙骨牡蛎总皂苷（SCLM）对 PC12 细胞的保护作用。

【原理】糖皮质激素是调节机体活动的一种重要的内分泌激素，它的作用几乎涉及人体的每一个器官，例如调节能量代谢、免疫功能、性功能、情绪反应等。皮质酮作为一种糖皮质激素，在临床前的研究中应用非常广泛，皮质酮能调节神经元存活、神经元的兴奋性、神经发生等，但是高含量的皮质酮能通过这些作用损伤大脑的神经元。SCLM 能显著抑制皮质酮诱导的 PC12 细胞的损伤。

【器材】圆底烧瓶；冷凝管；大孔树脂柱；旋转蒸发仪；96 孔平底细胞培养板；移液器（1 mL, 200 μL）及相应吸头；细胞培养箱；酶标仪。

【试剂】D101 大孔吸附树脂；石油醚；乙酸乙酯；正丁醇；皮质酮；PBS；DMEM；SCLM；氟西汀；MTT[溴化（4,5）-二甲基-2-噻唑基-2, 5-二苯基四氮唑]。

【细胞】NFG 分化过的 PC12 细胞。

【方法】

1. 柴胡加龙骨牡蛎汤总皂苷（SCLM）的制备　称取柴胡加龙骨牡蛎汤方中各药材（柴胡 62.4 g、黄芩 23.4 g、半夏 25 g、人参 23.4 g、生姜 23.4 g、大枣 6 枚、桂枝 23.4 g、大黄 31.2 g、茯苓 23.4 g、龙骨 23.4 g、牡蛎 23.4 g）制成水煎液，使用分液漏斗作为萃取工具，首先用石油醚萃取，按 1∶1 加入石油醚，适当摇匀，静置分层，收集上层萃取液，重复萃取 3 次，合并萃取液；水层继续用等量乙酸乙酯萃取摇匀，重复 3 次，合并萃取液；水层继续用等量正丁醇萃取，重复 3 次，合并萃取液。3 种有机溶剂萃取液均用旋转蒸发仪减压回收溶剂，回收有机溶剂时，在完全回收结束前，即剩余少量溶剂不回收，转入蒸发皿中，低温挥发剩余溶剂得浸膏。D101 大孔吸附树脂用 90 % 乙醇液浸泡 12 h，装柱，然后用 90% 乙醇液洗脱杂质，控制流速为 2 倍柱体积（BV）/h，洗至 1 mL 洗脱液与 3 mL 蒸馏水混合澄清为止；加 5% HCl 浸泡过夜，2BV 5% HCl 洗脱，水洗脱至 pH 中性；加 5% NaOH 浸泡过夜，2 BV 5% NaOH 洗脱，水洗脱至 pH 中性。将上述正丁醇萃取部位浸膏用蒸馏水充分溶解成均一溶液，吸附于已处理好的 D101 大孔树脂柱[萃取部分和树脂的体积比为 1∶（15~20）]吸附 12 h 后，分别以 30% 乙醇反复洗脱至无色，洗脱速度 5 mL/min。合并洗脱液，低温挥发 30% 乙醇洗脱部分得干粉。SCLM 用无血清培养基溶解，配成 50 μg/mL，用 0.25 μm 的微孔滤膜过滤除菌。

2. PC12 细胞培养及分组给药　用含 10% 胎牛血清的 DMEM 培养基（含青霉素钠 200 U/mL，链霉素 100 μg/mL，pH 7.4）将细胞稀释为每毫升悬液含 2×10^5 个细胞，接种于 96 孔培养板，每孔 100 μL，放入 CO_2 培养箱，37 ℃，5% CO_2 条件下培养 2~4 天，待细胞长满孔底后即用于实验。细胞分为以下 4 组，*n*=8/ 组。对照组（Control）单纯更换无血清 DMEM 培养基，不含任何药品；模型组加入含有 100 μM 皮质酮的无血清 DMEM 培养基；SCLM 组加入终浓度为 100 μM 皮质酮及 50 μg/mL 的 SCLM；阳性对照组每孔加入 100 μM 皮质酮及 10 μM 氟西汀，37 ℃培养 24 h。

3. MTT 法检测细胞活力　取 96 孔板内贴壁生长的 PC12 细胞，每孔加入终浓度为 0.5 mg/mL MTT，继续培养 4 h 后吸去 DMEM 培养基，每孔加入二甲基亚砜（DMSO）100 μL，振摇混匀 10 min，待孔内颗粒完全溶解后，在酶标仪 490 nm 处测定吸光度（A 490 nm）值。

【结果】将结果填入表 15-3 中。

表 15-3　柴胡加龙骨牡蛎总皂苷对皮质酮诱导 PC12 细胞损伤的保护作用

分组	剂量	皮质酮（μM）	吸光度（A 490 nm）
空白组			
模型组			
SCLM 组			
氟西汀组			

【注意事项】

1. 操作需规范，避免染菌。
2. 每孔细胞量需保持一致。

【思考题】

1. 分析造模原理及药物作用的可能机制。
2. 如何改进方法？

Experiment 3　Protective effects of SCLM against corticosterone-induced neuronal injury in PC12 cells

【Purpose】 To learn the method how to establish a modle of neuronal injury in PC12 cells and observe the protective effect of SCLM on PC12 cell.

【Principles】 Glucocorticoids have multiple functions in almost every tissue of the human body, such as regulation of energy metabolism (through increased gluconeogenesis, lipolysis and protein degradation), regulation of immune functions, sexuality and mood. Cortisol is known to regulate neuronal survival, neuronal excitability, neurogenesis, whereas high levels of cortisol may impairing brain functions. SCLM can significantly attenuates corticosterone-induced injury in PC12 cell.

【Equipments】 round-bottom flask, condenser pipe, macroporous resin column, rotary evaporators, 96-well culture plates, transferpettors (10 μL -1,000 μL), plastical tubes (1.5 mL, 5 mL), water bath, cell incubator, spectrophotometer.

【Reagents】 Dulbecco's modified eagle's medium (DMEM), D101 macroporous adsorption resin, petroleum ether, acetic ester, n-butanol, SCLM saponins (SCLM) extracted from a traditional Chinese medicine, Chaihu-jia-longgu-muli-tang (CLM), fluoxetine, 3-(4, 5-dimethylthiazol-2-yl)-2, 5-diphenyl tetrazolium bromide (MTT).

【Cell】 The pheochromocytoma cells (PC12).

【Methods】

1. Preparation of saponins　Each material were mixed to the given ratio and extracted with water. The filtrates were collected and mixed together, and then the solution was extracted successively with petroleum ether, acetic ester and n-butanol. The n-butanol soluble fraction was dried in vacuum at 40 ℃ into a brown powder, then the powder was dissolved in distilled water and eluted through macroporous absorption resin, first with distilled water in order to eliminate carbohydrates and other water soluble principles, then eluted with 30% ethanol repeatedly. The combined elutes of 30% ethanol were concentrated under reduced pressure at 40 ℃. Prior to treatment with PC12 cells, SCLM was dissolved and diluted with serum-free DMEM and was sterilized by filtration through 0.25 μm Millipore filter and stored at 4 ℃ .

2. Cell culture and evaluation of cell viability　The cells were seeded into 96-well plates at a density of 2×10^5 /mL and cultured in the medium consisting of 90% Dulbecco's Modified Eagle Medium (DMEM), 10% fetal calf serum, 200 kU/L benzyl penicillin and

100 mg/L streptomycin in a humidified incubator with 5% CO_2, 37 ℃ for 2~4 days. The cells were divided into four equal groups: control, control, 100 μM Cort, 10 μM Cort + SCLM (50 μg/mL), 100 μM Cort + FLU (10 μM), *n*=8 per group, 37 ℃ for 24 h.

3. Evaluation of cell viability In the MTT assay, after two washes with D-Hanks, the cells were incubated with 0.5 mg/mL MTT added to the growth medium for 4 h at 37 ℃ . The medium was then aspirated and the MTT reduction product, formazan, was dissolved in dimethyl sulfoxide (DMSO) and quantified spectrophotometrically at 490 nm (A490 nm values).

【Results】 Write down your data in the table 15-3.

Table 15-3 Effects of SCLM on corticosterone-induced injury in PC12 cells

Group	dose	CORT (μM)	absorbancy (A 490 nm)
control			
model			
SCLM			
Fluoxetine			

【Notes】

1. Operation should be subject to regulations to avoid contamination.

2. The quantity of cells per well should be keep the same.

【Questions】

1. Analyze the mechanisms of the preparation of model and the effect of SCLM on cell survival.

2. How will you improve the experimental design?

二、降压法

实验四　钩藤对麻醉大鼠血压的影响（直接测压法）

【目的】学习直接测定大鼠血压的方法；了解钩藤对大鼠血压的影响。

【原理】将动脉插管插入颈总动脉，动脉插管与压力换能器构成抗凝密闭系统，压力换能器与生物信号采集处理系统相连，记录动脉血压。钩藤为平肝息风之要药，主治肝阳偏亢，肝风上扰所致头痛，眩晕。通过本实验可证明钩藤的降压作用。

【器材】大鼠固定板；注射器；气管插管；动脉插管；静脉插管；动脉夹；手术丝线；手术器械；血压换能器；二道生理多用仪。

【试剂】1% 盐酸钩藤碱溶液；钩藤提取物（1 g/mL）；生理盐水；5% 枸橼酸钠溶液；3% 戊巴比妥钠溶液；1% 氯化乙酰胆碱溶液；盐酸肾上腺素（0.1 mg/mL）。

【动物】大鼠。

【方法】取大鼠，称重，戊巴比妥钠 35 mg/kg 腹腔注射麻醉后仰位固定于鼠台上，进行以下操作：

1. 气管插管　在颈部正中线切开皮肤约 3 cm，用止血钳分离两侧肌肉，露出气管，在气管下穿一细线，提起气管，作“⊥”形切口，向肺方向插入 Y 形气管插管，用细线扎紧固定，作呼吸通气用。

2. 颈动脉插管　根据动脉搏动找到颈动脉鞘，分离颈总动脉周围组织及迷走神经，使其游离，并在其下面穿两根线，远心端结扎，用动脉夹夹住近心端，在近线结处向心方向剪一“V”切口，插入充满枸橼酸钠溶液并连接压力换能器的动脉插管，结扎固定。

3. 静脉插管　在腹股沟处触及股动脉搏动处，纵向切开皮肤 3 cm，分离出股静脉，在其下穿两根线，远心端结扎，于线结处向心方向剪一“Λ”切口，插入有生理盐水的静脉插管，结扎固定，供输液、给药用。

另外分别给右侧颈总动脉和两侧迷走神经下穿上手术丝线，以备作加压反射及提拉迷走神经后切断之用。

以上操作完成，放开动脉夹，即可进行血压描计及给药观察。

按以下步骤进行实验：

（1）快速耐受性实验：待血压平稳后记录血压值。静注盐酸钩藤碱溶液 1 mL/100 g 体重，或钩藤提取物 2 mL/100 g 体重，记录降压值。待血压基本恢复用药前水平时，再次注射相同剂量的钩藤碱或提取物，比较两次降压值。

（2）对中枢性加压反射的影响：血压平稳后，将右侧颈总动脉上的手术丝线提起，立即用动脉夹夹住颈动脉，阻断血流 30 s，测两次加压反射的血压变化，再比较给药前后加压反射血压平均升高的差异。

（3）对乙酰胆碱的作用：描记颈动脉血压，静注乙酰胆碱 0.1 mL/kg。待血压恢复后，静注钩藤碱或钩藤提取物；在血压还未提升时，再注射相同剂量的乙酰胆碱，观察血压的变化。

（4）对肾上腺素的作用：描记颈动脉血压，静注盐酸肾上腺素 0.05 mL/kg，记录血压上升值。待血压恢复后，静注钩藤碱或钩藤提取物；在血压还未回升时，再注射相同剂量的肾上腺素，观察血压的变化。

（5）对迷走神经的影响：待血压平稳后记录血压值。静注盐酸钩藤碱溶液 1 mL/100 g 体重，或钩藤提取物 2 mL/100 g 体重，记录降压值。切断两侧迷走神经，血压稳定后再注射钩藤碱或钩藤提取物，观察血压的变化。分析钩藤对未切断迷走神经和切断迷走神经动物血压的影响有何不同。

【结果】实验结果按表 15-4 记录。

表 15-4　钩藤碱降压作用机理的分析

项目	血压(mmHg)					
	给药前		差值	给药后		差值
	处理前	处理后		处理前	处理后	
快速耐受						
加压反射						
乙酰胆碱						
肾上腺素						
迷走神经						

【思考题】钩藤的降压作用及其机理如何？

2. Experiment for pressuring blood pressure

Experiment 4　Effect of Uncaria rhynchophylla (UR) on blood pressure measured in anesthetic rats

【Purpose】 Study the method of testing rat BP directly and illustrate the effect of Uncaria rhynchophylla on blood pressure.

【Principles】 BP recordings are collected by biosignal scan and analysis system, connected with blood pressure transducer in anticoagulant obturator which is constituted by artery intubation and blood pressure transducer. Uncaria rhynchophylla（UR）, as the key medicine for calming the liver to extinguish internal wind, mainly treats patients with headache and dizzy caused by excessive Liver Yang and ascending Liver Wind. This study aims to observe the effect of UR on blood pressure.

【Equipments】 Banding rats board, Injector, Tracheal intubation, Artery intubation, Vein intubation, Artery clamp, Silk sutures, Instruments, Blood pressure transducer, Polygraph.

【Reagents】 Rhynchophylline HCL 1%, Uncaria rhynchophylla Extract（1 g/mL）, sodium, Citrate sodium 5%, pentobarbital sodium 3%, acetylcholine chloride1%, adrenalin HCL（0.1 mg/mL）.

【Animals】 Rats.

【Methods】 Place rats at banding board on their back till they are anesthetic by pentobarbital sodium（ip, 35 mg/kg）. Please perform this experiment in rats under pentobarbital anesthesia:

1. Tracheal intubation　create a small opening（about 3 cm in length）in the middle of neck cutis, and separate windpipe carefully from muscles around by hemostatic forceps, raise windpipe lightly to make a '⊥' cut in order to insert tracheal intubation heading for lung, then ligate it with silk suture for breathing smoothly.

2. Carotid artery intubation　isolate carotid artery and vagus nerve from surrounding organization, identified it by the pulse of artery. Then place two silk sutures under each and ligate one in the distal ends. Using artery clamp to occlude the proximal artery, make a small "V" creation in artery to insert intubatton filled with solution of citrate sodium, which is connected with blood pressure transducer. At last ligate to fix.

3. Vein intubation　Cut skin vertically（3 cm in length）along femoral veins（identified

it by the pulse) in groin and then separate femoral vein. Prepare two string under femoral vein and one is for ligating the distal ends of vein, the another is for tightening intubatton filled with normal sodium. Create a "Λ" opening at the vein. At last vein intubation which is offered to transfusion and administration is inserted heading for the heart.

Place silk sutures under right carotid artery and bilateral vagus nerve respectively to prepare tests of pressor reflect and severing vagus nerve.

After accomplishing upwards work, unloosen artery clamp and start immediately to record BP and administration.

The experiment proceeds according to following process:

(1) Experiment on tachyphylaxis: wait a moment for recording BP till it calms. Note values of depressing BP after intravenous injection of solution of Rhynchophylline HCL (1 mL/100 g weight) and extract of UR (2 mL/100 g weight). Injection solutions at same dose till BP go back to the pre-administration level. And then compare twice value of depressing BP.

(2) Experiment on pressor reflect of CNS: after BP calm, raise silk sutures at right carotid artery, clamp carotid with artery clamp to block blood for 30 s at once in order to detect the change after pressor test. Finally, compare the difference between before and after administration.

(3) Effect on acetylcholine: draw carotid blood pressure before and after injecting acetylcholine (0.1 mL/kg). Wait for a moment until BP calming, and you can study effects of solution of Rhynchophylline HCL and extract of UR on BP. Then inject acetylcholine again at same dose before BP ascending to compare difference.

(4) Effect on adrenalin: draw carotid blood pressure before and after injecting adrenalin (0.05 mL/kg). Wait for a moment until BP calming, and you can test effects of Rhynchophylline HCL and extract of UR on BP. Then inject adrenalin again at same dose before BP ascending to compare difference.

(5) Effect on vagus nerve: record BP after it calms. Note values of depressing BP after intravenous injection of Rhynchophylline HCL (1 mL/100 g weight) or extract of UR (2 mL/100 g weight). And inject them again after cutting down bilateral vagus nerve. Finally, please analyze effects of UR on BP after cutting down vagus nerve compared with normal.

【Results】Note the results according to the table 15-4.

Table 15–4 Analyzing the mechanism of Uncaria rhynchophylline on pressuring blood pressure

ITEM	Blood pressure (mmHg)					
	Pre–administration		Difference	Administration		Difference
	before	after		before	after	
Tachyphylaxis						
Oressor reflect						
Acetylcholine						
Adrenalin						
Vagus nerve						

[Qestions] What is the functional mechanism of Uncaria rhynchophylla?

第十六章　补益药实验

凡能补益人体气血，调节阴阳，提高机体抗病能力，消除虚弱证候的药物，称为补益药。补益药根据其作用和应用范围的不同分为补气药、补血药、补阴药和补阳药四类。传统常用的补益药有人参、黄芪、当归、熟地黄、麦冬、枸杞子、鹿茸、冬虫夏草等。现代药理学研究结果证明，这类药物的药理作用非常广泛，主要包括提高机体免疫功能、神经内分泌功能及中枢神经系统功能、促进物质代谢、延缓衰老、增强某些重要器官和系统的功能、抗肿瘤等。在研究补益药时，一般从影响免疫功能，抗应激能力，益智，促进造血功能，促进物质代谢，影响内分泌功能，延长寿命，促进消化、吸收功能等方面设计实验指标，并结合药物的具体功效和临床应用选择其他项目和指标进行实验。常用实验方法如下：

1. 免疫学实验

（1）影响非特异性免疫功能的实验方法：常选用小鼠腹腔巨噬细胞吞噬功能测定法、小鼠碳粒廓清法、小鼠免疫器官重量法等实验，观察药物对非特异性免疫功能的作用。

（2）特异性免疫功能实验—体液免疫功能的实验方法：常选用小鼠血清溶血素抗体测定法、鸡红细胞作免疫原的溶血素测定法、单向免疫扩散法等实验，观察药物对体液免疫功能的作用。

（3）特异性免疫功能实验—细胞免疫功能的实验方法：常选用二硝基氯苯（DNCB）所致小鼠迟发性皮肤过敏反应、小鼠外周血液中T淋巴细胞酶标记染色法等实验，观察药物对细胞免疫功能的作用。

2. 抗应激能力实验　实验方法主要包括耐缺氧、耐疲劳、耐高温、耐寒冷、抗辐射等。常选用小鼠耐缺氧能力、小鼠游泳时间、小鼠耐寒能力、小鼠耐高温能力等实验，观察药物抗应激能力的作用。

3. 益智实验　实验方法主要包括跳台、避暗、穿梭箱、爬杆、水迷宫、操作式条件反射和突触传递长时程增强（LTP）等。常选用药物对小鼠记忆获得障碍的影响（跳台法），药物对小鼠空间辨别能力的影响（迷宫法）等实验，观察药物的益智作用。

4. 促进造血功能实验　血虚动物模型的制备方法有：失血法、化学物质损伤法、辐射损伤法、营养法等。常选用药物对失血性血虚小鼠的补血作用观察，药物对乙酰苯肼所致小鼠血虚的补血作用等实验，观察药物促进造血功能的作用。

5. 促进物质代谢实验　常选用药物对小鼠超氧化物歧化酶（SOD）活性的影响（邻苯三酚法），药物对小鼠血浆过氧化脂质（LPO）的影响等实验，观察药物促进物质代谢的作用。

6. 其他　可根据补益药的具体功效和应用的特点，安排其他相关实验，如影响内分泌功能，延长寿命，促进消化、吸收功能等实验。

Chapter 16 Experiments on tonic

All the drugs that can tonify Qi and blood, adjust Yin-Yang, improve the disease resistance and eliminate the weakness are called tonic. According to their different effects and appliances, they are differentiated as invigorating vital energy, hematic tonic, invigorating yin and invigorating yang. Drugs like radix ginseng, radix astragali, angelicae sinensis, prepared rehmannia root, ophiopogonis tuber, barbary wolfberry fruit, cartialgenous and Chinese caterpilar fungus are traditional tonic in common use. It has been proved that the pharmaceutical effects of these drugs are quite extensive, including improving the organic immunocompetence, neuroendocrine function and central nervous system ability, promoting energy metabolism, slowing the aging process, enhancing the function of some important organs and systems, inhibiting tumor growth, and so on. While conducting research on tonic, we often design experiments following the guideline of their effects such as influencing on organic immunocompetence, anti-hyperirritability, improving intelligence, promoting hematopoiesis and physical metabolizing, regulating endocrine function, prolonging longevity, enhancing digesting and absorbing food, and so on. Considering their respective effects and clinical applications, we carry out the experiments aiming at some other items and targets as well. Regular experiments are as follows:

1. Immunological experiments

(1) Non-specific immunity experiments: macrophage phagocytosis, carbon particles clearing, miceimmune organ weight.

(2) Specific immunity-humoral immunity experiments: usually carry out the mensuration of antibody of serum haemolysin in mice, haemolys in mensuration about chicken red blood cell used as immunogen, single radil immunodiffusion method.

(3) Specific immunity-cellular immunity experiments: delayed hypersensitivity induced by dinitrochlorobenzene (DNCB) in mice, enzyme labeled staining method of the peripheral blood T lymphocytes in mice.

2. Anti-stress experiments　Hypoxia tolerance, fatigue resistance, high temperature tolerance, cold resistance, antiradiation, and so on. Usually carry out the experiments on mice, including the competent of bearing hypoxia, counting swimming time, the competent of heat or cold-resistance, to inspect the anti-stress capability of the drug.

3. Intelligence development experiments　Mainly including step-down test, avoiding darkness, shuttle box, pole test, watermaze, operant conditioned reflex and long-term potentiation (LTP) and so on. Usually carry out the effect on impairment of learning and memory in mice (step-down test), the effect on spatial discrimination ability in mice (Morris Water Maze), to inspect the intelligence development effect of the drug.

4. Hematopoietic function promoting experiments　To develop the blood-deficiency modelincludes bloodletting, chemical damage, radiation injury, alimentation, and so on. Usually carry out the experiments to observe the blood tonifing effect on blood deficiency mice caused by bleeding or acetyl phenylhydrazine, to inspect the effect of promoting hematopoietic function of the drug.

5. Promoting metabolism experiments　Usually carry out the experiments about the effects on superoxide dismutase (SOD) activity and lipid peroxidase (LPO) level in mice to inspect the promotion of metabolism effect of the drug.

6. Others　According to the specific effects and applications of each kind of tonic, to arrange some other correlative experiments, such as ones that inspect the effects of endocrine function, extending lifespan, promoting absorption and digestion, and so on.

实验一　人参对小鼠游泳时间的影响

【目的】观察人参对小鼠游泳时间的影响，掌握抗疲劳作用药物的常用筛选方法。

【原理】人参具有抗疲劳作用，可以延长小鼠的游泳时间，故以游泳时间作为小鼠疲劳的指标，可以考察人参的抗疲劳作用。

【器材】天平；50 cm × 30 cm × 25 cm 的玻璃缸；负重物；温度计；小鼠灌胃针；秒表。

【试剂】人参水煎液 2.5 g/mL；单蒸水。

【动物】ICR 小鼠，雌雄各半，体重 18~22 g。

【方法】玻璃缸内加水至水深 20 cm，水温保持在（20 ± 0.5）℃。取 4 只 ICR 小鼠，雌雄各半，称重，标记，随机分为两组。给药组每只灌胃人参水煎液 0.25 mL/10 g，对照组每只灌胃等容量的单蒸水，给药后 30 min 在小鼠尾部系 2 g 的重物（小鼠体重 10% 的负荷）。将给药组及对照组小鼠每次取出一只，分别放入玻璃缸内游泳，立即计时并注意观察小鼠开始游泳至体能耗竭，即小鼠头部沉入水中 10 s 不能浮出水面时，停止计时，记录小鼠游泳时间。

综合全实验室的结果，分别算出两组的平均游泳时间。将给药组与对照组比较并进行统计学处理。

【结果】实验结果按表 16-1 记录。

表 16-1　人参对小鼠游泳时间的影响

组别	动物数	剂量（g/kg）	游泳时间（s）
对照组			
人参水煎液组			

【注意事项】

1. 小鼠应该单只游泳，如果两只以上同时游泳，会影响实验结果。
2. 严格控制水温。

【思考题】结合所学的中药学及药理学知识，解释人参抗疲劳的可能机制。

Experiment 1　The effect of Panax ginseng on swimming time in mice

【Purpose】To examine the effect of P. ginseng on swimming time in mice. Grasp the commonly used screening methods of anti-fatigue drugs.

【Principle】Take the swimming time of mice as the index of tiredness.The present study was performed to investigate the anti-stress ability of P. ginseng on load swimming test in mice.

【Equipments】electronic balance, glass trough (size: 50 cm × 30 cm × 25 cm), load steel ring (2 g), thermometer, injector forintragastric administration, stopwatch.

【Reagents】Aqueous extract of Panax ginseng (2.5 g/mL), water.

【Animals】ICR mice, weighing 18-22 g, half male and half female.

【Methods】Add water into the glass trough (50 cm × 30 cm × 25 cm) until to depth of 20 cm, temperature of the water maintained at (20 ± 0.5) ℃.

Four mice (half male and half female), weighed and marked, divided into control and P. ginseng groups. Water/ P. ginseng (0.25 mL/10 g) was orally administered 30 minutes before the swimming test was preformed. A load of steel ring weighing 2 g was attached to the proximal end of the tail. Each mouse was allowed to swim till exhausted in a glass trough. The end point was taken when the mice drowned and “Swimming time” for each mouse was noted. The mean swimming time for each group was calculated and the data was statistically analyzed.

【Results】Record the results according to the table 16-1.

Table 16-1　Effect of aqueous extract of Panax ginseng on the swimming time in mice

Groups	No. of mice	Dose (g/kg)	Swimming time (s)
Control			
Panax ginseng			

【Notes】

1. Each time only one mouse can be swim in one glass trough, too many mice in one trough may lead to the mice climb and push with each other, then the results may be affected.

2. The temperature of water should be strictly controlled.

【Questions】Combined with your knowledge of TCM and pharmacology, think about what might be the antifatigue mechanisms of Panax ginseng.

实验二　当归补血汤对失血性“血虚”小鼠的补血作用

【目的】学习失血性血虚动物模型的制备方法，并观察当归补血汤的补血作用。

【原理】血虚证多为失血过多，人为的放血可使血红蛋白（Hemoglobin, HB）的含量及红细胞计数（red blood count, RBC）显著降低，类似临床血虚症状。当归补血汤具有补血调血之功效，为补血调经的主方。

【器材】手术剪；眼科镊；0.5 mL 小塑料管；干棉球；血细胞计数板；灌胃针等。

【试剂】当归补血汤（浓度为 1 g/mL）；单蒸水。

【动物】雄性 ICR 小鼠，体重 18~22 g。

【方法】取小鼠，随机分为正常对照组、模型对照组、当归补血汤组，除正常对照组不放血外，其余两组小鼠用锋利的手术剪在距小鼠尾尖 0.5 cm 处剪断放血 0.5 mL，测各组 HB 和 RBC。24 h 后眼眶取血测 HB 和 RBC，并随即灌胃给予当归补血汤 0.2 mL/10 g，正常对照组和模型对照组给予等量单蒸水。连续给药 7 天，第 8 天给药后 30 min，眼眶取血测 HB 和 RBC。

【结果】实验结果按表 16-2、16-3 记录。

表 16-2　当归补血汤对失血性血虚小鼠 HB 含量的影响

模型对照组	动物数	剂量（g/kg）	HB（g/L）		
			失血前	失血后	给药后
正常对照组					
模型对照组					
当归补血汤组					

表 16-3　当归补血汤对失血性血虚小鼠 RBC 的影响

组别	动物数	剂量（g/kg）	RBC（/L）		
			失血前	失血后	给药后
正常对照组					
模型对照组					
当归补血汤组					

【注意事项】

1. 取血应准确控制取血量。

2. 注意用棉球及时止血。

【思考题】

1. 分析、讨论实验结果，如与理论不符请说明原因。

2. 当归补血汤补血作用的机理是什么？还可用哪些方法证明？

Experiment 2 Bloodtonifing effect of Danggui Buxue Tang (DBT) in hemopenia mice induced by bloodletting

【**Purpose**】Master the method of developing mice model of hempenia induced by bloodletting and observe the bloodtonifing effect of DBT.

【**Principle**】Excessive loss of blood can cause blood-deficiency syndrome. Bloodletting is accompanied by a decrease in the amount of hemoglobin (HB) and red blood count (RBC), in the blood. DBT exerts nourish blood and anti-dysmenorrheic actions.

【**Equipments**】surgical scissor, ophthalmic forcep, plastic tube (0.5 mL), dry cotton ball, blood cell count plate, injector for intragastric administration.

【**Reagents**】Danggui Buxue Tang (1 g/mL), water.

【**Animals**】Male mice, weighing 18~22 g.

【**Methods**】After weighed and marked, mice were divided randomly into the following groups: normal group, control group and DBT group. Except the mice in the normal group, mice in the other two groups were cut at 0.5 cm from the base of the tail for bleeding until 0.5 mL blood were collected, then measure HB and RBC. 24 hours later, measure HB and RBC again. DBT was orally administered 0.2 mL/10 g for 7 days, normal and control mice were orally given an equal volume of vehicle in the same schedule. On the eighth day, collect blood and measure HB and RBC.

【**Results**】Record the results of experiment in the tables 16-2、16-3.

Table 16–2 Effect of 'Angelicae Sinensis Decoction for Supplementing Blood' on the content of HB in hemopenia mice

Group	No. of mice	Dose (mg/kg)	HB (g/L)		
			Before bleeding	After bleeding	After drug administered
Normal					
Control					
DBT					

Table 16–3　Effect of ‘Angelicae Sinensis Decoction for Supplementing Blood’ on the number of RBC in hemopenia mice

Group	No. of mice	Dose (mg/kg)	RBC (/L)		
			Before bleeding	After bleeding	After drug administered
Normal					
Control					
DBT					

【Notes】

1. The amount of collected blood should be accurately controlled.

2. Use the dry cotton balls to stanch in time.

【Questions】

1. Analysis the results of the experiment, if the results are different from the theory, please think deeply about the possible reasons.

2. Try to explain the mechanisms of blood to nifing effect of “Angelicae Sinensis Decoction for Supplementing Blood” . Are there any other methods that could also certificate it?

实验三　免疫功能实验：人参对 DNCB 所致小鼠皮肤迟发型变态反应的影响

【目的】学习测定整体动物免疫功能的实验方法，观察人参对小鼠免疫功能的影响。

【原理】2,4- 二硝基氯苯（DNCB）是小分子半抗原，将其涂布于皮肤上，可与皮肤内的角蛋白及胶原蛋白结合成全抗原，从而刺激 T 淋巴细胞转化成致敏淋巴细胞，再分布于全身皮肤内。10~14 天后动物对此类物质便产生过敏性，再以 DNCB 攻击，即可见攻击部位形成迟发型皮肤过敏反应。

【器材】手术剪；镊子；试管；移液器；100 μL 微量注射器；1 mL 注射器；玻璃漏斗；721 型分光光度计；乳胶手套等。

【试剂】人参水煎液 2.5 g/mL；2,4- 二硝基氯苯（DNCB）；硫化钡；伊文思蓝（Evans）；丙酮；生理盐水等。

【动物】ICR 小鼠，雌雄各半，体重 18~22 g。

【方法】取 ICR 小鼠雌雄各半，按体重和性别随机分为两组，给药组从致敏当日起每日灌胃人参水煎液 0.2 mL/10 g，对照组给予等容积蒸馏水，连续给药 10 天。致敏前 1 天，用硫化钡糊脱去颈背部毛。致敏当天给药后，将 0.5 g/mL DNCB 丙酮溶液 2 μL/ 只滴于已脱毛的小鼠颈部皮肤上致敏，10 天后，在致敏部位的皮肤上滴 0.025 g/mL DNCB 丙酮溶液 20 μL/ 只进行攻击。24 h 后小鼠尾静脉注射 1% 伊文思蓝 0.1 mL/10 g，30 min 后处死小鼠，取下背部蓝染皮肤，剪碎，置试管中，用 1∶1 丙酮生理盐水混合液 5 mL 浸泡 24 h，将浸泡液过滤，取滤液用 721 分光光度计在 610 nm 处测定光密度。

【结果】实验结果按表 16-4 记录。

表 16-4　人参对小鼠 DNCB 迟发型过敏反应的影响

组别	动物数	剂量（g/kg）	皮肤反应（OD）
蒸馏水			
人参水煎液			

【注意事项】DNCB 也可使人致敏，产生迟发型皮肤过敏反应，因此致敏或攻击时，实验者必须戴手套操作。

【思考题】如何用人参对免疫功能的影响解释本实验的结果？

Experiment 3　Immunological experiment: the effect of ginseng on delayed cutaneous hypersensitivity reaction in mice caused by DNCB

【Purpose】 To study the method of detecting immune function in mouse model, to inspect the influence of ginseng in cellular immunity.

【Principle】 when coated on skin, 2,4-dinitrochlorobenzene (DNCB), a small molecular hapten, can turn into antigen by combining with keratinose and collagen protein, consequently activate T lymphocytes to sensitize T lymphocytes which then distribute to skin all over the body. 10~14 days later, when attacked again with DNCB, it could cause allergic reaction in the attacked area of skin. Then delayed cutaneous hypersensitivity reaction occurs.

【Equipments】 surgical scissor, forcep, test tube, pipettor, 100 μL microinjector, 1 mL injector, glass funnel, 721 spectrophotometer, latex gloves.

【Reagents】 aqueous extract of ginseng 2.5 g/mL, 2,4-dinitrochlorobenzene (DNCB), barium sulphide, Evans, acetone, normal saline (NS).

【Animals】 ICR mice, weighing 18~22 g, half male and half female.

【Methods】 After weighed and marked, ICR mice (half male and half female) were divided randomly into two groups: control group and ginseng group. One day before sensitization, barium sulfide is used to remove cervicodorsal hair. Then aqueous extract of ginseng isorally administered 0.2 mL/10 g for 10 days continuously. Control mice are orally given an equal volume of vehicle in the same schedule. On the day of sensitization, after intragastric administrated, each mouse was sensitizated by dropping 2 μL of 0.5 g/mL DNCB acetone solution on the cervicodorsal skin without hair. 10 days later, each mouse is dropped 20 μL of 0.025 g/mL DNCB acetone solution on the sensitization skin to attack again. After 24 h, mice are intravenously injected 1% Evans 0.1 mL/10 g. 30 min later, mice are sacrificed and cut the cervicodorsal blue stainedskin down, then mince it and put it into test tubes. Soak it in 5 mL acetone-NS (1 ∶ 1) mixture for 24 h. To filter the soak solution and measure the optical density of the filtrate at 610 nm with 721 spectrophotometer.

【Results】 Record the results in the table 16-4.

Table 16-4 The effect of ginseng on delayed cutaneous hypersensitivity reaction in mice caused by DNCB

Group	No. of mice	Dose (g/kg)	Delayed Cutaneous Hypersensitivity Reaction (OD)
Control			
Ginseng			

【Notes】DNCB can also cause human delayed hypersusceptibility, when sensitization or challenge, the operator must wear gloves.

【Questions】How to explain the result in the experiment with the regulatory effect of ginseng on immunologic function ?

第十七章　虚证动物模型和补虚药实验

补虚药（补益药）是指能治疗虚证的一类药物。为探索“虚证”的本质，研究补虚药及方剂的作用，需要建立模拟中医“虚证”的动物模型。

阴虚和阳虚动物模型和补阴、补阳药实验

研究阴虚、阳虚“证”的动物模型，并用补阴药进行验证，是探讨中医阴虚、阳虚“证”的实质和中药药理的一个手段和途径。目前主要有以下几种激素、药物及手术造成阴虚、阳虚证动物模型：

1. 肾上腺皮质激素　因皮质激素使用的剂量和时间不同，可造成“阴虚”和“阳虚”两类模型。早期为“阴虚”阶段，应用补阴药有改善作用；后期为“阳虚”阶段，应用补阳药有改善作用。

（1）皮质激素阴虚模型：短程大剂量应用皮质激素，可使动物体内皮质激素突然升高。如成年小白鼠或大白鼠以可的松或氢化可的松每天 1~1.25 mg/ 只灌胃，3~5 天内动物血浆环磷腺苷（cAMP）水平升高。此时用滋阴药生地、龟板等可起一定保护作用，可使 cAMP 降低。

（2）皮质激素阳虚模型：大剂量皮质激素给予动物 7~10 天后，出现“阳虚”现象。如给小白鼠灌胃或肌肉注射醋酸可的松或醋酸氢化可的松 0.5~1 mg/ 只 / 天，5~7 天后，动物即出现体重减轻，活动减少，反应迟钝，蜷曲拱背等形寒肢冷的“阳虚”表现。增加给药量，病情更加重，甚至致死。助阳药附子、肉桂合剂及淫羊藿、肉苁蓉、仙茅组成的方剂对此类阳虚型动物有保护作用。

2. 甲状腺激素　临床上甲状腺机能亢进患者多数出现阴虚证候，甲状腺机能减退者多出现阳虚证候，对动物给予甲状腺激素可造成甲亢“阴虚”型模型；若抑制甲状腺激素合成和分泌，可造成甲减“阳虚”型模型。

（1）甲亢阴虚型：用三碘甲状腺氨酸钠（T_3）0.9 mg/kg 给小鼠灌胃，连续 5 天，或将药物按 0.5 mg/kg 给大鼠皮下注射，隔天 1 次共 3 次，动物均可逐渐出现体重减轻，体温

升高等甲亢“阴虚”证状。对此类模型,用滋阴药生地龟板合剂能降低β受体数量和血浆 cAMP 水平,改善“阴虚”症状,但不降低血清 T_3、T_4 水平;知母能降低红细胞、肾、肝组织的 Na^+-K^+-ATP 酶活性。

（2）甲减阳虚型:给动物喂一段时间甲状腺激素合成抑制剂甲基硫氧嘧啶或他巴唑,使甲状腺合成和分泌甲状腺激素减少,血清 T_3、T_4 水平降低,动物出现形寒肢冷、饮水量减少,体重减轻等甲减“阳虚”证候,用附子、肉桂合剂能升高血浆儿茶酚胺及 cAMP 水平,增加肾脏组织β受体数量,降低细胞对 M 胆碱能激动剂反应性;右归丸等能提高血浆甲状腺素水平。

3. 氨基导眠能　以肾上腺皮质激素阻滞剂氨基导眠能灌喂小鼠,可使小鼠出现形寒肢冷的“阳虚”症状,血浆皮质醇减少。助阳药可减轻此“阳虚”症状,使肾上腺组比较低 cAMP 水平及血浆皮质醇水平升高,减轻肾上腺组织病理性改变。此模型属肾上腺皮质机能抑制的“阳虚”型动物模型。

4. 羟基脲　核苷酸还原酶抑制剂羟基脲能抑制 DNA 的合成,使核酸代谢低下。每天以羟基脲按 7.5 mg/ 只给小鼠灌胃,连续 7 天,动物会出现形寒肢冷的“阳虚”证候。助阳药淫羊藿、肉苁蓉合剂可拮抗羟基脲的这一作用,从而促进 DNA 的合成,起到保护动物的效果。

5. 利血平　按 750 mg/kg 剂量将利血平注射于小鼠,数分钟内即可见其皮肤温度下降,表现出形寒肢冷的“阳虚”证候。附子、肉桂、干姜、仙茅、肉苁蓉和山茱萸等能不同程度地增加该模型动物下丘脑的去甲肾上腺素（NE）、纹状体的多巴胺（DA）、脑干 5- 羟色胺（5-HT）水平,附子、肉桂合剂能升高利血平化小鼠血浆 cAMP 水平。而泻心火药黄连则能降低利血平化小鼠的下丘脑 NE 和脑干 5-HT 含量。“阳虚”的出现可能与动物神经递质有关。

6. 手术法　肾血管狭窄型高血压:用银丝夹夹闭大鼠一侧肾动脉,可造成肾血管狭窄型高血压。动物醛固酮升高,脑组织脑啡肽减少,心肌肥厚伴有左心室羟脯氨酸浓度升高。助阳药附子、肉桂使病理变化加剧,滋阴药六味地黄汤则具有改善作用,因而认为这可能属于“阴虚”模型。

7. 其他阴虚证造模方法

（1）超负荷运动的造模:雄性 SD 大鼠强迫游泳 6 周,每周 5 天,每天 1 次,日游泳时间由 10 min 逐日增加至第 5 周末 120 min。水深 60 cm,水温（30 ± 2）℃。认为其模型为“阴虚内热证”。

（2）长期激怒的造模:采用雄性 SD 大鼠,体重 200~240 g,从实验第 1 天起将大鼠双后肢束缚,成对倒吊于笼内,以引起明显激怒,表现为粗叫、撕咬,首次激怒 20 min,以后每隔 1 天,增加 10 min。造模时间均为共 20 天。认为其模型为“肝肾阴虚证”。

（3）特殊环境的造模:大鼠置于人工气候室内进行热应激 3 h 处理,大鼠表现为耳、爪、尾等潮红、大量流涎、呼吸急促、四肢伸展、呈昏睡状态。认为其模型为“热损伤阴虚证”。

（4）毒素造模:雌或雄性日本大耳白兔,实验前 18 h 开始禁水禁食,然后在自然清醒状态下,由耳静脉注射速尿注射液,剂量 2.5 mL/ kg, 1 h 后同法注入等量速尿, 2 h 后再以大肠杆菌内毒素按 0.5 μg/ kg 耳静脉注射。认为其模型为“温病阴虚热盛证”。

Chapter 17　Animal models of asthenia syndrome and experiments for tonifying drugs

Tonifying drugs are used to treat the asthenia syndrome. To explore the nature of asthenia syndrome, investigate the pharmacological actions of drugs and complex prescriptions for reinforcing asthenia syndrome, it is important to establish the animal models mimicking the asthenia syndrome in Chinese medical science.

Animal models of YIN or YANG asthenia and experiments for reinforcing YIN or YANG

Investigating the animal models of YIN or YANG asthenia syndrome and validating these models with drugs for tonifying YIN or YANG is one of the approaches to studying the nature of the syndrome of YIN or YANG asthenia in Chinese medical science and pharmacology of TCM. At present, the models could be prepared by using some hormones, drugs or surgical operations.

1. Adrenocortical hormones　The difference in doses and times of corticosteroid exposure could result in the establishment of YIN or YANG asthenia model. In the earlier period the animals show signs of YIN asthenia which can be reduced by treating with drugs for reinforcing YIN, and during the later period the models exhibit the characteristics of YANG asthenia which are counteracted by drugs for reinforcing YANG.

(1) Corticosteroid-induced YIN asthenia model. Short period and high dose of application of corticosteroid could increase the corticosteroid level in animals. For example, 3~5 days after administration of adult mice or rats with 1~1.25 mg cortisone or hydrocortisone, the plasma adenosine cyclophosphate (cAMP) is increased, which could be antagonized by drugs for tonifying YIN such as Rehmannia Dride Rhizome and Terrapin Shell.

(2) Corticosteroid-induced YANG asthenia model. 7~10 days after administration of

high dose of corticosteroids, animals show the symptoms of YANG asthenia. For example, the cold symptoms of body weight loss, action reduction, responses dullness and body crimps are observed in mice 5~7 days after intramuscular injection with 0.5~1 mg /mouse/day of cortisone acetate or hydrocortisone. If the dose is increased, the symptoms aggravate and even lead to the death of animals. Drugs for tonifying YANG such as Aconite Root, Cinnamon Misture, Herba Epimedii, Caulis Cistanchis and Rhizoma Curculiginis could protect animals from the disease.

2. Thyroid hormones Clinically, YIN asthenia syndromes appear in most patients with hyperthyreosis, while YANG asthenia syndromes appear in most patients with hypothyreosis. The YIN asthenia model is prepared in animals by administration of thyroid hormones, and hypothyroidism-based YANG asthenia model is obtained by inhibiting the synthesis and secretion of thyroid hormones.

(1) Hyperthyroidism-based YIN asthenia model: After the mice are orally administered with 0.9 mg /kg of liothyronine sodium (T_3) for 5 days, or rats are treated with subcutaneous injection of 0.5 mg/kg T_3 3 times at one day interval, the YIN asthenia syndromes such as body weight loss and body temperature increase appear gradually. Drugs for reinforcing YIN, such as Rehmannia Dride Rhizome and Terrapin Shell could decrease β-receptor number and plasma cAMP level, improve the YIN asthenia syndromes without downregulation of serum T_3 and T_4 levels. Anemarrhenae could lower the Na^+-K^+-ATPase activity in red blood cells (RBCs), kidney and liver.

(2) Hypothyroidism-based YANG asthenia model: As a thyroid hormone inhibitor, thyreostat or thiamazole inhibit thyroid hormones secretion and lower blood T_3 and T_4 accompanied with YANG asthenia symptoms such as cold body and limbs, reduced drinking water and body weight loss in animal after oral treatment. Aconite Root and misture of Cinnamon increase plasma catecholamine and cAMP levels and β- receptor number in kidney, downregulate the responses of cells to M-receptor agonists. YOUGUIWAN increases the tetraiodothyronine concentration in plasma.

3. Aminoglutethimide Mice treated orally with aminoglutethimide, a blocker of adrenal cortex hormone, show the YANG asthenia symptomes such as cold body and limbs and decreased concentration of plasma hydrocortisone. Drugs for tonifying YANG could relieve the symptoms, restore the decreased cAMP and hydrocortisone levels in plasma, improve the pathological changes in the adrenal gland. Therefore, this is a YANG-asthenia animal model with hypofunction of the adrenal cortex.

4. Hydroxycarbamide Hydroxycarbamide, an inhibitor of ribonucleotide reductase, could reduce nucleic acid metabolism by inhibiting DNA synthesis. Mice would show YANG asthenia symptoms of cold body and limbs after oral treatment with 7.5 mg hydroxycarbamide per mouse for 7 days. Epimedium and mixture of Caulis Cistanchis, drugs for reinforcing YANG, could promote DNA synthesis, protect animals from the damage by antagonizing the

action of hydroxycarbamide.

5. Reserpine Injection of 750 mg/kg reserpine into mice could induce the YANG asthenia symptoms indicated by decreased skin temperature within a few minutes. Aconite Root, Cinnamon, Zingiberis, Rhizoma, Curculiginis, Rhizoma, Caulis Cistanchis and Asiatic Cornelian Cherry Fruit could increase the noradrenaline (NE) level in hypothalamus, dopamine (DA) level in striatum and 5-HT level in the brain stem to some extent. Coptidis Rhizoma, a drug of purging the sthenic heart-fire, can decrease the NE level in hypothalamus and 5-HT level in the brain stem of reserpinized mice, while Aconite Root and Cinnamon misture can increase the plasma cAMP level in reserpinized mice. Thus, this type of YANG asthenia model is associated with the alterations of neurotransmitters in animals.

6. Surgical operation Renovascular hypertension model, which is induced by occlusion of the renal artery with silver wire clip, shows increased aldosterone level, decreased enkephalin content in brain tissue, myocardial hypertrophy accompanied with an increased hydroxyproline concentration in the left ventricle. Aconite Root and Cinnamon, drugs for tonifying YANG, aggravate the symptoms, while Rehmanniae Decoction of Six Ingredients, complex prescription of drugs for reinforcing YIN, and ameliorate the syndrome. Thus, this model is regarded as a model of YIN asthenia.

7. Other methods for the preparation of YIN-asthenia model

(1) Overloading-exercise-induced asthenia model: Male SD rats are forced to swim in water (60 cm deep and 30 ℃ temperature) for 6 weeks (5 days every week, 1 time/day, and the swimming time increases from 10 minutes at first to 120 minutes at the end of the fifth week). The model is looked as the type of YIN asthenia generating intrinsic heat.

(2) Long-term-rage-induced model: Male SD rats, weighed 200~240 g, are enraged by being hang up upside down with the two hind limbs tied together from the first day of the experiment. The animals would shout and bite each other. The enraging time is 20 min on the first day, and increased by 10 min every other day for 20 days. This model is regarded as a type of hepatic and renal YIN deficiency.

(3) Specific-environment-induced model: Rats are taken in the controlled environment chamber to suffer heat treatment for 3 h. Then rats will show the appearance of red ears, claws and tails, a great deal of dribbling, breathlessness, limbs stretching and being at deep slumber. This model is looked as the YIN asthenia syndrome of heat-related-casualty.

(4) Toxin-induced model: After deprivation of food and water for 12 h, rabbits are injected with 2.5 mL/kg frusemide through the ear vein for two times at 1 h intervals. After 2 h, rabbits are intravenously injected with 0.5 μg/ kg endotoxin derived from Escherichia coli. The model is looked as the seasonal febrile disease-related extreme heat with YIN asthenia.

实验一　生地、龟板对甲亢“阴虚”型小白鼠血浆 cAMP 水平的影响

【目的】学习甲状腺激素致甲亢“阴虚”动物模型的制备方法，观察滋阴药对此模型血浆中 cAMP 的影响。

【原理】给予人剂量甲状腺素后，小鼠出现甲状腺功能亢进，机体耗氧量增加，心肌、脑及肾脏组织等细胞的 β 受体数量增加，cAMP 系统对异丙肾上腺素刺激的反应和血浆 cAMP 水平都升高。生地、龟板能使升高的反应趋向正常，降低升高的 cAMP 水平。

【器材】液体闪烁计数器；减压抽滤装置；冷冻离心机；微量注射器；微量移液器；小烧杯；离心管；玻璃试管；液体闪烁杯；冰瓶；滴管；注射器及注射针头。

【药品和试剂】环磷酸腺苷（cAMP）放射免疫分析试剂盒［内含醋酸缓冲液母液；抗 cAMP；抗血清原液；^{3}H-cAMP；标准 cAMP；三乙胺；醋酐；磷酸缓冲液干粉；人血清白蛋白；微孔滤膜；0.05 mol/L 的 EDTA 钠盐水溶液；1 mol/L 的 $HClO_4$；2 mol/L 的 KOH；甲苯或二甲苯（含 4 g/L 的 PPO 闪烁液）］；冰；L- 甲状腺素钠盐；异丙肾上腺素；生地加龟板水煎液合剂（各 1 g/mL）。

【动物】小白鼠。

【方法】取体重约 22 g 的同性同窝小白鼠随机分为 3 组，每组 10 只。

甲亢“阴虚”组：每天皮下注射 L- 甲状腺素钠盐 0.4 mg/ 只，共 4 天。

甲亢“阴虚”加生地龟板组：造模前 1 天开始灌胃生地龟板合剂 10 g/kg，共 5 天。造模方法同甲亢“阴虚”组。

对照组：每天灌等量水，共 5 天。

断头采血前 10 min 每鼠皮下注射 1 次 100 μg/kg 异丙肾上腺素。

血浆样品处理、标准曲线制作及 cAMP 的测定方法按所购试剂盒使用说明书进行。

【结果】甲亢“阴虚”组的血浆 cAMP 水平升高，生地龟板合剂则使之降低。参照表 17-1 记录。

表 17-1　生地、龟板合剂对甲状腺素致甲亢“阴虚”型小鼠血浆 cAMP 的影响

分组	动物数（只）	异丙肾上腺素（μg/kg）	血浆 cAMP（mol/L）
对照组			
甲亢“阴虚”组			
“阴虚”+ 生地龟板组			

【注意事项】

1. 给予甲状腺激素的天数必须以动物耗氧量明显升高,出现“阴虚”证候为指标。

2. cAMP 水平也可以应用 cAMP 酶联免疫吸附试剂盒(cAMP ELISA KIT)检测。

【思考题】

1. 分析和讨论血浆 cAMP 测定结果,并说明其意义。

2. 为什么用甲状腺素制作“阴虚”动物模型?试评价本模型。

Experiment 1 Effects of Rehmannia Dride Rhizome and Terrapin Shell on the plasma cAMP Level in Mice with YIN Asthenia

【Purpose】 Learn the method of preparing thyroid hormone-induced YIN asthenia model and observe the effects of drugs for notifying YIN on the plasma cAMP level.

【Principles】 After administration of high dose of tetraiodothyronine, mice show the symptoms of hyperthyreosis along with increased oxygen consumption and β -receptor number in cardiomyocytes, brain and kidney, and a stronger response of cAMP system to isoprenaline and higher level of plasma cAMP. Rehmannia Dride Rhizome and Terrapin Shell could downregulate the increased responsibility and decrease the elevated cAMP level.

【Equipments】 Liquid scintillation counter, vacuum filtration system, refrigeration centrifuge, microinjectors, micropippetes, little beakers, centrifuge tubes, glass tubes, liquid scintillating disc, ice container, dropper, syringe and needles.

【Drugs and reagents】 Cyclic adenosine monophosphate (cAMP) radioimmunoassay kit (contains stock solution of acetate buffer, anti-cAMP, antiserum stock solution, 3H-cAMP, standard cAMP, triethylamine, acetic anhydride, powder of phosphate buffer, human serum albumin, millipore filter, 0.05 mol/L EDTA sodium solution, 1 mol/L HClO4, 2 mol/L KOH, methyl benzene or dimethyl benzene containing 4 g/L of PPO scintillation fluid), ice, L-thyroxine sodium, isoprenaline, misture of Rehmannia Dride Rhizome and Terrapin Shell (1 g/mL respectively).

【Animals】 Mice.

【Methods】 Mice of the same sex weighing about 22 g are divided into 3 groups at random, 10 animals per group. Mice in hyperthyreosis-based YIN asthenia group is subcutaneously injected with 0.4 mg/mouse L-thyroxine sodium for 4 days. Mice in groups of hyperthyreosis-based YIN asthenia treated with Rehmannia Dride Rhizome and Terrapin Shell are orally given with 10 g/kg the misture for 5 days from one day before model preparation. Mice in normal control is given a gavage of water for 5 days.

10 min before blood collection by decapitation, all the mice are subcutaneously injected with 100 μg/kg isoprenaline. The sample treatment, standard curve preparation and the cAMP assay are performed according to the operating instructions in the kit.

【Results】 The plasma cAMP level increases in Hyperthyreosis-based YIN asthenia mice. Misture of Rehmannia Dride Rhizome and Terrapin Shell downregulate the high level of cAMP. Data are filled in table 17-1.

Table 17–1　Effects of Rehmannia Dride Rhizome and Terrapin Shell on the plasma cAMP level in mice with tetraiodothyronine–induced YIN asthenia

Group	Animal number	Isoprenaline (μg/kg)	Plasma cAMP (mol/L)
Normal control			
Hyperthyreosis-based YIN asthenia			
YIN asthenia group treated with misture			

【 Notes 】

1. The period of thyroid hormone administration is decided by the appearances of significant increased oxygen consumption and other classical symptoms of YIN asthenia.

2. The cAMP level is also able to be measured by using cAMP ELISA KIT.

【 Questions 】

1. Analyze the results of plasma cAMP assay and explain its importance.

2. Why is the YIN asthenia model prepared by tetraiodothyronine treatment? Try to evaluate this model.

实验二 附子肉桂对他巴唑致甲减“阳虚”型小白鼠血浆 cGMP 水平的影响

【目的】了解他巴唑致甲减“阳虚”动物模型及助阳药附子、肉桂合剂对此模型血浆 cGMP 的影响。

【原理】灌胃给予小鼠甲状腺激素合成抑制剂他巴唑之后,甲状腺激素合成和分泌减少,出现甲状腺功能减退。细胞 cGMP 系统对 M 受体激动剂氨甲酰胆碱反应性升高,血浆 cGMP 水平升高。附子和肉桂能降低 cGMP 系统的反应性,从而降低 cGMP 水平。

【器材】液体闪烁计数器;减压抽滤装置;冷冻离心机;微量注射器;微量移液器;小烧杯;离心管;玻璃试管;液体闪烁杯;冰瓶;滴管;注射器及注射针头。

【药品和试剂】附子;肉桂水煎液合剂(各 1 g/mL);0.3 g/L 他巴唑溶液;氨甲酰胆碱;^{3}H-cGMP 放射免疫试剂盒。

【动物】小白鼠。

【方法】取体重约 22 g 的同性同窝小白鼠,随机分为 3 组,每组 10 只。

对照组:每天灌胃水。

甲减“阳虚”组:每天灌胃他巴唑溶液 6 mg/kg 体重,直至造模成功(通常需 2~3 个月,动物才出现形寒肢冷、耗氧量减少等“阳虚”证候)。

甲减“阳虚”加附子、肉桂组:每天灌胃他巴唑溶液 6 mg/kg 体重,直至造模成功。随后每天灌胃附子、肉桂合剂 1 mL/ 只,连续 10~14 天后进行实验。

断头采血前 6 min 给每只小鼠皮下注射 1 次氨甲酰胆碱 400 μg/kg。

血浆样品处理、标准曲线制作及 cGMP 测定步骤均按所购试剂盒说明进行。

【结果】甲减“阳虚”组 cGMP 水平升高,附子、肉桂合剂使之降低。按表 17-2 记录。

表 17-2 附子、肉桂合剂对他巴唑致甲减“阳虚”型小鼠血浆 cGMP 的影响

分组	动物数(只)	氨甲酰胆碱(μg/kg)	血浆 cGMP(mol/L)
对照组			
甲减“阳虚”组			
“阳虚”+附子肉桂组			

【注意事项】

1. 动物出现形寒尾冷和耗氧量减少等指征,方为“阳虚”造模成功。
2. cAMP 水平也可以应用 cAMP 酶联免疫吸附试剂盒(cAMP ELISA KIT)检测。

【思考题】

1. 分析和讨论本实验的血浆 cGMP 测定结果,并说明其意义。
2. 为什么用他巴唑制作“阳虚”动物模型?试评价本模型。

Experiment 2　Effects of Aconite Root and Cinnamon on plasma cGMP level in hypothyroidism-based YANG asthenia Mice induced by thiamazole

【Purpose】 Learn the method of preparing the hypothyroidism-based YANG asthenia model induced by thiamazole, and observe the effects of Aconite Root and Cinnamon on the plasma cGMP level.

【Principles】 As an inhibitor of thyroid hormone synthesis, thiamazole inhibits the synthesis and secretion of thyroid hormones. Exposure of mice to thiamazole lead to the symptoms of hypothyroidism. The response of the cGMP system in cells to carbaminoylcholine, an M-receptor agonist, increases and results in a higher level of plasma cGMP. Aconite Root and Cinnamon can reduce the cGMP level by downregulating the response of the cGMP system.

【Equipments】 Liquid scintillation counter, vacuum filtration system, refrigeration centrifuge, microinjectors, micropippetes, little beakers, centrifuge tubes, glass tubes, liquid scintillating disc, ice container, dropper, syringe and needles.

【Drugs and reagents】 Misture of Aconite Root and Cinnamon (1 g/mL of Aconite Root and Cinnamon respectively), 0.3 g/L thiamazole solution, carbaminoylcholine, cyclic guanosine monophosphate (cGMP) radioimmunoassay kit.

【Animals】 Mice.

【Methods】 The same sex mice weighing about 22 g are divided into 3 groups at random, 10 animals per group. Normal control mice are orally administered with water every day. The mice in the group of hypothyroidism-based YANG asthenia (model) are orally administered with 6 mg/kg thiamazole every day until the model is established (It would be spent 2~3 months that the animals show YANG asthenia symptoms of cold body and limbs, and low oxygen consumption). During the process of thiamazole treatment , mice are given a gavage of 1 mL misture of Aconite Root and Cinnamon for 10~14 days. 6 min before blood collection by decapitation, all the mice are subcutaneously injected with 400 μ g/kg carbaminoylcholine. The sample treatment, standard curve preparation and the cGMP assay are performed according to the operating instructions in the kit.

【Results】 The plasma cGMP concentration increases in mice with hypothyroidism-based YANG asthenia. Treatment with Misture of Aconite Root and Cinnamon can lower the increased cGMP. Data are filled in table 17-2.

Table 17-2 Effects of misture of Aconite Root and Cinnamon on plasma cGMP level in mice with hypothyroidism-based YANG asthenia induced by thiamazole

Group	Animal number	Carbaminoylcholine (μg/kg)	Plasma cGMP (mol/L)
Control			
Hypothyroidism-based YANG asthenia			
YANG asthenia and treated with misture			

【Notes】

1. The appearance of cold body and limbs and decreased oxygen consumption suggests the successful establishment of YANG asthenia model.

2. The cGMP level is also able to be measured by using cAMP ELISA KIT.

【Questions】

1. Analyze the results of plasma cGMP assay and explain its meanings.

2. Why is the YANG asthenia model prepared by thiamazole administration? Try to evaluate this model.

“气虚”动物模型和补气药实验

气虚在临床上极为常见。据临床观察,气虚是人类几乎所有疾病在一定阶段上共有的基本特征,常见于慢性消耗性疾病或急性病恢复期及老年体衰弱患者。不同原因所导致的气虚,依脏腑病理表现不同,具体辨证为“心气虚”、“脾气虚”、“肾气虚”、“肺气虚”等。近年来研究人员从基础和临床两方面对各类气虚证进行了研究,发现气虚证可表现为神经系统、呼吸系统、循环系统、消化系统、内分泌系统、免疫系统等各个系统机能活动的衰退。目前有关气虚动物模型的研究仍很不够,尚缺乏理想的模型。现仅选择部分研究工作简介如下。

1. 家兔气虚模型　根据中医临床辨证经验,贫血多有气虚表现。将家兔放血,使其贫血而可表现气虚症状。实验用健康成年家兔,体重 1.7~2.5 kg,每天由耳动脉、耳静脉或心脏放血 10 mL 左右,形成人工慢性贫血而造模。气虚家兔表现精神萎钝、嗜睡、四肢蜷缩,肌张力减低,体温稍高,血细胞压积下降、总蛋白略低,舌质苍白、胖嫩、湿润,与气虚病人的临床症状大致相符合。

2. 大白鼠气虚模型　根据中医过度劳倦有伤形体的理论,迫使大白鼠连续游泳两周,造成其体力逐步衰弱而致“气虚”,出现血液流变学及血细胞形态的明显异常。与正常对照组动物比较,气虚大鼠表现为全血比黏度和血浆比黏度显著增高,红细胞电泳时间明显延长,红细胞压积增高等。补气药人参和黄芪等对此具有改善作用。

Animal model of deficiency of vital energy and experiments relevant to drugs for invigorating vital energy

Clinically, deficiency of vital energy (QI deficiency) is a common syndrome. According to clinical observation, deficiency of vital energy might be the same fundamental characteristic of all diseases developing to some stage, and is common in older patients of weakness or in chronic wasting disease and in the restoration period of acute diseases. Deficiency of vital energy induced by different factors could be differentiated according to the pathological changes of entrails into deficiency of heart-QI, deficiency of spleen-QI, deficiency of kidney-QI and deficiency of lung-QI, et al. Preliminary basic and clinical studies on various types of QI deficiency suggest that the syndrome of QI deficiency is related to the deteriorations of nervous system, respiratory system, circulation system, digestive system, endocrine system and immune system. At present, studies about models of QI deficiency are still limited and the ideal models are not available. Thus, just some experimental work in exploration stage is briefly introduced as follows.

1. Rabbit model of QI deficiency According to the clinical experience of differentiation of symptoms and signs in Chinese medical science, symptoms of QI asthenia appear in anaemia patients. Anaemia rabbits obtained by bleeding could show symptoms of QI deficiency. Healthy adult rabbits, weighed 1.7~2.5 kg, are used in the model preparation of chronic anaemia by bloodletting from arteria auricularis, ear vein or heart. Rabbits with QI deficiency exhibit the symptoms of weak spirit, drowsiness, twisted limbs, hypomyotonia, slightly higher of body temperature, lower volume of packed blood cells, slightly lower of total protein, and accompanied with pale, fat, tender and moistening texture of tongue, most of which accord with that of patients with QI deficiency.

2. Rat model of QI deficiency According to the theory of Chinese medical science that excessive exhaustion is detrimental to the body, rat model of QI deficiency is developed by forcing rats to swim for two weeks, leading to the gradual weakness in physical strength. Compared with normal animals, the model rats show the symptoms of the significantly increased whole blood viscosity (ratio) and plasma viscosity (ratio), obviously prolonged erythrocyte electrophoretic time and elevated volume of packed red blood cells, and accompanied with immune dysfunction. Ginseng and Radix Astragali, drugs for invigorating vital energy, could be helpful for the recovery from the asthenia syndrome.

实验三　大白鼠“气虚”模型和黄芪、人参的补气作用

【目的】了解劳倦过度所致“气虚”动物模型的建立以及补气药黄芪、人参的作用。

【原理】根据中医过度劳倦有伤形体的理论，迫使大鼠连续游泳，使其处于极度的应激状态，体力逐步衰弱而致“气虚”。气行则血行，气虚则血虚，故此模型动物可出现血液流变学方面的改变。补气药对此种动物可能具有保护作用。

【器材】恒温水槽；注射器；大鼠灌胃针头；毛细管黏度计；细胞电泳黏度计时器；离心机。

【药品和试剂】黄芪水煎液 2 g/mL；人参水煎液 0.25 g/mL；1% 肝素。

【动物】大白鼠。

【方法】取 180~200 g 大白鼠 40 只，雌雄兼用，随机分为 4 组，每组 10 只。

（1）游泳劳损造模组：每鼠每天灌胃自来水 5 mL/kg；

（2）游泳劳损加黄芪组：每鼠每天灌胃黄芪水煎液 10 g/kg；

（3）游泳劳损加人参组：每鼠每天灌胃人参水煎液 1.25 g/kg；

（4）正常对照组：仅灌胃水，不迫使游泳。

前 3 组大鼠灌胃水或药液 40 min 后，放入恒温水槽[水温（43 ± 0.5）℃、水深 35 cm]中游泳，以每只大鼠出现自然沉降的时间为其游泳耐疲劳的时间。当全组 50% 大鼠出现自然沉降时，全组大鼠均停止游泳。如此连续 14 天，第 15 天不进行游泳，给水或给药 40 min 后以乙醚麻醉大鼠，眼静脉丛取血，加肝素抗凝。用玻璃毛细管黏度计测定全血比黏度和血浆比黏度；用细胞电泳黏度计时器在恒温 25 ℃、电压为 40 V 的条件下，测定 10 个红细胞，每个红细胞泳动 165 μm 所需要的时间为红细胞的电泳时间；用离心机于 3 000 rpm 离心 30 min，所得值为红细胞压积。正常对照组第 15 天给水 40 min 后同法测定上述指标。

【结果】游泳劳损组大鼠全血黏度、血浆黏度及全血还原黏度明显增高，而红细胞电泳时间显著延长。黄芪和人参对上述发生明显变化指标皆有不同程度改善。参照表 17-3 记录。

表 17-3　补气药对“气虚”动物血液流变学指标的影响

分组	动物数	全血黏度（比）	血浆黏度（比）	全血还原黏度（比）	红细胞电泳时间（s）	红细胞压积（%）
游泳劳损造模组						
游泳劳损加黄芪组						

（续表）

分组	动物数	全血黏度（比）	血浆黏度（比）	全血还原黏度（比）	红细胞电泳时间（s）	红细胞压积（%）
游泳劳损加人参组						
正常对照组						

【思考题】

1. 分析和讨论各实验组的结果，并说明其意义。

2. 试结合活血化瘀药的药理作用，说明活血化瘀药与补气药合用治疗血瘀证的理论的意义。

Experiment 3 Rat model of QI deficiency and the invigorating-vital-energy actions of Ginseng and Radix Astragali

【Purpose】 Learn the method of establishing overstrain-induced Qi-deficiency model, and observe the effects of Ginseng and Radix Astragali on vital energy.

【Principles】 According to the theory of Chinese medical science that excessive exhaustion is detrimental to body, rats are forced to continuously swim for some time to an exceeding stress extent, resulting in QI deficiency because of gradual weakness in physical strength. Invigoration of QI promotes blood flow, while QI deficiency leads to the blood deficiency. The model animals could show the hemorheological changes. Drugs for invigorating vital energy could protect the animals from the exceeding damages.

【Equipments】 Thermostatic water bath, syringes, lavage pinhead, capillary viscometer, time counter of cell electrophoresis and viscosity, centrifuger.

【Drugs】 Radix Astragali decoction 2 g/mL, Ginseng decoction 0.25 g/mL, 1% heparin.

【Animals】 Rats.

【Methods】 Female or male rats weighing 180 g to 200 g, are divided into 4 groups at random, 10 animals per group.

(1) Rats in the model group are orally administered with 5 mL/kg water.

(2) Rats for the Radix Astragali treatment re orally administered with 10 g/kg Radix Astragali decoction.

(3) Rats for ginseng treatment are orally administered with 1.25 g/kg ginseng decoction.

(4) Rat in the normal control group are orally administered with 5 mL/kg water without being forced to swim.

Rats in the first three groups are put into the thermostatic water bath [water temperature is (43 ± 0.5) ℃, 35 cm deep] to swim. The antifatigue time is that from the beginning of swimming to the time rats sink naturally. When 50% of animals sink, all the animals in this group stop swimming. The procedure is repeated for 14 days. On the 15th day, rats are anesthetized with ether and blood is collected from the retro-orbital plexus 40 min after the drug exposure and treated with heparin. The whole blood viscosity and plasma viscosity are measured by capillary viscometer. Erythrocyte electrophoretic time is the mean time of 10 RBCs spent in electrophoresis for 165 μm, which is obtained by time counter of cell electrophoresis and viscosity under the conditions of constant temperature of 25 ℃ and 40 V of voltage. The volume of packed red blood cells is recorded after centrifuge at 3,000 rpm for 30 min. Rats in normal control group are treated as the method above except for swimming.

【Results】 In model group, the whole blood viscosity, plasma viscosity and whole blood reduced viscosity increase obviously, while the erythrocyte electrophoretic time increases significantly, but these changes can be prevented by Ginseng and Radix Astragali treatment. Please fill the data in the table 17-3.

Table 17-3 Effects of drugs for invigorating vital energy on the hemorheological indexes in QI deficiency model rats

Group	Animal number	Whole blood viscosity (ratio)	Plasma viscosity (ratio)	Whole blood reduced viscosity (ratio)	erythrocyte electrophoretic time (s)	Volume of packed RBCs (%)
Normal						
Model						
Radix Astragali						
Ginseng						

【Questions】

1. Analyze and discuss the results and explain the meanings.

2. Illustrate the theoretical significance of combined use of drugs for invigorating blood circulation and eliminating stasis and drugs for invigorating vital energy.

“血虚”动物模型和补血药实验

血虚多因失血过多或脾胃功能衰弱，血液生化之源不足，或因瘀血阻滞而新血不生等引起。其症状为面色苍白或萎黄，唇、舌、指甲淡而无华，头晕眼花，心悸失眠、手足麻木、脉细数无力。这些症状与现代医学所讲的贫血一致，因此，采用造成贫血的方法可以造成“血虚”模型。造模方法一是失血过多，包括出血与溶血；二是生血不足，可用化学因素，如烷化剂，或物理因素，如 ^{60}Co 照射，造成骨髓造血功能抑制。联合注射溶血剂乙酰苯肼和烷化剂环磷酰胺的方法也较常用。此外，还可采用食物中营养不足（如维生素 B_{12} 缺乏），或营养吸收障碍而造成“血虚”证。

Animal models of blood deficiency and experiments of antanemic

Blood deficiency is mainly resulted from excessive hemorrhage, weak functions of the spleen and stomach, short of the source of vital function, or deficiency of fresh blood because of the stagnation of blood stasis. The symptoms include pale or etiolated face, lip, tongue and nail, dizziness and dim eyesight, palpitation and insomnia, deadlimb, and fine, quick and powerless pulses, all of which are the same as that of anaemia in modern medicine. Therefore, blood deficiency models could be established by the methods of preparing anaemia models, such as excessive loss of blood, hemogenesis impairment induced by chemical agents or irradiation. Combined use of hemolytic agent acetylphenylhydrazine and alkylating agent cyclophosphamide is commonly adopted. Furthermore, nutrition deprivation (such as deficiency of Vit B_{12}) or malabsorption of nutrition also induces the syndrome of blood deficiency.

实验四　当归对失血性、溶血性“血虚”小白鼠的补血作用

【目的】了解失血法及溶血法造成的“血虚”动物模型及补血药的作用。

【原理】人工造成小鼠失血，使血液中红细胞（RBC）减少，血红蛋白（Hb）降低，而补血药使之趋于正常。

乙酰苯肼（Acetylphenyl hydrazine，APH）能破坏RBC而造成溶血性“血虚”。APH是强氧化剂，对RBC膜具有缓慢的进行性氧化损伤，并干扰RBC中的葡萄糖-6-磷酸脱氢酶（G-6-PDH），进而使还原型辅酶II（NADPH）生成障碍，谷胱甘肽生成减少，使RBC膜稳定性遭破坏，高铁血红蛋白不易还原而堆积，凝集成变性的珠蛋白小体（海氏小体），促使RBC破裂致Hb降低，RBC减少。

【器材】剪刀；镊子；注射器；10 mL刻度离心管；抗凝管；红细胞压积管；玻璃毛细管；pH吸管；10 mL量筒；20 μL微量移液器；分光光度计；低速离心机；天平；小烧杯。

【药品和试剂】红细胞稀释液；1%HCl；当归水浸液（0.2 g/mL）。

【动物】小白鼠。

【方法】小鼠随机分为5组，正常对照组每天灌胃水25 mL/kg；失血对照组用毛细管由眼眶静脉丛放血10滴/天，连续5天，从放血当天开始灌胃水25 mL/kg，连续7天；失血并给药组除放血5天外，从放血当天开始灌胃当归水浸液25 mL/kg，连续7天。末次给药1.5 h后，采血于抗凝管内，混匀备用。溶血组于第1、4天两次皮下注射1%APH生理盐水溶液100 mg/kg，同失血组灌胃水；溶血并给药组除注射APH外，灌胃当归水浸液25 mL/kg，连续7天，同上法制备抗凝血。

Hb测定：10 mL离心管中加入1%HCl 0.2 mL，再加20 μL抗凝血，混匀，10 min后加蒸馏水至5 mL，混匀，在分光光度计414 nm处测定光密度值（OD_{414}）。

RBC压积测定法（Wintrobe法）：将余下的抗凝血加于压积管中，3 000 rpm离心10 min，读RBC高度 a 及总高度 b，求100 mL血液中RBC的含量：$(a/b) \times 100\%$。

【结果】与正常对照组比较，失血性及溶血性血虚模型小鼠RBC压积及Hb吸收度皆显著降低。当归对此变化有明显改善效应。参照表17-4记录。

表 17-4 当归对“血虚”小鼠 RBC 及 Hb 的影响

分组	RBC 压积（%）	Hb（OD_{414}）
正常对照组		
失血组		
失血并给药组		
溶血组		
溶血并给药组		

【思考题】试评价常用的几种血虚证动物模型，并探讨当归的补血作用。

Experiment 4 Antanemic effect of Angelica Root on blood-loss or haemolysis-induced blood deficiency in mice

【Purpose】 Learn the method of the preparation of blood deficiency models via blood loss and haemolysis, and observe the effect of hematicum (Angelica Root).

【Principles】 In mice of blood loss by the man-made method, the population of red blood cells (RBC) and hemoglobin (Hb) content decrease. Antanemics could restore the changes.

Acetylphenyl hydrazine (APH) can destroy RBCs and induce haemolysis blood deficiency. APH, a strong oxidant with chronical and progressive oxidative damage to membranes, interferes the function of phosphate dehydrogenase (G-6-PDH) in RBCs, induces dyspoiesis of reduced coenzyme II (reduced form of nicotinamide-adenine dinucleotide phosphate, NADPH), downregulates the systhesis of glutathione and reduces the membrane stability of RBC. As a result, the produced ferrihemoglobin accumulates and agglutinates into denatured hematohiston, leading to erythrolysis and subsequent decreases of both Hb content and RBCs population.

【Equipments】 Scissors, forceps, syringes, graduated centrifuge tube of 10 mL volume, anticoagulation tubes, hematocrits, glass capillary, pH pipette, micropipette of 20 μL volumes, spectrophotometer, conventional centrifuge, balance, little bakers.

【Drugs and reagents】 Dilution solution of RBCs, 1% HCl, Angelica Root infusion (0.2 g/mL).

【Animals】 Mice.

【Methods】 Mice are randomized into 5 groups. Animals in normal control group are orally administered with 25 mL/kg water. Model mice of blood loss are exanguinated 10 drops of blood per day for 5 days from the plexus venosus of fossa orbitalis, and orally administered with water as normal mice from the first day of blood loss for 7 days. Mice of blood loss and treated with the Angelica Root infusion are exanguinated as the model mice and administered with 25 mL/kg Angelica Root infusion for 7 days. 1.5 h after the last administration, blood is collected in an anticoagulation tube until use. Haemolysis model are prepared by subcutaneous injection of 100 mg/kg 1% APH on day 1 and day 4 for two times and mice are administered with water for 7 days from day 1. Haemolysis mice treated with drug are exposed to Angelica Root infusion for 7 days.

Hb assay: 0.2 mL 1% HCl is added into a 10-mL centrifuge tube prior to the addition of

20 μL anticoagulated blood, followed by the addition of 5 mL distilled water 10 min later. The optical density value (OD_{414}) is measured with spectrophotometer.

Volume of packed RBCs assay (method of Wintrobe): The remained anticoagulated blood is added into hematocrit, centrifuged for 10 min at 3,000 rpm. The *a*, height of RBCs, and *b*, the overall height, are recorded, and the hematocrit is calculated as (a/b) × 100%.

[Results] The hematocrit and Hb content in blood deficiency mice of blood loss or haemolysis decrease significantly in comparison to that of normal control mice, and Angelica Root could antagonize the changes. Data are filled in the table 17-4.

Table 17–4　Effect of Angelica Root on the hematocrit and Hb content in mice with blood deficiency

Group	Volume of packed RBCs (%)	Hb (OD_{414})
Normal control		
Blood loss group		
Blood loss group treated with Angelica Root		
Haemolysis group		
Haemolysis group treated with Angelica Root		

[Question] Evaluate the commonly used animal models of blood deficiency and discuss the antanemic action of Angelica Root.

实验五　女贞子的抗突变作用

【目的】学习微核实验方法，观察女贞子的抗突变作用。

【原理】微核实验是毒理学中常用筛选化学致突变剂的方法之一。微核是由染色体遗落下来的断片演变而成。由于化学性、物理性或生物性因子作用于细胞周期的合成前期（G1 期或 S 期）引起染色单体断裂，无着丝点的染色体断裂片和染色单体的断片遗落在细胞质中，在细胞分裂末期之后，这些断片形成规则的一个或几个比主核小的次核称为微核。这些断片就是微核的主要来源。此外，完整的染色体由于纺锤体功能失调也可形成的微核。在骨髓中无核的红细胞有嗜多染红细胞和成熟红细胞两种。在正常情况下嗜多染红细胞占多数。由于毒性物质影响了骨髓红细胞，尤其是嗜多染红细胞（Polychromatic erythrocytes，PCEs），使其中的比例失衡，所以在微核试验中常以嗜多染红细胞进行计数。

女贞子有滋阴补血、扶正固本的作用，其主要活性成分之一为齐墩果酸，能保护骨髓红细胞的染色体。

【器材】1 mL 注射器；小鼠灌胃针头；解剖剪；镊子；钝大头针；解剖板；纱布；显微镜（带油镜头）；载物片；镜头油（香柏油）。

【药品和试剂】环磷酰胺；女贞子煎剂 0.5 ~1 g/mL；小牛血清；Giemsa 应用液；二甲苯；甲醇；pH6.4 磷酸盐缓冲液。

【动物】小白鼠。

【方法】小鼠分为 3 组，从骨髓涂片前 7~10 天开始，每天给第 1 组小鼠灌胃 1 次 25 g/kg 女贞子煎剂，直至实验当天为止，第 2、3 组小鼠灌胃等体积水。实验前 30 h 及 6 h，第 1 组及第 2 组小鼠分别腹腔注射环磷酰胺 50 mg/kg 各 1 次。第 3 组小鼠设为正常对照，腹腔注射生理盐水代替环磷酰胺，0.5 mL/ 只。然后按微核实验方法，取材，骨髓涂片，进行微核计数、嗜多染红细胞（PCE）及正染红细胞（RBC）计数，比较 3 组小鼠微核率与 PCE 百分率。

微核实验方法：

1. 骨髓涂片　小鼠脱颈椎处死，切开皮肤、肌肉，取出股骨，用纱布或软纸擦净，纵向剪去股骨 1/4，用钝的大头针挑出骨髓，放在已滴好一滴小牛血清的载玻片上（血清宜滴在载玻片的一端），另用一块边缘整齐的厚载玻片放在血清上轻轻地按摩，让骨髓团块完全分散均匀，然后以 45°~50° 角进行推片，在空气中晾干。

2. 固定　将涂片放入甲醇中固定 5~10 min，晾干。

3. 染色　直接在 Giemsa 应用液中，染色 10~30 min，取出染片放入 pH6.4 磷酸盐缓冲液中反复冲洗，在空气中晾干或置于 37 ℃恒温箱中烘干。

4. 封片　将晾干或烘干的染色片放入二甲苯中 5~10 min，取出，滴上一滴光学树脂胶，盖上盖玻片，制片完毕。

5. 微核的观察　微核的形态多数是圆形单个的，边缘光滑整齐，嗜色性与核质一致，大小约占细胞的 1/20~1/15，偶尔有肾形、环形、马蹄形、椭圆形等。用 Giemsa 染色后微核呈紫红色或蓝紫色。先以低倍镜、高倍镜粗检，选择细胞分散均匀、细胞完整、染色好的区域，在油镜下（1 000 倍计数）计数。嗜多染红细胞（PEC，呈灰蓝色或浅蓝色）和成熟红细胞（RBC，呈粉红色或橘红色）。

每只动物选择性计数嗜多染红细胞或红细胞中带有微核的细胞出现率，一般以千分率表示。一个嗜多染红细胞中出现两个或更多个微核，仍按一个微核细胞计算。

$$\text{微核率‰}=\frac{\text{含微核的PCE数}}{\text{PCE数}}\times 1\,000‰ \qquad （式 17-1）$$

$$\text{嗜多染红细胞\%(PCE\%)}=\frac{\text{PCE数}}{\text{PCE数+RBC数}}\times 100\% \qquad （式 17-2）$$

【结果】环磷酰胺注射小鼠微核率明显升高，灌胃给予女贞子后明显降低环磷酰胺诱导的骨髓红细胞微核率。数据记入表 17-5。

表 17-5　女贞子对小鼠微核形成的影响

分组	剂量	PCE 数	微核细胞数	微核率（‰）	PCE%
正常组					
环磷酰胺					
女贞子 + 环磷酰胺					

【注意事项】

1. 骨髓涂片关键在于使细胞分散均匀，否则细胞成堆，影响观察。
2. 若染色太浅，宜重放 Giemsa 应用液中重染。
3. 玻片、滴管、注射器等保持干净。
4. 若细胞分布很不均匀或细胞变形破碎就不宜计数。

【思考题】试分析环磷酰胺致突变及对骨髓抑制作用以及女贞子的抗突变作用。

Experiment 5 The antimutagenic Effect of Glossy Privet Fruit

【Purpose】Learn the method of micronucleus test and observe the antimutagenic effect of Glossy Privet Fruit.

【Principles】Mammalian micronucleus test in erythrocytes is one of the frequently used methods in toxicology for screening chemical mutagens. Micronuclei are developed from the fragments derived from chromosome. Briefly, chemical, physical or biological factors, acting on presynthetic phase (G1 phase or S phase) of the cell cycle, result in the breakage of chromatids. During telophase, the acentric fragments derived from chromosomes or chromatids remain in the cytoplasm and form one or more regular secondary nucleus (nuclei) called micronucleus (micronuclei) which are smaller than a main nucleus. Thus, these fragments are the main source of micronuclei. The other source is the whole chromosomes, which form micronuclei because of the spindle apparatus dysfunction.

In the bone marrow, akaryotic cells include polychromatic erythrocytes and mature erythrocytes. Generally, polychromatic erythrocyte is the majority. Toxic substances might affect bone marrow erythrocytes, especially polychromatic erythrocytes, and therefore interfere the cell proportion. Generally, polychromatic erythrocytes are recommended for enumeration in micronucleus assay.

Glossy Privet Fruit, containing the active component oleanolic acid, can nourish YIN and the blood and enhance healthy energy, and therefore protect the chromosome of bone marrow erythrocytes from the toxic factors.

【Equipments】 Syringes (1 mL), lavage pinhead for mice, dissecting scissors, forceps, mutic pin, dissection plate, gauze, microscope (with oil len), slides, cedar oil.

【Drugs and reagents】Cyclophosphamide, Glossy Privet Fruit decoction (1 g/mL), calf serum, Giemsa Application solution, dimethyl benzene, methanol, phosphate buffer (pH6.4).

【Animals】Mice.

【Methods】Mice are divided into 3 groups. 7 to10 days before the preparation of bone marrow smears, mice in the first group are orally administered with Glossy Privet Fruit decoction (25 g/kg), once a day, until the day to prepare smears. Mice in the other two groups are treated with the an equal volume of water. At 30 h and 6 h before the micronucleus assay, 50 mg/kg cyclophosphamide is applied to the first two groups of mice by intraperitoneal injection, the third group of mice are regarded as the normal control and injected with saline. Then, bone marrow smears are prepared and the numbers of micronucleated erythrocytes, polychromatic erythrocytes and normochromatic erythrocytes are recorded. The frequencies of micronucleated erythrocytes and polychromatic erythrocytes are evaluated according to the procedure of micronucleus test and compared among these three groups.

Procedures of micronucleus test.

1. Preparation of bone marrow smears　Mice are killed by cervical dislocation. After the skin and muscle being cut open, the femur is isolated and cleared off the adherent connective tissue. One fourth of the femur is cut off longitudinally and the bone marrow is squeezed out by inserting a mutic pin into the bone marrow cavity and put into a drop of calf serum on a glass slide (the serum should be dropped on one side of the slide). The marrow in the serum is dispersed well-distributed by slight massage with the edge of a thick glass slide, then is pushed along the slide by the angle of 45°~50° and allowed to air dry.

2. Fixation　Marrow smears are put into methanol for 5~10 minutes and dried in the air.

3. Staining　Marrow smears are put into Giemsa application solution for 10~30 minutes, then rinsed with phosphate buffer (pH 6.4) several times and dried in the air or in the thermostat at 37 ℃ .

4. Mounting　The smears are immersed into dimethyl benzene for 5~10 minutes, then a drop of optical resin glue is added on the smear before the latter is covered with a cover glass.

5. Observation of micronuclei　Most micronuclei are single and round, with smooth and regular edge and the same chromaticity as nuclear hyaloplasm. The size of a micronucleus is 1/20~1/15 of the cell. Occasionally, micronuclei appear with the shape of kidney, ring, horseshoe or ellipse. After put into Giemsa solution, micronuclei are stained prunosus or amethyst. Before counting, the smears are roughly inspected under low and high power lens to select the fields where the cells are intact, evenly spread and well stained, then cells in these fields are counted under oil len (1,000 times). Polychromatic erythrocytes (PEC) : gray-blue or light blue; Mature erythrocytes (RBC) : pink or reddish yellow.

The frequency of micronucleated erythrocytes is generally indicated in permillage. If two or more micronucleus are observed in the same cell, the number of micronucleated erythrocytes is still regarded as one.

$$\text{Frequency of micronucleated PEC ‰} = \frac{\text{Population of micronucleated PCE}}{\text{Population of PCE}} \times 1{,}000\text{‰}$$

(formula 17-1)

$$\text{Frequency of PCE \%} = \frac{\text{Population of PEC}}{\text{Population of PEC+Population of RBC}} \times 100\%$$

(formula 17-2)

【**Results**】Mice treated with Glossy Privet Fruit show a decreased frequency of micronucleated erythrocyte in bone marrow. Data are filled into the table 17-5.

Table 17-5 Effect of Glossy Privet Fruit on the formation of micronucleus in mice

Group	Dose	PCE number	Micronucleated erythrocyte number	Frequency of micronucleated erythrocyte (‰)	PCE%
Normal control					
Cyclophosphamide					
Glossy privet fruit					

【**Notes**】

1. The key point of preparation of bone marrow smear lies in the even spread of cells, otherwise the cells pile up and interfere the observation.

2. The marrow smears should be stained once more in Giemsa solution if the staining is too light.

3. The slides, dropper and syringes should be clean.

4. The fields where the cells spread unevenly or are deformed and broken into pieces should not be included in the counting.

【**Question**】Analyze the mutagenic and myelosuppressive effects of cyclophosphamide and the antimutagenic action of Glossy Privet Fruit.

实验六 当归芍药散对东莨菪碱记忆损伤小鼠学习记忆的影响

【目的】学习东莨菪碱所致记忆损伤模型的制备；观察当归芍药散对模型小鼠学习记忆的改善作用。

【原理】东莨菪碱诱导小鼠记忆损伤模型，利用跳台实验评价小鼠学习记忆能力。通过测定跳台实验的潜伏期与错误次数评定小鼠的记忆损伤程度，当归芍药散具有明显抗炎、抗氧化作用，延长小鼠跳台实验的潜伏期、减少错误次数，改善学习记忆能力。

【器材】被动回避反应箱。

【试剂】当归芍药散（当归∶芍药∶川芎∶白术∶茯苓∶泽泻 =1∶1.34∶1.34∶1.34∶1.34∶1）。

【动物】雄性小鼠，体重 18~22 g。

【方法】

1. 东莨菪碱记忆损伤模型的制备以及分组及给药　选择 18~22 g 雄性 ICR 小鼠 30 只，按体重随机分组，分为空白组、模型组、DSS 组（0.4 g/kg）。除空白组外，各组小鼠腹腔注射东莨菪碱（1 mg/kg），空白组小鼠注射生理盐水最为对照；DSS 组分别按体重灌胃对应剂量的 DSS，空白组和模型组灌胃对应体积的蒸馏水，连续 7 天后进行行为学检测。

2. 跳台实验　被动回避反应箱，底板设有铜栅，可通交流电，电压为 36 V。铜栅的一角放置一个橡胶平台作为安全区，小鼠可停留在平台上回避电击。末次给药 1 h 后开始进行学习训练。训练前先将小鼠放入箱中自由活动 3 min，熟悉环境，然后接通铜栅电源，持续 3 min，记录第一次跳下平台的潜伏期和 3 min 内的错误次数（动物跳下平台次数），以此作为学习成绩。24 h 后测验，记录动物第一次跳下平台的潜伏期和 3 min 内的错误次数，以此作为记忆成绩。

【结果】将结果填入表 17-6 中。

表 17-6　当归芍药散对东莨菪碱记忆损伤小鼠模型的改善作用

分组	错误次数	潜伏期
空白组		
模型组		
DSS 组		

【注意事项】

1. 行为学检测应注意外界因素的影响。

2. 熟练小鼠的灌胃方式。

【思考题】

1. 分析造模原理及药物作用的可能机制。

2. 如何改进方法？

Experiment 6 Protective effects of Danggui-Shaoyao-Sanon scopolamine-induced learning and memory deficits in mice

【Purpose】To investigate the effects of Dangui-Shaoyao-San on scopolamine-induced learning and memory deficits in mice and study how to prepare the model.

【Principles】The learning and memory deficits that induced by scopolamine in mice can be measured by step-down test through recording the latent phase and the frequency of stepping down the platform. DSS has significant anti-inflammatory and anti-oxidant activity, thereby can relieve the learning and memory deficits in mice that induced by scopolamine.

【Equipments】Equipments for mice step-down test.

【Reagents】Danggui-Shaoyao-San.

(Danggui : Shaoyao : Chuanxiong : Baizhu : Fuling : Zhexie =1 : 1.34 : 1.34 : 1.34 : 1.34 : 1)

【Animals】Mice (male), weighing 18~22 g.

【Methods】

1. Animals and drug administration 30 mice (18~22 g) were randomly divided into 3 groups (normal, model and DSS 0.4 g/kg, n=10). Scopolamine (1 mg/kg) is injected subcutaneously daily expect for the normal group. In addition, apart from the normal and model group, the remaining mice are administrated DSS by gavage daily for 7 days.

2. The Step-Down test In the step-down test, animals were placed in the equipment to adapt to the environment for 3 min, then 36 V electric current was applied. Error response was determined if mice jumped to copper bars after electric shock and correct response was determined if mice jumped back to the safe area. This training was performed for 3 min and the test started 24 h later. The latent phase and times of stepping down the platform are recorded.

【Results】Write down your data in the table17-6.

Table 17-6 Protective effects of Danggui-Shaoyao-San on learning and memory deficits in mice induced by scopolamine

Grouping	Times of error response	latent phase
Normal		
Model		
DSS		

【Notes】

1. Pay attention to the external factor when the experiment going.

2. Be familiar with the drug administration of mice.

【Questions】

1. Analyze the mechanisms of the preparation of model and the effect of Danggui-Shaoyao-San.

2. How will you improve the experimental design?

“脾虚”动物模型和补脾药实验

脾虚是脾病的主要证候。据临床所见，脾虚患者的消化系统功能减退，肠道菌失调，免疫功能、代谢水平、内分泌功能和血浆环磷酸腺苷（cAMP）含量等均偏低。由此可见中医的“脾”是与消化功能相关的多功能单位。自从口服大黄煎剂复制出“脾虚”证动物模型后，研究人员采用不同致虚证因子复制“脾虚”模型，这对进一步研究脾虚证的本质及阐明某些方药的作用机制起到重要作用。现将目前复制“脾虚”动物模型的常用方法简介如下。

实验可选用大鼠、小鼠、金黄地鼠、豚鼠和家兔等，其中以小鼠应用较多。根据致病因素不同，常用者有以下几种：

1. 苦寒中药法　利用泻下药大黄、番泻叶等给动物大量灌胃。因大黄等药性苦寒，过量能伤元气，耗阴血，损脾胃，使脾失健运、泄泻而致虚。例如给小鼠灌胃生大黄水煎液 1 g/mL，0.6~1.0 mL/ 只，每日 1 次，连续 7 天 ~9 天可造成小鼠“脾虚”模型。

2. “饮食失节”及“生化乏源”法　根据中医饮食失节，过食肥甘，饥饿、烦渴等均可伤元气、损脾胃 的理论，采用饮食失节及半饥饿或限量营养的方法，复制“脾虚”模型。例如仅给小鼠喂食甘兰，每两天加喂 1 次猪油，9 天后可造成饮食失节“脾虚”模型。

3. 利血平法　临床研究表明，脾虚泄泻证患者多有植物神经功能紊乱，副交感神经功能偏亢，表现为胃肠蠕动加快，消化液分泌增加以及吸收功能障碍等。利血平可以耗竭动物体内的单胺类递质（主要是去甲肾上腺素和 5- 羟色胺），降低脑内和外周神经中单胺类递质的含量，使副交感神经功能相对偏亢。一定剂量的利血平能使动物引起与中医脾虚证类似的症状。小鼠每日皮下注射 0.15~0.3 mg/kg 体重的利血平，连续 10~14 天，可出现脾虚症状。

4. 其他方法　可以采用过度疲劳（例如跑步或游泳）联合“饮食失节”等方法造模。

上述模型动物均程度不等地出现体重减轻，食量减少，毛枯槁无光泽，行动迟缓无力，嗜卧，体温降低、耐寒力差、便溏及脱肛等。目前临床关于脾虚证的辨证标准是：大便溏泻，食后腹胀而喜按，面色萎黄，食欲减少，肌瘦无力。具备其中 3 项者即可辨证为脾虚证。上述模型动物的主要表现类似于中医临床的脾阳虚或脾气虚，基本符合中医理论的论述。

Animal model of Splenic Asthenia and experiments relevant to drugs for reinforcing the Spleen

Splenic asthenia is the main syndrome of splenetic disease. According to clinical observation, symptoms such as hypofunction of the digestive system, intestinal dysbacteriosis, decrease in immune function, metabolic level, endocrine function and cyclic adenosine monophosphate (cAMP) level are common in patients with splenic asthenia, which suggests that the spleen in Chinese medical science consists of multi-units relevant to digestive functions. After the animal model of splenic asthenia is established by oral administration of Rhubarb decoction, researchers have applied different deficiency syndromes–induced methods to prepare the models of splenic asthenia, which is beneficial to the study of the nature of splenic asthenia and interpretations of the mechanisms of some drugs and prescriptions. The commonly-used methods for preparation of the models of splenic asthenia are briefly presented as below.

Rat, mouse, golden hamster, guinea pig and rabbit can be adopted in the experiments, and mouse is widely used. According to different factors inducing splenic asthenia, there are several methods generally used for model preparation.

1. Exposure to bitter cold traditional Chinese medicine　Eliminates such as Rhubarb and Folium Sennae are orally administered to animals. Excess use of these drugs with the nature of bitterness and cold could hurt vigour, consume the YIN-blood, and therefore results in splenic asthenia by inducing dys-splenism and diarrhoea. For example, the mouse model could be obtained by treating of mice orally with the decoction of Rhubarb (1 g/mL), 0.6~1.0 mL/mouse, for 7 to 9 days.

2. Intemperate food taking or nutrition deficiency　According to the theory in Chinese medical science that the intemperance of taking food , hyperphagia of fat and sweet, starvation and dipsosis are harmful to the vigour, the spleen and stomach, the methods of the intemperance of taking food, semistarvation or limitation of nutrition could be applied to establish the model of splenic asthenia. For example, mice are orally administered only with cabbage, and with additional swine fat every two days. After 9 days, the model of intemperance of taking food could be produced successfully.

3. Reserpine treatment　The clinical studies indicate that functional disorder of autonomic nerve and domination of the parasympathetic nerve often appear in the patients with the symptoms of splenasthenic diarrhea who show increasing secretion of digestive juice

and disturbance of absorptive function. Reserpine could exhaust monoamine transmitters (including NE and 5-HT), lower the content of monoamine transmitters in the brain and peripheral nerve, which results in the excessive function of parasympathetic nerve. Thus, reserpine can be used to induce the symptoms in animals similar to that of splenasthenic syndrome described in Chinese medical science. Mice might show the symptoms of splenic asthenia after subcutaneous treatment with 0.15~0.3 mg/kg of reserpine for 10~14 days.

4. Other methods Combination of overfatigue (such as running or swimming) and intemperate taking food.

All the animal models described above display the symptoms of body weight loss, reduced appetite, dry and broom hair, sluggish and weak action, long time of lying state, decreased body tempcrature, weak cold endurance, loose stool and archoptosis. At present, the standards of differentiation of symptoms and signs in splenasthenic syndrome include loose stool, abdominal distention, relief with pressure, complexion etiolate, weak appetite and weak and powerless muscle. If three of these standards are satisfied, it is differentiated as the splenasthenic syndrome. The main appearance of the model animals described above is similar to that of insufficiency of spleen-YANG or deficiency of spleen-QI in clinical Chinese medical science, which is in line with the description in the theory of Chinese medical science.

实验七　小白鼠"脾虚"模型复制和附子理中汤的作用

【目的】学会用中药大黄建立"脾虚"模型的方法；观察附子理中汤对此模型的调理作用。

【原理】大黄药性苦寒，过度使用能损伤元气、耗阴血，损脾胃，使脾失健运，泄泻致虚。研究表明，大黄口服后，结合型蒽苷到达大肠，在细菌酶的作用下，还原成蒽酮或蒽酚，刺激肠黏膜，并抑制 Na^+ 转运至细胞，水分滞留肠腔；肠道被扩张，刺激肠壁而致泻下。同时大黄可抑制消化酶的活性，导致动物食欲不振，消化不良，体重下降，造成"脾虚"证。附子理中汤具有温中祛寒、补气健脾的功效，对此模型有改善作用。

【器材】电子秤；冰箱；注射器；小鼠灌胃针头；眼科镊；眼科剪等。

【药品和试剂】生大黄煎液 1 g/mL；大黄合剂（大黄 6 g，芒硝 1 g，水煎成 5 mL）；附子理中汤（附子、党参、白术和干姜各 1 g，炙甘草 6 g，水煎成 6 mL）。

【动物】小鼠。

【方法】小鼠随机分成 6 组：大黄致"脾虚"组、大黄合剂致"脾虚"组、脾虚治疗组及正常对照组各两组。

1. 耐寒机能测定　大黄致"脾虚"组小鼠每天灌胃生大黄煎液 0.8 mL~1.0 mL，连续 8 天；药物治疗组除灌胃大黄煎液外，每天灌胃附子理中汤 0.5 mL/ 只。正常对照组仅灌胃等体积水。于实验第 9 天将三组动物同时放入饲养盒内，置于零下 3~5 ℃冰箱中，每隔 30 min 观察动物死亡数。持续 3 小时。

2. 免疫机能测定　治疗组每天灌胃大黄合剂 0.7 mL，连续 18 天。第 8 天加灌胃附子理中汤煎液 0.5 mL/ 只，连续 11 天。"脾虚"组则灌胃大黄合剂及水；正常对照组仅灌胃水。于灌胃后的第 15 天腹腔注射 0.2 mL/ 只 10% 绵羊红细胞进行免疫。免疫后 4 天（第 19 天）处死动物，解剖，取脾脏作用溶血空斑（Plaque forming cell, PFC）实验和 E 玫瑰花结实验（Erythrocyte rosette formation test, ERFC）。

【结果】脾虚组动物死亡数明显增多，附子理中汤治疗组有一定改善；脾虚组动物脾重降低，PFC 及 ERFC 明显降低，附子理中汤则表现出显著改善作用。数据记入表 17-7A 及表 17-7B。

表 17-7A　附子理中汤对脾虚小鼠耐寒机能的影响

分组	动物数（只）	冷冻 3 h		平均每鼠存活时间（h）
		死亡数	死亡率（%）	
正常对照组				
脾虚组				
附子理中汤组				

表 17–7B　附子理中汤对脾虚小鼠脾细胞 PFC、ERFC 的影响

分组	动物数（只）	平均脾重（mg）	PFC/10^6 脾细胞	ERFC/10^6 脾细胞
正常对照组				
脾虚组				
附子理中汤组				

【注意事项】

1. 本实验易受温度的影响，在 4~24 ℃范围内，淋巴细胞形成花结的程度较高，故放置 4 ℃冰箱较为合适。37 ℃时花结易解离，在沉淀物中需加入等量 1% 戊二醛，置 4 ℃冰箱固定 10~20 min，然后取出染色。据报道，淋巴细胞在接触红细胞之前预温（37 ℃ 1 h）可提高 E 玫瑰花结形成度。

2. 用生理盐水代替 Hank's 液洗涤淋巴细胞，不影响 E 玫瑰花结形成度，但 pH 应保持 7.2。

【思考题】

1. 分析各实验组的结果，并说明其意义。

2. 试述大黄致脾虚动物模型的理论根据及附子理中丸的复健作用和原理。

【附】

1. 溶血空斑实验（PFC）　测定方法采用平皿法。将免疫 4~5 天的动物放血处死。取脾脏，用 pH7.2 的 Hank's 液制备脾细胞悬液，细胞浓度应调整到 1×10^7/mL。取试管置于 45~48 ℃恒温水浴中，每管加入 2.5 mL 融化的 7 g/L 琼脂糖（用含 5 g/L 水解乳蛋白的 Hank's 液配制，调 pH 为 7.2~7.4），再依次加入 3 : 5 稀释的绵羊红细胞 0.1 mL、脾细胞悬液 0.1 mL（约含 1×10^6 个脾细胞）。迅速混匀，立即倒入直径 9 cm 的无菌培养皿中，水平放置待琼脂糖凝固。每个处理设置 3 个平皿。

将平皿置 37 ℃温箱内孵育 1 h，每个平皿加入 1 : 5（用 Hank's 液稀释）稀释的新鲜豚鼠血清 1 mL，使其均匀地覆盖整个琼脂糖平皿表面。继续温育 30 min 即可见溶血空斑。若空斑不清晰，则再在室温下放置 30 min。

弃去平皿中的豚鼠血清，加入 3% 的甲醛或 2.5% 戊二醛溶液固定。显微镜下分别计数每个平皿（1×10^6 细胞）内的溶血空斑。显微镜下可见每个空斑由抗体形成细胞及其周围的透明区组成。分别计算对照组、模型组和药物处理组每 10^6 脾细胞中的溶血空斑均值。

2. E 玫瑰花结形成实验（ERFC）　取 0.25 mL 淋巴细胞悬液（约 3×10^5 个淋巴细胞）置离心管中，加入 1% 绵羊红细胞悬液 0.25 mL，混匀，放入 37 ℃水浴保温 5 min，用 500~800 rpm 离心 5 min，置 4 ℃冰箱 2~4 h 或过夜。弃去上清，加入 Hank's 液及新配制的 Giemsa 染液各 0.2 mL，混匀，置于 4 ℃冰箱或冰浴中 30 min。然后将 1 滴细胞悬液置血细胞计数板中，显微镜下观察计数。镜下可见淋巴细胞和多形核白细胞呈蓝色，绵羊红细胞不着色。凡黏附 3 个以上绵羊红细胞的淋巴细胞称 ERFC。计数大格淋巴细胞与 ERFC，计算 ERFC 形成百分率，再按下式计算 T 淋巴细胞总数：

$$T\text{ 淋巴细胞总数}/\text{mm}^3=(\text{白细胞总数}/\text{mm}^3)\times\text{淋巴细胞百分率}\times\text{ERFC 形成百分率}\qquad(\text{式 }17\text{–}3)$$

Experiment 7　The establishment of the Splenic Asthenia model in Mouse and the pharmacological action of Fuzilizhongtang

【**Purpose**】Learn the method of preparation of splenic asthenia model induced by Rhubarb, and observe the pharmacological action of Fuzilizhongtang.

【**Principles**】Excessive use of Rhubarb, a TCM with bitter cold nature, could hurt vigour, consume the YIN-blood, injure the spleen and stomach and results in splenic asthenia by inducing dys-splenism and diarrhoea. After oral administration of Rhubarb, the combined type of anthra glycoside reaches the large intestine where it is reduced into anthrone or anthranol by the action of bacterial enzyme. Anthranol might stimulate the intestinal mucosa, inhibit Na+ transport into cells, and detains the water in enteric cavity, therefore results in decanta by dilating and stimulating the intestinal tract. Moreover, Rhubarb could also induce the splenic asthenia syndrome with the symptoms of anepithymia, dyspepsia and body weight loss by inhibiting the activity of digestive enzymes. Fuzilizhongtang has the efficiency of warming middle energizer to dispel cold, invigorating vital energy and the spleen, leading to the improvement of asthenia syndrome.

【**Equipments**】Electronic scale, refrigerator, syringes, pinhead of intragastric administration for mice, pincette and eye scissors.

【**Drugs and reagents**】Crude Rhubarb decoction（1 g /mL）, Rhubarb misture（Rhubarb 6 g, Mirabilite 1 g, decocted into 5 mL）, Fuzilizhongtang（1 g of Aconite Root, Radix Codonopsitis, Atractylodes Macrocephala and Zingiberis, Rhizoma respectively, prepared RADIX GLYCYRRHIZAE 6 g, decocted into 6 mL）.

【**Animals**】Mice.

【**Methods**】Mice are divided into 6 groups at random. One splenic asthenia group treated with Rhubarb, the other splenic asthenia group treated with Rhubarb misture, 2 groups of treatment and two sets of normal control.

1. Determination of cold-resistant function　Mice in the group of Rhubarb-induced splenic asthenia are treated orally with crude Rhubarb decoction 0.8~1.0 mL per mouse for 8 days. Except being treated with Rhubarb as the first group, the second group of mice are also given a gavage of Fuzilizhongtang for 8 days. Normal control mice are treated with the an equal volume of water. On day 9, three groups of mice in breeding cages are put into refrigerator at 3~5 ℃ temperature. The death rate is recorded every 30 min for a total time of 3 hours.

2. Immune function assay Mice in the treatment group are orally administered with 0.7 mL Rhubarb misture for 18 days. The Fuzilizhongtang is administered from the 8th day, 0.5 mL per mouse, for 11 days. Model mice are administered Rhubarb misture and water, and mice in normal control are treated only with water. On the 15th day of the experiment, mice are immuned via intraperitoneal injection with 0.2 mL per mouse of sheep erythrocytes (10 %). 4 days after immunization (the 19th day of initiation of the experiment), mice are killed and the spleen is isolated for plaque-forming cell (PFC) assay and Erythrocyte rosette formation cell (ERFC) assay.

【Results】 After treatment of low temperature, the death rate in splenic asthenia increases obviously, which is blunted by treatment with Fuzilizhongtang. In the second set of experiment, body weight, numbers of PFC and ERFC decrease significantly in model mice, which are antagonized by Fuzilizhongtang. Data are filled in table 17-7A and 17-7B.

Table 17-7A Effect of FUZILIZHONGTANG on cold-resistant function in mice with splenic asthenia

Group	Animal number	Low temperature treatment for 3 h		Mean survival time (h)
		Number of dead mouse	Death rate (%)	
Normal control				
Splenic asthenia				
Fuzilizhongtang				

Table 17-7B Effect of Fuzilizhongtang on the frequency of PFC and ERFC in mice with splenic asthenia

Group	Animal number	Mean weight of spleen (mg)	PFC/10^6 splenocytes	ERFC/10^6 splenocytes
Normal control				
Splenic asthenia				
Fuzilizhongtang				

【Notes】

1. The experiment is sensitive to the temperature, at the range of 4~24 ℃, the frequency of erythrocyte rosette formation cells is higher, so it is better to keep cells in 4 ℃ refrigerator. At 37 ℃, the formed rosette is easy to disaggregate, therefore, the an equal volume of glutaric dialdehyde (1%) should added into the segment for 10~20 min fixation at 4 ℃ followed by staining. It has been reported that preincubation at 37 ℃ for 1 h would raise the frequency of ERFC.

2. Saline can replace Hank's solution to wash lymphocytes without influencing the erythrocyte rosette formation under the condition of pH7.2.

【Questions】

1. Analyze the result of each group and explain its significance.

2. Try to explain the theory basis of Rhubarb-induced splenic asthenia model and the effect and underlying mechanisms of Fuzilizhongtang.

【Appendix】

1. Hemolytic plaque assay (plaque-forming cell assay)(PFC)　The assay is carried out in triplicate flat plates. The animals are killed on the fifth day after immunization with SRBC. The spleen is removed, and a single cell suspension of 10^7 cells/mL was prepared in Hank's solution. 2.5 mL colliquative agarose (7 g/L, prepared with Hank's solution containing 5 g/L of lactoalbumin hydrolysate) is added into the tube and kept in a thermostatic water bath (45~48 ℃), then 0.1 mL SRBC (3 : 5 solution) and 0.1 mL splenocyte suspension are added inorder. Cells are mixed quickly and pushed into a culture dish (9 cm diameter) until solidification.

After 1 h of incubation, 1 mL fresh guinea pig serum diluted with Hank's solution by 1∶5 is added into the culture dish and cover the whole surface of the agarose. The plaques might appear after an incubation of 30 min. Another 30-min incubation would be necessary if the plaques are not clear.

Then guinea pig serum is removed prior to the fixation with 3% formaldehyde or 2.5% glutaral. Plaques are counted under a light microscope and expressed as PFC per 10^6 spleen cells. The plaque is composed of the antibody-forming cell and the peripheral bright zone. The mean value of the plaque numbers of each group is recorded .

2. Erythrocyte rosette formation cell (ERFC) assay　0.25 mL lymphocyte suspension (about 3×10^5 splenocytes) is added into a centrifuge tube and mixed with 0.25 mL of 1% SRBC. After incubation at 37 ℃ for 5 min, cells are centrifuged at 500~800 rpm for 5 min, then kept in 4 ℃ -refrigerator for 2~4 h or overnight. The supernatant is discarded, followed by the addition of 0.2 mL Hank's solution and fresh Giemsa staining solution respectively. Cells are kept at 4 ℃ or in an ice bath for 30 minutes. A drop of the cell suspension is added onto a counting plate for the ERFC counting under the microscope. Lymphocytes or polymorphonuclear leukocytes are stained blue and SRBCs are stainless. A lymphocyte is looked as an E rosette—formation cell when it is adhered with more than three SRBCs. Count the lymphocytes and ERFCs in the large grills and calculate the percentage of ERFC. The population of T cells is obtained by formula 16-4.

Population of T cells/mm^3 = (total white blood cells /mm^3) × percentage of lymphocyes × percentage of ERFCs　(formula 17-3)

第十八章　抗衰老实验

Chapter 18　Anti-aging experiments

实验一　何首乌醇提物对小鼠脑内单胺氧化酶活性的影响

【目的】掌握单胺氧化酶 -B 活性测定方法，观察何首乌醇提物对单胺氧化酶 B 的抑制作用。

【原理】以苄胺作为底物，在 MAO-B 的作用下生成苄醛，用环己烷提取，在 242 nm 下测定吸光度值。

$$RCH_2-NH_2+O_2+H_2O \xrightarrow{MAO} RCHO+NH_3+H_2O$$

【试剂】8 mmol/L 苄胺；0.1 mol/L 磷酸缓冲液（pH7.6）；10% 高氯酸；环己烷；何首乌醇提物（取其粗粉 2.5 kg 用 5 倍量乙醇提取 3 次，减压回收乙醇，得提取物 285 g，作为供试药物，备用）。

【动物】老龄小鼠 20 只，雄性。

【方法】

1. 取小鼠 20 只，随机分为 2 组，一组给予何首乌醇提物（200 mg/kg），一组给予生理盐水作为对照组。给药 5 天。

2. 末次给药后 1 h，取小鼠全脑加入 10 倍体积遇冷的 0.1 mol/L 磷酸缓冲液（pH7.6）制成匀浆，超声，在 5 000 r/min 下离心，取上清液。

3. 上清液在 10 000 r/min 下离心 30 min，取沉淀，用磷酸缓冲液将沉淀重新悬浮即为粗酶。

4. 取上述粗酶悬浮液 0.5 mL 加入底物苄胺（8 mmol/L）0.3 mL，用 0.1 mol/L 磷酸缓冲液（pH7.6）补足至 3 mL，在 37 ℃下孵育 3 h 后，空白样品中加入苄胺 0.3 mL，之后加入 10% 高氯酸 0.3 mL 终止反应。

5. 加环己烷 3 mL 提取，在 5 000 r/min 下离心 10 min，取上清液于 242 nm 下测定吸

光度（A）值。

步骤 4、5 操作程序如下：

	空白管	测定管
酶液	—	0.5 mL
8 mmol/L 苄胺	—	0.3 mL
0.1 mol/L 磷酸缓冲液	3.0 mL	补足到 3.0 mL
	37℃下保温 3 h	
8 mmol/L 苄胺	0.3 mL	—
10% 高氯酸	0.3 mL	0.3 mL
环己烷	3 mL	3 mL

【结果】酶活性以每 3 h 生成苄醛 nmol 表示，或以 3 h 产生 0.01 个吸光度为一个活性单位，即每小时的单位 / 毫克蛋白质。酶液蛋白质含量按 Lowry 法测定。

【注意事项】为了消除酶液中存在的单胺底物的干扰，空白样品在保温前不加苄胺，保温后再加。

【方法评价】该方法成本较低、操作简便，但样品处理较麻烦，不如同位素法灵敏准确。

【思考题】试述 MAO-B 活性与衰老的关系。

Experiment 1 The effect of ethanol extract of Tuber Fleeceflower Root on the monoamine oxidase-B in aged mice brain

【Purpose】Master the method of testing the activity of MAO-B, observe the inhibition effect of the ethanol extract of Tuber Fleeceflower Root on MAO-B by.

【Principles】Use benzyl amine as the substrate to produce benzyl aldehyde under the action of MAO-B, extract it with cyclohexane, and measure absorbance values at 242nm.

$$RCH_2\text{–}NH_2 + O_2 + H_2O \xrightarrow{MAO} RCHO + NH_3 + H_2O$$

【Reagents】8 mmol/L benzyl amine, 0.1 mol/L phosphate buffer (pH 7.6), 10% perchloric acid, cyclohexane, ethanol extract of Tuber Fleeceflower Root (2.5 kg powder, extracted 3 times with 5 times volume of ethanol, vacuum distillation the extract, and obtain extracted material 285 g as the test drugs).

【Animals】20 old mice, 18~22 g, male.

【Methods】

1. 20 aging mice are randomly divided into two groups, give the ethanol extract of Tuber Fleeceflower Root to the first group, and give the physiological saline to the second group as the control group.

2. Drugs are administered to mice for 5 days. Take out the whole brain of the mice one hour after the last administration, put it into a container, add the cool phosphosphoric acid buffer (0.1 mol/mL) 10 times of the volume to prepare the homogenate by sonication. After, centrifuging it (5 000 r/min for 15 minutes), the supernatant is collected.

3. Centrifuge the supernatant (10 000 r/min) for 30 minutes, take out the deposit, suspend it with the phosphoric acid buffer, and thus the coarse enzyme is made.

4. Add 0.3 mL benzyl amine (8 mmol/L) into the suspension (0.5 mL), add 0.1 mol/L phosphoric acid buffer (PH7.6) to 3 mL, warm the reactive system at 37 ℃ for 3 hours, add 0.3 mL benzyl amine into the blank sample, then add 10% perchloric 0.3 mL to stop the reaction.

5. Extract it by 3 mL cyclohexane, centrifugate it at 3 000 r/min for 10 minutes, take out the suspension to detect the absorbance (A) at 242 nm.

The operations of 4,5 are as follows:

	The blank tube	The test tube
Enzyme	—	0.5 mL
8 mmol/L benzyl amine	—	0.3 mL
0.1 mol/L phosphoric	3.0 mL	Add to 3.0 mL
	Warm it for 3 hours at 37 ℃	
8 mmol/L benzyl amine	0.3 mL	—
10% perchloric	0.3 mL	0.3 mL
Cyclohexane	3 mL	3 mL

【Results】Observe the activity of the enzyme with the productive benzaldehyde in 3 hours, or consider 0.01 absorption produced in 3 hours as an activity unit, which is the protein produced each hour. Use Lowry's method to test the content of the enzyme.

【Notes】Don't add the benzyl amine in the blank sample before warming it to avoid the interferences of the monoamine in the enzyme solution.

【Evaluation】Due to its low cost and simple operation, it is suitable for screening MAO-B inhibitors. But it is troublesome to dispose the samples, and its sensitivity and accuracy are less than the isotope test.

【Questions】Talk about the relationship between the activity of MAO-B and aging.

实验二 果蝇寿命试验

【目的】熟悉果蝇寿命试验方法，观察药物枸杞的延缓衰老作用。

【原理】枸杞中含有枸杞多糖、胡萝卜素、维生素 B1 和 B2、维生素 C、烟酸、钙、磷、β-谷甾醇、亚油酸等，这些有效成分决定了枸杞具有抑制脂肪在肝细胞内沉积和促肝细胞新生的作用，降低胆固醇的作用，枸杞子能提高生命效率，增强体质，延缓机体生理衰老过程，增强免疫能力和延长寿命，在临床上能达到较好的疗效。

果蝇是一种真核多细胞昆虫，其成长、发育、繁殖和衰老与人类基本相似，且具有高度纯种、生命周期短、繁殖能力强、饲养简便等特点，实验条件易控制，短期内可获得结果，常应用于衰老实验研究。除观察平均寿命以外，其飞翔能力和交配能力也可供参考。

【器材】果蝇培养箱；紫外灭菌灯；各种大小试管。

【试剂】枸杞；乙醚。

【动物】果蝇。

【方法】实验果蝇饲料：玉米粉 20 g，蔗糖 10 g，琼脂粉 3 g，酵母粉 4 g，苯甲酸 0.6 g，水 180 mL。饲养条件：繁殖和实验用果蝇均饲养在（25 ± 1）℃、相对湿度 45%~65% 的温箱中。将果蝇分成对照组和给药组分设雌雄两组，每组 60 只分别装入孵出 24 h 的雌雄果蝇，培养基厚度 3 cm，采用纱布封口，隔天更换培养基一次。逐日记录死亡数，直至全部死亡。

【结果】以果蝇存活时间的总和除以成虫的总数量得到该组的平均寿命，并规定每组果蝇半数死亡所需天数为半数死亡时间，最后一个死亡的存活天数为该组最高寿命。

将结果填入表 18-1 中，药物组与对照组各指标进行 t 检验，评价药物的作用强度。

表 18-1 枸杞子对果蝇寿命的影响

组别	性别	样本数（只）	平均生存时间（小时）	最长寿命（天）
对照组	♂			
	♀			
给药组	♂			
	♀			

【注意事项】

1. 防止果蝇落在基质表面，翅膀被粘住而加快死亡。
2. 防止培养基被细菌、霉菌污染。
3. 及时清除死蝇和更换培养基，防止老蝇钩挂在死蝇以及试管壁上。

【思考题】

1. 为何选用果蝇作为寿命试验的对象？
2. 试述枸杞子的抗衰老机制。

Experiment 2　Longevity test of drosophila

【Purpose】Be familiar with the method of longevity test on drosophila and observe the macrobiotic effects of Lycium barbarum L.

【Principles】Wolfberry contains LBP, carotene, vitamins B1 and B2, vitamin C, niacin, calcium, phosphorus, β-sitosterol, linoleic acid, etc. These active ingredients determine the wolfberry has a role in inhibiting fat deposition in the liver , promoting hepatocyte regeneration, and reducing blood cholesterol. Wolfberry fruit can improve the life efficiency, improve physical fitness, slow down the body's physiological aging process, enhance immunity and prolonging life, demonstrating its beneficial effects on enhancing health.

Drosophila, a eukaryotic multicellular insect, which share the similar growth stages with human beings, has important characteristics such as highly purebred, short life cycle, high reproductive capacity, easy feeding, etc. Because it is easy to control the experimental conditions and acquire results in short time, drosophilae have been used for aging researches. In addition to observing the average lifespan of drosophila, flying ability and mating ability are also available for reference.

【Equipments】incubator for drosophila, sterilamp, tubes of various sizes.

【Reagent】wolfberry extract, ether.

【Animals】Drosophila.

【Methods】The food for the drosophila: 20 g cornmeal, 10 g sucrose, 3 g agar, 4 g yeast powder, 0.6 g benzoic acid and 180 mL water. Feed conditions: drosophila for reproduction and experiment must be bred in the warm incubator with the temperature of 25 ± 1 ℃ and the relative humidity of 45%~65%. Divide drosophilae into two groups: control group and the treatment group. Each group has two test tubes with culture medium 3cm in thickness, which is replaced every other day. Put 60 male and 60 female drosophilae hatched within 24 hours in each tube, seal the test tube with carbasus. Write down the number of dead drosophila every day till all of them die.

【Results】Average longevity comes by dividing total survival time with the number of mature ones. Half-lethal time refers to the time (hours) in which 50% of the drosophilae in each group die and the longest life-span is the time (days) in which the last one in each group dies.

List the data in the table 18-1, do statistical t-test to the indicators of two groups and evaluate the effective intensity of the drugs.

Table 18-1 Effect of wolfberry on the longevity of drosophila

Group	Sex	Number	average survival time (H)	longest life-span (D)
Control	♂			
	♀			
Drug	♂			
	♀			

[Notes]

1. Prevent the drosophila from falling on the surface of the basic medium as it can accelerate their death by sticking their wings.

2. Prevent the medium from being polluted by bacteria and moulds.

3. Replace the medium and clear up dead bodies in time to prevent the old ones from sticking to dead bodies and feces.

[Questions]

1. Why is drosophila chosen as the subject in the longevity test experiment?

2. Try to describe the anti-aging mechanism of wolfberry fruit.

实验三　白藜芦醇对小鼠肝脏脂质过氧化的影响

【目的】了解抗氧化实验，探讨白藜芦醇抗脂质过氧化的生物活性

【原理】活性氧（ROS）是一系列氧代谢物的总称，包含超氧阴离子，羟自由基，过氧化氢。活性氧的累积是氧化代谢必不可少的过程。活性氧具高反应性，可以造成DNA，蛋白质和脂肪酸的损害，进而导致脂质过氧化。许多疾病（衰老、肿瘤、动脉硬化）的发生与脂质过氧化有密切的关系。白藜芦醇是一种多酚类化合物，具有抗氧化、衰老等生物活性。

【器材】常规手术器械；5 mL玻璃离心管；离心机；恒温热水器；酶标仪；移液器。

【试剂】白藜芦醇；硫酸亚铁；L-半胱氨酸；硫代巴比妥酸；三氯醋酸。

【动物】小鼠，18~22 g。

【方法】小鼠禁食12小时，颈椎脱臼处死，摘取肝叶，以4 ℃预冷的磷酸缓冲液（pH 7.4）清洗，滤纸吸干，称重，剪碎，按1 ∶ 9的比例加入预冷的磷酸缓冲液（pH7.4），匀浆，离心（5 000转/min，5 min）取上清，即得肝组织匀浆液。按下列步骤进行操作：

	空白组	对照组	药物组
肝组织匀浆液	1 mL	1 mL	1 mL
白藜芦醇（1 mmol/L）	150 μL（缓冲液）	150 μL（缓冲液）	150 μL
硫酸亚铁（0.67 mmol/L）	150 μL（缓冲液）	150 μL	150 μL
L-半胱氨酸（10 mmol/L）	50 μL（缓冲液）	50 μL	50 μL
混匀，37 ℃温育 30 min			
10%三氯醋酸	1 mL	1 mL	1 mL
混匀			
0.67%TBA 硫代巴比妥酸（TBA）法	1 mL	1 mL	1 mL
沸水浴15 min，流动水冷却			
离心（3 000转，15 min），取上清，以缓冲液调零，在532 nm处测定OD值			

【结果】实验结果填入表 18-2 中。

表 18–2　白藜芦醇对小鼠肝脏脂质过氧化的影响

组别	样本数	浓度(mmol/L)	OD
空白组			
对照组			
药物组			

【注意事项】

1. 制作匀浆前肝组织尽量剪碎,匀浆时,时间和频率应每次保持一致。
2. 每次取匀浆时,应摇动烧杯使所取匀浆浓度一致。

【思考题】脂质过氧化与衰老之间是什么关系?

Experiment 3　The effect of resveratrol on lipid peroxidation in rat liver homogenate

【Purpose】

1. Study the methods involved in antioxidant capacity tests.

2. Evaluate the effect of resveratrol on FeSO(4)-L-Cys-induced lipid peroxidation in rat liver homogenate.

【Principles】Reactive oxygen species (ROS) is a general term for a series of oxygen metabolites, which includes superoxide anions, hydroxyl radicals and hydrogen peroxides. The ROS generates in normal metabolism, whereas increased or accumulated ROS can damage DNA, proteins and fatty acids, leading to lipid peroxidation. Studies have shown that lipid peroxidation is associated with many metabolic disorders, such as aging, atherosclerosis, etc. Resveratrol, a polyphenolic compounds, is considered shown to be an potent antioxidative agent.

【Equipments】surgical scissors, 5 mL glass tubes, centrifuge, Water heater thermostat, microplate Reader, transferpettors.

【Reagents】Resveratrol, ferrous sulfate, L-cysteine, thiobarbituric acid, acetocaustin.

【Animals】Mice (male or female) weighing 18~22 g.

【Method】Fasted mice are killed by cervical dislocation, the liver lobes are removed and washed with 4 ℃ cold phosphate beffer (pH 7.4, N.S or PBS) and put on a fliter paper, weighed. About 1 g of liver tissue is cutted into pieces and homogenized with the pre-cooled phosphate buffer (according to the ratio of 1g: 9 mL buffer). The homogenate is centrifuged at 5000 rpm for 5 min, and the supernatant is obtained, i.e., the liver homogenate. The FeSO (4)-L-Cys-induced lipid peroxidation reaction is performed as follows:

	blank	control	Resveratrol
liver homogenate	1 mL	1 mL	1 mL
resveratrol (1mmol/L)	150 μL (buffer)	150 μL (buffer)	150 μL
ferrous sulfate (0.67mmol/L)	150 μL (buffer)	150 μL	150 μL
L-cysteine (10 mmol/L)	50 μL (buffer)	50 μL	50 μL

（续表）

	blank	control	Resveratrol
	shaked, incubated in 37 ℃ for 30 min		
10%trichloroacetic acid（TDA）	1 mL	1 mL	1 mL
	Shaked		
0.67% thiobarbituric acid（TBA）	1 mL	1 mL	1 mL
	incubated in boiling water bath for 15 min, cooled with flowing water		
	centrifuged at at 3,000 rpm, 15 min, determined OD at 532 nm		

【Result】Record the results of experiment in the table 18-2.

Table 18-2　The effect of resveratrol on lipid peroxidation in rat liver homogenate

Group	number	Concentration（mmol/L）	OD
blank			
control			
resveratrol			

【Notes】

1. The liver must be sheared into pieces as small as possible before the preparation of the homogenate. The time and frequency must be kept in consistence in the preparation.

2. Each time when homogenate is taken, shake the beaker to make the compound mixed together to obtain consistent concentration.

【Question】What's the relationship between lipid peroxidation and caducity?

实验四 小鼠耐缺氧实验

【目的】掌握小鼠耐常压缺氧实验方法，观察人参对小鼠耐常压缺氧的作用。

【原理】缺氧是一种紧张性刺激，可引起机体产生各种应激性反应。脑、心脏缺氧是死亡的主要原因。许多抗衰老药物可通过增加心肌供血或降低心肌耗氧，改善心肌能量代谢而延长小鼠缺氧条件下的存活时间。

【器材】150 mL 广口玻璃瓶；秒表；天平；凡士林；钠石灰。

【试剂】人参水煎液 0.25 mL/10 g。

【动物】小鼠 30 只，体重 18~20 g，性别相同。

【方法】将小鼠随机分成三组，每组 10 只，分别放入容积相同（150 mL）的密闭广口瓶中，瓶内装有等量的钠石灰（25 g）以吸收水和二氧化碳。瓶盖涂以凡士林，放入小鼠后将瓶密闭，以秒表观察小鼠呼吸停止时间。每次实验均设空白对照组和阳性药（人参水煎液 0.25 mL/10 g）对照组。

【结果处理】计算各组小鼠死亡时间平均数（$\bar{x} \pm SD$），T 检验比较组间显著性。

【注意事项】

1. 所用容器必须密封，不漏气，而且容量相等。
2. 为防止钠石灰受潮，故每次实验应开启封口。
3. 小鼠体重、性别及室温不同，实验结果均有差异。

【方法评价】本方法简单易行，可作初筛基本方法。

【思考题】本实验中钠石灰的作用是什么？

Experiment 4 Hypoxia tolerance test of mice

【Purpose】Master the method for hypoxia tolerance test of mice and observe the effect of ginseng on hypoxia tolerance in mice.

【Principle】Hypoxia, a kind of tension stimulus, can cause various kinds of irritability actions. Hypoxia of brain and heart is the main cause for death. Many anti-aging drugs can lengthen the survival time of mice in anoxic condition by improving myocardial energy metabolism and increasing blood supply in the heart or reducing oxygen consumption.

【Equipments】150 mL wide-mouthed glass bottle, stopwatch, balance,

【Reagents】vaseline, sodium lime, ginseng water decoction 0.25 mL/10 g

【Animals】30 mice, 18~20 g, male or female.

【Method】Divide the mice into three groups with 10 mice in each, put them into a wide mouthed bottle (150 mL) with equal sodium lime (25 g) in it to absorb water and CO_2. The lid of the bottle is smeared with vaseline. After putting the mice in, close tightly the lid and calculate the time of respiratory arrest by using stopwatch . Set controls of negative group and positive group (ginseng water decoction 0.25 mL/10 g , ig) for each experiment.

【Results】Calculate the average dead time of each group ($\bar{x} \pm SD$), do statistical t-student test to see significance between groups.

【Note】

1. The containers must be sealed tightly without air leak,and they must have equal volume.

2. In order to prevent the sodium lime from being affected with damp, he seal must be opened in each experiment.

3. Experiment data varies with different weight, sex and room temperature.

【Evaluation】This method is easily manipulated and therefore usually used for initial screening as basic approach.

【Questions】What is the function of sodium lime in the experiment?

实验五 免疫器官重量法

【目的】掌握免疫器官重量法，观察药物对免疫器官重量的影响。

【原理】免疫增强剂使免疫器官（胸腺、脾脏）增重，而免疫抑制剂则相反。用该法可观察药物对已知免疫抑制剂所致免疫器官减重的对抗作用。

【器材】天平；常规手术器械。

【试剂】环磷酰胺。

【动物】小鼠 20 只，体重 18~22 g，雌雄不限。

【方法】

1. 造模　进行小鼠免疫抑制模型的制备。取小鼠 20 只，随机分成空白对照组（给生理盐水）、待试药物组、环磷酰胺组及待试药物＋环磷酰胺组，待试药物每天给药一次，连续 6 天，在给予待试药物后第四天开始腹腔注射环磷酰胺 50 mg/kg（对照组除外），连续 3 天，造成动物免疫抑制模型。

2. 观察疗效　末次给药后次日，眼眶放血。动物脱臼处死后，剥取脾脏、胸腺，称重。脏器重量以 mg/10 g 体重表示。随后进行组间 t 检验，比较组间差异的显著性。

【结果】将结果填入表 18-3 中。

表 18-3　待试药物组对免疫器官的影响

分组	剂量（g/kg）	动物数	脾脏指数（mg/10 g）	胸腺指数（mg/10 g）
空白对照				
待试药物组				
环磷酰胺及待试药物组				
环磷酰胺组				

【注意事项】

1. 必须用年轻小鼠。
2. 胸腺和脾脏必须分离干净。

【方法评价】

1. 此法比较简单，可供中药初筛，已知许多补益中药对免疫器官有增重作用。
2. 实验结果如与其他指标所得结果平行，则比较可靠。

【思考题】为什么本实验用环磷酰胺引起免疫功能抑制后再观察待试药的作用？

Experiment 5 The assay to weight the immune organs

【Objective】Master the assay to weight immune organs, and observe the effect of drug on the the weight of immune organs.

【Principle】The weight of immune organs (thymus, spleen) can be increased by immunopotentiators, while immunosuppressive drugs act in the opposite way. By this method we can observe the antagonistic effect of drugs on the immune organs' weights which are decreased by immunosuppressive drugs.

【Equipments】balance, surgical scissors

【Reagents】Cyclophosphamide

【Animals】20 mice, 18-22 g, male or/and female

【Methods】

1. The preparation of immunosuppressive mice model Divide 20 mice into four groups at random: control group (only saline is administered), test drug group, cyclophosphamide group, and the cyclophosphamide plus the test drug group. Give the drug once a day for six days. On the fourth day after administration, mice are administerated with 50 mg/kg cyclophosphamide intraperitoneally (except the control group) for three consecutive days, leading to immunosuppression.

2. Observe curative effect The next day of the last time of administration, blood was collected from the orbital sinus, pick out the eyeballs to collect blood and excavate, and then the spleen and thymus are isolated for weighing after killing by cervical dislocation. The weight the organs is expressed as the weight in terms of mg/10 g body weight, then do the statistical calculations by inter-group t-test and compare the differences between the comparison groups to see if they have statistical significance.

【Results】Write down your data in the table 18-3.

Table 18-3 Effects of test drug on the immune organs

Group	dose (g/kg)	Animal number	Spleen (mg/10 g)	Thymus (mg/10 g)
Control group				
Test drug group				

(Continued)

Group	dose (g/kg)	Animal number	Spleen (mg/10 g)	Thymus (mg/10 g)
the cyclophosphamide plus the test drug group				
cyclophosphamide group				

[Notes]

1. Young mice must be used.

2. Thymus and spleen must be parted clearly.

[Evaluation]

1. This method can be easily manipulated, and it can be used to initially screen the traditional Chinese herbs. Many known beneficial herbs have weight-increasing effect on immunological organs.

2. If the results are parallel with other indicators, they are more reliable.

[Question] Why do we observe the effect of the test drug when immunological function is inhibited by cyclophosphamide?

附　录

附录 1　常用生理溶液的成分和配制

成分	任氏液	洛氏液	任 - 洛氏液	台氏液	克氏液	邵氏液	戴克降氏液
NaCl（g）	6.5	9.0	9.0	8	6.9	1.65	9.0
KCl（g）	0.14	0.42	0.42	0.2	0.35	0.46	1.42
$CaCl_2$（g）	0.12	0.24	0.24	0.2	0.28	0.05	0.06
$NaHCO_3$（g）	0.2	0.10~0.30	0.5	1.0	2.1	2.52	0.5
NaH_2PO_4（g）	0.006 5			0.065		0.25	
KH_2PO_4（g）	0.2		0.5	1	0.16		0.5
$MgCl_2$（g）						0.022	
$MgSO_4 \cdot 7H_2O$（g）				0.26	0.29		
Glucose（g）	2	1~2.5	1.0	1.0	2		0.5
蒸馏水加至（mL）	1 000	1 000	1 000	1 000	1 000	1 000	1 000

附录 2　常用实验动物的最大给药剂量

（单位：mL）

动物	灌胃	皮下注射	肌肉注射	腹腔注射	静脉注射
小鼠	0.8~1.0	1.5	0.2	1.0	0.8
大鼠	6~8	2.0	1.0	5.0	4.0
豚鼠	10	2	2	10	10
兔	150~200	10	2.0	5.0	10
猫	120~150	10	2.0	5.0	10
蛙	淋巴囊注射最大量为 1 mL				

Supplement 1 The composition and preparation of normal physiological fluids

Composition	Ri nger solution	Locke solution	Ringer-Locke's solution	Trycd e's solution	Krebs solution	Theroton solution	De-Jalon's solution
NaCl(g)	6.5	9.0	9.0	8	6.9	1.65	9.0
KCl(g)	0.14	0.42	0.42	0.2	0.35	0.46	1.42
$CaCl_2$(g)	0.12	0.24	0.24	0.2	0.28	0.05	0.06
$NaHCO_3$(g)	0.2	0.10~0.30	0.5	1.0	2.1	2.52	0.5
NaH_2PO_4(g)	0.006 5			0.065		0.25	
KH_2PO_4(g)	0.2		0.5	1	0.16		0.5
$MgCl_2$(g)						0.022	
$MgSO_4 \cdot 7H_2O$ (g)				0.26	0.29		
Glucose(g)	2	1~2.5	1.0	1.0	2		0.5
Distilled water added to(mL)	1 000	1 000	1 000	1 000	1 000	1 000	1 000

Supplement 2 The maximum dose of drug given in experimental animals

(单位: mL)

Animal	p.o.	i.h.	i.m.	i.p.	i.v.
mouse	0.8~1.0	1.5	0.2	1.0	0.8
rat	6~8	2.0	1.0	5.0	4.0
guinea pig	10	2	2	10	10
rabbit	150~200	10	2.0	5.0	10
cat	120~150	10	2.0	5.0	10
frog	1 mL in saccus lymphaticus injection				

参 考 文 献

[1] 徐叔云,卞如濂,陈修主编.药理学实验方法学.北京:人民卫生出版社,2002.

[2] 钱之玉主编.药理学实验与指导.北京:中国医药科技出版社,2003.

[3] 丁启龙,李运曼主编.生理学实验与指导.北京:中国医药科技出版社,2004.

[4] 陈奇主编.中药药理研究方法学.北京:人民卫生出版社,1993.

[5] 陈奇主编.中药药理实验方法.北京:人民卫生出版社,1994.

[6] 魏伟,吴希美,李元建主编.药理实验方法学.北京:人民卫生出版社,2010.

[7] 国家药典委员会. 中华人民共和国药典(一部).北京:化学工业出版社,2010.

[8] 王璟,莫传丽,却翎,等.苍耳子不良反应研究进展.中草药,2011,42(3):613-616.

[9] 吴秀珍.苍耳子慢性中毒导致心肌损害、肝功能损害14例.医学理论与实践,1996,9(7):312.

[10] 何芙莉,闫姝,张小波,等.苍耳子小鼠最大耐受量实验观察.中国中西医结合外科杂志,1998,4(2):107-108.

[11] 龙绍疆,胥林波,顾健,等.关木通的表观毒代动力学参数的测定.中药药理与临床,2003(1):19-20.

[12] 丁英钧,王彦田.关木通肾毒性与剂量时间相关性及复方配伍减轻其毒性的实验研究(硕士毕业论文).石家庄:河北医科大学,2003.

[13] Liu Guoqing, Luo Jiabo. Effects of Mahuang Decoction in Different Combinations on Diaphor etic Function in Rats. New Drug for Chinese Material Medica and Clinical Pharmacology, 1995, 16(5): 318-320.

[14] Sun J, Zhang L, Song J, et al. Pharmacokinetic study of salvianolic acid A in beagle dog after oral administration by a liquid chromatography–mass spectrometry method: A study on bioavailability and dose proportionality. Journal of Ethnopharmacology, 2013, 148: 617-623.

[15] Zhao J, Su C, Yang CP, et al. Determination of ginsenosides Rb1, Rb2, and Rb3 in rat plasma by a rapid and sensitive liquid chromatography tandem mass spectrometry method: Application in a pharmacokinetic study. Journal of Pharmaceutical and Biomedical Analysis, 2012, 64-65: 94-97.

[16] B Zhang, XM Zhu, JN Hu, et al. Absorption Mechanism of Ginsenoside Compound K and Its Butyland Octyl Ester Prodrugsin Caco-2 Cells. Journal of Agricultural and Food Chemistry, 2012, 60: 10278-10284.

[17] Rajic A, Akihsa T. Inhibition of trypsin and chymotrypsin by anti-inflammatory triterpenoids from Compositae flowers. Planta Medica, 2001, 67(7): 599-604.

[18] Zang X, Shang M, et al. A-type proanthocyanidins from the stems of Ephedra sinica (Ephedraceae) and their antimicrobial activities. Molecules, 2013, 18(5): 5172-5189.

[19] Tang J, Zhou X, et al. Effects of ephedra water decoction and cough tablets containing ephedra and liquorice on CYP1A2 and the pharmacokinetics of theophylline in rats. Phytotherapy Research, 2012, 26(3): 470-474.
[20] Bielory L. Complementary and alternative interventions in asthma, allergy, and immunology. Annals of Allergy, Asthma & Immunology, 2004, 93: S45-S54.
[21] Wang L, Zhao D Q, Liu Y H.GC-MS analysis of the supercritical CO_2 fluid extraction of Ephedra sinica roots and its antisudorific activity. Chemical Communications, 2009, 45: 434-435.
[22] Lumpkin E A, Caterina M J.Mechanisms of sensory transduction in the skin.Nature, 2007, 445 (7130): 858-865.
[23] Frosini M, Sesti C, et al. A specific taurine recognition site in the rabbit brain is responsible for taurine effects on thermoregulation. British Journal of Pharmacology, 2003, 139(3): 487-494.
[24] Jilge B, Kuhnt B, et al. Circadian thermoregulation in suckling rabbit pups. Journal of Biological Rhythms, 2000, 15(4): 329-335.
[25] Liu K, Luo T, Zhang Z, et al. Modified Si-Miao-San extract inhibits inflammatory response and modulates insulin sensitivity in hepatocytes through an IKK β/IRS-1/Akt-dependent pathway. Journal of Ethnopharmacology, 2011, 136(3): 473-479.
[26] Shao L, Liu K, Huang F, et al. Opposite effects of quercetin, luteolin, and epigallocatechingallate on insulin sensitivity under normal and inflammatory conditions in mice.Inflammation, 2013, 36(1):1-14.
[27] Weili Zhu, Shiping Ma, Rong Qu, et al. Antidepressant Effect of Baicalin Extracted from the Root of Scutellariabaicalensis in Mice and Rats. Pharmaceutical Biology, 2006, 44(7): 503-510.
[28] Weili Zhua, Shiping Maa, Rong Qu, et al. Antidepressant-like effect of saponins extracted from Chaihu-jia-longgu-muli-tang and its possible mechanism. Life Sciences, 2006, 79(8):749-756.
[29] Weili Zhu, Shiping Ma, Rong Qu, et al. Antidepressant-like Effect of Paeonol. Pharmaceutical Biology, 2006, 44(3):229-235.
[30] 侯家玉 . 中药药理学 . 北京 : 中国中医药出版社, 1994.
[31] Wang Chan, Dai Yue, Chou Guixin, et al. Effects of total alkaloids from Radix Linderae on adjuvant induced arthritis in rats. Pharmacology and Clinics of Chinese Material Medica, 2006, 22(3, 4): 63-66.
[32] Yao X, Ding Z, Xia Y, et al. Inhibition of monosodium urate crystal-induced inflammation by scopoletin and underlying mechanisms. International Immunopharmacol, 2012, 14(4): 454-462.
[33] Luo Y, Liu M, Xia Y, et al. Therapeutic effect of norisoboldine, an alkaloid isolated from Radix Linderae, on collagen-induced arthritis in mice. Phytomedicine, 2010, 17(10): 726-731.
[34] 陈奇主编 . 中药药理研究方法学 . 3 版 . 北京 : 人民卫生出版社, 2011.
[35] 李仪奎主编 . 中药药理实验方法学 . 2 版 . 上海 : 上海科学技术出版社, 2006.
[26] Somuncu S, Caglayan O, Cakmak M, et al. The effect of indwelling catheter on OH-proline in the urethral wound: An experimental study. Journal of Pediatric Urology, 2006, 2(3): 182-184.
[37] 魏伟 , 吴希美 , 李元建主编 . 药理实验方法学 . 4 版 . 北京 : 人民卫生出版社, 2010.
[38] 刘颖 , 纪超 , 吴伟康 . 附子多糖保护缺氧 / 复氧乳鼠心肌细胞及其抗内质网应激的机制研究 . 中

国病理生理杂志，2012, 28（3）: 459-463.
[39] Wang S, Tian S, Yang F, et al. Cardioprotective effect of salvianolic acid A on isoproterenol-induced myocardial infarction in rats. European Journal of Pharmacology, 2009, 615（1）: 125-132.
[40] Ellis M, Gwynne RM, Bornstein JC. S11.5 Nutrient induced segmentation is mediated by serotonin and cholecystokinin in isolated guinea pig small intestine. Autonomic Neuroscience, 2009, 149（1-2）: 42.
[41] Ji CX, Fan DS, Li W, et al. Evaluation of the anti-ulcerogenic activity of the antidepressants duloxetine, amitriptyline, fluoxetine and mirtazapine in different models of experimental gastric ulcer in rats. European Journal of Pharmacology, 2012, 691（1）: 46-51.
[42] Jin L, Qin L, Xia D, et al. Active secretion and protective effect of salivary nitrate against stress in human volunteers and rats. Free Radical Biology and Medicine, 2013, 57: 61-67.
[43] Wang F, Miao M, Zhang Y, et al. Effects of fufangyimucao oral liquid on acute ache model mice. Neural Regeneration Research, 2007, 2（6）: 372-375.
[44] 黄继汉，黄晓晖，陈志扬，等．药理试验中动物间和动物与人体间的等效剂量换算．中国临床药理学与治疗学，2004（9）: 1069-1072.
[45] 陈奇．中药药理实验．贵阳：贵州人民出版社，1988.
[46] 田金洲，王永炎，徐意，等．血瘀证动物模型的种类、评价与研究．北京中医药大学学报，2006, 29（6）: 396-400.
[47] 孙荏苒，张满云，陈勤．桔梗皂苷胶囊抗炎止咳平喘作用研究．中药药理与临床，2010, 26: 27-29.
[48] 赵益，朱卫丰，刘红宁，等．贝母辛平喘作用及机制研究．中草药，2009, 40: 597-601.
[49] Assayag EI, Beaulieu MJ, Cormier Y. Bronchodilatory and Anti-Inflammatory Effects of ASM-24, a Nicotinic Receptor Ligand, Developed for theTreatment of Asthma. PLoS One, 2014, 9: e86091.
[50] Weili Zhu, Shiping Ma, Rong Qu, et al. Antidepressant-like effect of saponins extracted from Chaihu-jia-longgu-muli-tang and its possible mechanism. Life Sciences, 2006, 79（8）: 749-756.
[51] Qi B, Liu L, Zhang H, et al. Anti-fatigue effects of proteins isolated from Panaxquinquefolium. Journal of Ethnopharmacology, 2014, 153（2）: 430-434.
[52] Wang J, Sun C, Zheng Y, et al. The effective mechanism of the polysaccharides from Panax ginseng on chronic fatigue syndrome. Archives of Pharmacal Research, 2014, 37（4）:530-538.
[53] Xu YX, Zhang JJ. Evaluation of anti-fatigue activity of total saponins of Radix notoginseng. Indian Journal of Medical Research, 2013, 137（1）:151-155.
[54] Yang M, Chan GC, Deng R, et al. An herbal decoction of Radix astragali and Radix angelicaesinensis promotes hematopoiesis and thrombopoiesis. Journal of Ethnopharmacology, 2009, 124（1）:87-97.
[55] Gao QT, Cheung JK, Li J, et al. A Chinese herbal decoction, DangguiBuxue Tang, prepared from Radix Astragali and Radix AngelicaeSinensis stimulates the immune responses. Planta Medica, 2006, 72（13）:1227-1231.
[56] Kang S, Min H. Ginseng, the 'Immunity Boost': The Effects of Panax ginseng on Immune System. Journal of Ginseng Research, 2012, 36（4）:354-368.
[57] Choi JH, Jin SW, Park BH, et al. Cultivated ginseng inhibits 2,4-dinitrochlorobenzene-induced atopic dermatitis-like skin lesions in NC/Nga mice and TNF-α/IFN-γ-induced TARC activation in HaCaT

cells. Food and Chemical Toxicology, 2013, 6: 195-203.

[58] Sohn EH, Jang SA, Lee CH, et al. Effects of korean red ginseng extract for the treatment of atopic dermatitis-like skin lesions in mice. Journal of Ginseng Research, 2011, 35 (4): 479-486.

[59] 董晓华,张丹参,房杰 . 大黄酚对东莨菪碱致小鼠学习记忆障碍的作用及脑内 NO 和 NOS 的影响 . 河北北方学院学报 (医学版), 2009, 26 (1): 7-9.

[60] 冯学花,梁肖蕾 . 当归化学成分与药理作用的研究进展 . 广州化工 , 2012, 40 (22): 16-18.

[61] 付晓伶,方肇勤 . 阴虚证动物模型的造模方法及评析 . 上海中医药大学学报 , 2004, 18 (2): 51-54.

[62] 彭杨,张万萍,程鹏,等 . 雷沙吉兰对小鼠肝和脑组织中单胺氧化酶活性的影响 . 重庆医科大学学报 , 2013, 38 (6): 577-579.

[63] 杨秀伟 . 何首乌醇提物对易老化小鼠肝脏和脑单胺氧化酶活性的影响 . 中国中药杂志 , 1996, 21 (2): 48-49.

[64] 程桂花 . 枸杞子抗衰老作用的临床研究 . 中国医药指南 , 2012, 10 (34): 287-288.

[65] 徐曼妮,张欣文,徐思红 . 枸杞胶囊对果蝇的延缓衰老作用 . 同济大学学报 (医学版), 2001, 23 (5): 356-359.

[66] 付玉荣,王跃 . 衰老机制的研究进展及应用 . 国外医学: 老年医学分册 , 2003, 24 (4): 147-150.

[67] 李永涛,费洪新,沈雷,等 . 白藜芦醇对衰老昆明小鼠肝细胞作用机制的探讨 . 中国医药导报 , 2010, 7 (6): 25-27.

[68] 林松毅,殷涌光,刘静波,等 . 人参等复方中药功能液对小白鼠的抗缺氧作用 . 吉林大学学报 (工学版), 2005, 36 (1): 106-110.

[69] 陈洁君,黄萍,成金乐,等 . 黄芪破壁粉粒增强免疫功能及抗疲劳作用的研究 . 西北药学杂志 , 2013, 28 (3): 287-289.

[70] 刘善庭主编 . 药理学实验 . 北京 : 中国医药科技出版社, 2006.

[71] 谭毓治主编 . 药理学实验指导 . 北京 : 科学出版社, 2012.